Visions of Rogers' Science-Based Nursing

Visions of Rogers' Science-Based Nursing

Elizabeth Ann Manhart Barrett, Editor

Pub. No. 15-2285

National League for Nursing

Reprint 1.5M-0992-036950

The views expressed in this publication represent the views of the authors and do not necessarily reflect the official views of the National League for Nursing.

Cover photo by Lick Observatory
Neg. no. 315928
Courtesy Department Library Services
American Museum of Natural History

Printed in the United States of America

Contents

Contributors

Martha Raile Alligood, PhD, RN
  Associate Professor and
  Chair, Department of Psychophysiological Nursing
  University of South Carolina, College of Nursing
  Columbia, SC
Elizabeth Ann Manhart Barrett, PhD, RN
  Associate Professor and
  Director of Graduate Studies
  Hunter-Bellevue School of Nursing
  Hunter College of the City University of New York
  New York, NY
  and
  Private Nursing Practice
  New York, NY
Marie Boguslawski, PhD, RN
  Private Practice
  New York, NY
Howard K. Butcher, MScN, BSN, BS, RN
  Clinical Nurse Specialist-Psychiatry/Mental Health
  The Psychiatric Institute of Washington, DC
  Washington, DC
Cynthia Caroselli-Dervan, MS, RN, PhD Candidate
  Instructor
  Hunter-Bellevue School of Nursing
  Hunter College of the City University of New York
  New York, NY

W. Richard Cowling III, PhD, RN
Associate Professor and Chair
Department of Developmental Nursing
College of Nursing, University of South Carolina
Columbia, SC

Maureen B. Doyle, MEd, RN, CS, PhD Candidate
Assistant Professor
Division of Nursing, Dominican College
Blauvelt, NY

Mary Anne Hanley, MA, RN
Clinical Instructor
Division of Nursing
Lehman College of the City University of New York
Bronx, NY

Mary Dee McEvoy, PhD, RN
Coordinator, Oncology Nursing Services
Cancer Center, Hospital of the University of Pennsylvania
Former Robert Wood Johnson Clinical Nurse Scholar
School of Nursing
University of Pennsylvania
Philadelphia, PA

Mary Madrid, MA, RN, CCRN, PhD Candidate
Clinical Nurse Associate
New York University Medical Center
New York, NY

Violet M. Malinski, PhD, RN
Assistant Professor
Hunter-Bellevue School of Nursing
Hunter College of the City University of New York
New York, NY

Gean M. Mathwig, PhD, RN
Professor and Director, Baccalaureate Nursing Program
Division of Nursing, New York University
New York, NY

Thérèse C. Meehan, PhD, RN
Assistant Director of Nursing for Research
New York University Medical Center
New York, NY

Jeanne Lynch Paletta, PhD, RN
Associate Professor, Department of Graduate Nursing

Seton Hall University
South Orange, NJ
Nora I. Parker, PhD, RN
Professor Emerita
Faculty of Nursing
University of Toronto
Toronto, Ontario, Canada
J. Mae Pepper, PhD, RN
Chairperson of the Department of Nursing and
Director of the Graduate Program
Department of Nursing, Mercy College
Dobbs Ferry, NY
John R. Phillips, PhD, RN
Associate Professor
Division of Nursing
School of Education, Health, Nursing, and Arts Professions
New York Univeristy
New York, NY
Angela Racolin, MA, RN, PhD Candidate
Nurse Clinician, Oncology
Memorial Sloan-Kettering Hospital
New York, NY
Katherine E. Rapacz, MS, RNC, PhD Candidate
Frances Payne Bolton School of Nursing
Case Western Reserve University
Cleveland, OH
Marilyn M. Rawnsley, DNSc, RN
Professor
Teachers College, Columbia University
New York, NY
Francelyn Reeder, PhD, RN, CNM
Assistant Professor
School of Nursing
University of Colorado Health Sciences Center
Denver, CO
Judith A. Rizzo, MA, RN, PhD Candidate
Assistant Director of Nursing
New York University Medical Center
New York, NY
Martha E. Rogers, ScD, RN, FAAN

Professor Emerita
Division of Nursing,
School of Education, Health, Nursing, and Arts Professions
New York University
New York, NY
Ardis R. Swanson, PhD, RN
Associate Professor
Division of Nursing
School of Education, Health, Nursing, and Arts Professions
New York University
New York, NY
Suzanne D. Thomas, PhD, RNC
Assistant Professor
College of Nursing
University of Tennessee, Memphis
Memphis, TN
Patricia C. Walsh, MA, RNC, CNNA, PhD Candidate
Director, Home Care Department
Good Samaritan Hospital
Suffern, NY
Patricia Winstead-Fry, PhD, RN
Professor of Nursing
University of Vermont
Burlington, VT
Alice Adam Young, PhD, RN
Dean and Professor, School of Nursing
Washburn University
Topeka, KS

Editor's Note

A change in some of the definition of terms and the change of "four-dimensionality" to "multidimensionality" were received from Dr. Rogers immediately before this book went to press. The changes are reflected in Dr. Rogers' work in Chapter 1, Chapter 25, and the Glossary. However, the new terminology had not been created at the time the other authors wrote their chapters and, thus, is not reflected in their work.

To Martha E. Rogers
From all of us who have known and loved you
as our teacher, our mentor, our colleague, our friend

Foreword

The Science of Unitary Human Beings had its seminal origins in the writings of Martha E. Rogers 30 years ago. Ten years earlier nursing had made its first concerted efforts as a profession to fund nursing research by its members. In 1952, an official journal, *Nursing Research*, was established. In 1962, Dr. Rogers proposed nursing science to be unique and advocated its perspectives through the journal *Nursing Science*.

Today *Nursing Science* has a variety of faces which are expressed in the use of unique and borrowed, quantitative and qualitative, paradigmatic and preparadigmatic language. As a unique science, however, nursing science was advocated by Martha E. Rogers in the 1960s as *essential* for a discipline that was to realize its own contributions to the human sciences and to the actualization of a learned profession that could be empowered to provide compassionate service to humankind. There was knowledge in nursing to know and the discipline was obligated to develop and share it.

Human science, as conceived by Wilhem Dilthey in the 19th century, was an advance beyond natural science for inquiry into understanding the history, expressions, and achievements of human beings; however, Dilthey continued to use natural science world views and tenets to reach his goals. As a result, humans remained separated from their environments and from a continuity of self in the practice of testing research traditions.

Nursing science is the bridge between human science and human evolution into the 21st century. Rogerian science is human science at its best. Elizabeth Barrett's book testifies to the reasons why Rogerian science-based nursing is relevant to an age yearning and groping for an optimistic, negentropic world view in the face of contrary world views that perpetuate entropic messages of a world deconstructing. In the desire for hope, nursing is at the forefront!

An evolutionary perspective of the type envisioned by Teilhard de Chardin aptly describes Dr. Rogers' philosophy as a negentropic, optimistic continuity of life process unfolding in a universe of integral humans and environment. Such vision is exceedingly relevant to the global culture becoming manifest in the 21st century.

In 1971, Dr. Rogers' *Introduction to the Theoretical Basis of Nursing* captured my attention and became a preoccupation and inspiration during graduate education. It was the first nursing theory I had read that challenged all ways of knowing commonly engaged in my life as an existential nurse in the universe. The human sentience described and advocated by Dr. Rogers included a thinking, feeling, and perceiving that ranged from ordinary sense perception to extrasensory perception and mystical awareness. The insights which this view then opened were astounding and beckoned forth the "ancient" and "not yet" in me. It is a view that requires each of us to engage in knowing participation while being deeply embedded in mutual process in our respective and relative human-environmental fields. As Dr. Rogers proposed, we have to be there ourselves to "see" and to "know" the wondrous creative potential that continuously emerges before us as we live our lives.

In 1986, Dr. Malinski's *Explorations on Martha Rogers' Science of Unitary Human Beings* gave evidence of the life of scholarship that had developed, extending Dr. Rogers' conceptual systems through basic research and applied research in nursing science. The refinement of postulates and principles present an ever more coherent system of explanation that enhances the understanding of unitary human beings in the environment and provides the foundation for scholarship in advancing knowledge for the discipline of nursing. I continue to be inspired by this vision.

In 1990, *Visions of Rogers' Science-Based Nursing*, by Dr. Barrett, represents yet another evolutionary moment in Rogerian science that is paradoxically more tangible and yet transcendent for the 21st-century reflective, becoming nurse.

Baccalaureate, master's, and doctorally prepared nurses alike will find this resource exceptionally helpful for conceptual and practical endeavors. Nursing students of the 21st century will find this collection of scholarship and learned practice, Rogerian science-based nursing, a necessary companion on their voyage into their profession. The inherent links between Rogers' postulates and principles of homeodynamics have been presented in exceptionally clear, relevant human situations, recognizable to the attentive eye for purposes of education, research, and practice.

Common labels and jargon are largely avoided in these pages and words that enhance clarity of thought and creativity are carefully expressed. These pages are simply inspiring and challenging! A Foreword is not a fit substitute for a careful reading of the book, but rather serves to enliven the readers' expectations of themselves to "see" themselves in the four-dimensional world recreated here through a Rogerian perspective. Enjoy the adventure!

This work signals the increasing relevance of Rogerian science to a diverse, sophisticated world. Its challenge is to present an optimistic world view that recognizes the primacy of the life process on land, sea, and sky.

Central to Rogerian science is the view that the life process occurs throughout all change and chaos as an ordered unity. The continuity and endurance of the life process exceeds human choice and will, error or chance, and paradoxically manifests the source and principle of life ever new. The mandate to nursing is to provide knowledgeable, compassionate service to all humankind in light of this central focus on the life process. This book's unique purpose, therefore, is to refine human pattern seeing capacities and to illuminate the relevance of Rogerian science-based nursing to the 21st century and beyond.

Its greatest claim is that research conceived and implemented from an optimistic vision of a world becoming, that inspires the clearest imagination, wit, perception, and intellect, can also compassionately maximize human creative potential.

Its special contribution is education and practice based on an optimistic world view, and compassionate commitment to people that anticipate order in chaos through knowing participation. Such a view empowers the hopeless, inspires the despairing, and provides resilience through uncertainty and surprise. Its legacy is to view change as opportunity, four-dimensionality as freedom to create, and death as transition, in life ever new.

Francelyn Reeder, PhD, RN, CNM

Preface

Never doubt that a small group of
thoughtful, committed citizens
can change the world; indeed it's
the only thing that ever has.
Margaret Mead

Ten years ago this book could not have been written. Make no mistake about it, the winds of change are blowing. A quiet revolution is brewing in nursing; it is a revolution triggered by emergence of the unique knowledge of nursing science.

An ancient proverb says, "Without vision, the people perish." Throughout her career, Rogers has provided the vision for nursing to flourish. As a strong voice in the nursing revolution, Rogers, despite considerable opposition, implemented a radically new view of nursing. Her aim was to advance nursing as a basic science and as a learned profession. Regardless of audience or contradictory views, the courage of Rogers' convictions never waivered. It is, indeed, difficult to imagine what nursing would look like today without Martha Rogers.

This book is about Rogers' vision to establish nursing as a scientific art. Precisely, the aim is to provide a few pieces of a vast puzzle concerning people and their world, thereby contributing to an understanding of Rogerian science as a continuously evolving body of knowledge (product) and as a route to knowledge (process) for the 21st century.

The book was conceived amidst the excitement of the Third Rogerian Conference. Some chapters were originally presented at that conference in June 1988 at New York University. Those papers were revised for inclusion in this book; many others were added. This anthology then attests to both the potential of people to evolve imaginatively and to nursing's participation in shaping a visionary experience of health. Some of the authors are second-generation Rogerian theorists who continuously update and integrate new developments in nursing science.

This book casts a wide net since it is intended for a vast audience. Undergraduate and graduate students, educators, administrators, researchers, and those who directly deliver nursing services will appreciate its contents. The book is organized into five sections. However, research, education, and practice interface in Rogers' science-based nursing; boundaries are artificial.

Unit I presents the most recent thinking and newest developments. Rogers updates the Science of Unitary Human Beings. Phillips proposes a new theory of human field image.

Unit II, science-based practice, is a major focus of the book. Rogerians respect theory and research for the ways in which they can nourish and enlighten practice. The challenge is to use the information to describe and explain human and environmental fields and their ever-changing manifestations. The authors practice in a variety of settings; they are people of creative imagination engaged in the art of using Rogerian practice methodology; that is, pattern manifestation appraisal and deliberative mutual patterning through innovative unitary human field practice modalities. Undergraduate students, in particular, will delight in finding satisfaction of their often-voiced request for relevance to the "real world of practice."

Unit III presents science-based research from the perspective of (1) current issues in the conduct, process, and continuing evolution of Rogerian modes of inquiry and (2) current studies, their critiques by colleagues, and accompanying responses of researchers. Graduate students will be challenged to engage in scholarly debate of the evolving ideas concerning theory development, methods, and linkages from the abstract system to the design. Three major studies concern (1) testing Rogers' theory of the emergence of paranormal phenomena, (2) exploring the relationship of temporal experience and human time (including development of a research instrument to measure temporal experience), and (3) examining the patterning of time experience and human field motion during the experience of pleasant guided imagery.

Unit IV, science-based education, is concerned with both curriculum (what we teach) and pedagogy (how we teach it) in baccalaureate, master's, and doctoral programs. Nursing faculty will be particularly interested in the historical review of the early experiences of using the Science of Unitary Human Beings to guide curriculum design as well as the exploration of ongoing issues. Creative approaches in Rogerian education are illustrated through use of an original board game to solve the classroom issue of student facility in using the language of Rogerian science. Insights regarding ongoing challenges in using the system as a basis for doctoral dissertation research will be useful for faculty and graduate students.

Futurists in nursing and beyond will find Unit V, visions of the future, particularly compelling in its playful encounter with tomorrow's reality. Malinski describes the experience of astronauts and cosmonauts during their sojourns in outer space within the scholarly framework of the Science of Unitary Human Beings. She proposes a Rogerian perspective for the nursing practice modalities of therapeutic touch, imagery, and meditation as essential preparation for space exploration of outer space. Dialogue with Rogers closes this phase of our visionary adventure by answering questions posed by the eternal student in each of us. The horizon she envisions is limitless, and so too is her optimism about nursing's creative potential amidst unending change.

It is our hope that this book, alive with ideas and information, will participate in the quiet revolution in nursing by contributing state-of-the-science and state-of-the-art knowledge of Rogers' Science of Unitary Human Beings. When nurses everywhere, in unity through diversity, use nursing knowledge for the betterment of humankind, the revolution will transform health care.

Using the metaphor of vision, this book issues a clarion call to dreamers and pragmatists alike. Come, see with us. For now, dear readers, the book is yours.

Elizabeth Ann Manhart Barrett, Editor

Editorial Review Panel[1]
Maureen B. Doyle
Mary Madrid
Violet M. Malinski
Angela Racolin
Patricia C. Walsh

---

[1]Editor's Note: It is with deep appreciation that I acknowledge the members of the Editorial Review Panel for their valuable assistance in the editing of the manuscripts including mine. Their knowledge of Rogerian science as well as their collegiality was an inspirational experience for me.

E.A.M.B.

Unit I

The Science of Unitary Human Beings

The science of nursing is an emergent—a new product. The term *nursing*, used to signify a learned profession, is a noun, not a verb. By definition, then, "nursing" specifies an organized body of abstract knowledge specific to its central purpose.

Martha E. Rogers

1

Nursing: Science of Unitary, Irreducible, Human Beings: Update 1990

Martha E. Rogers

The countdown for the 21st century has begun. New facts and ideas continue to generate syntheses for new world views. Genetic engineering engenders a mechanistic explanation of life and spawns ethical issues that far exceed Aldous Huxley's (1932) *Brave New World.* Concomitantly, "caring" has become an "in" word as the public is told that the mother who cares gives her child Castoria and the wife who cares feeds her spouse Nutragrain. Major American contemporary health problems are iatrogenesis, nosocomial conditions, and nosophobia. Toxic terrorism is rampant with the health fields frequently providing the terrorists themselves.

Entrepreneurship marks one of the fundamental changes in today's economy. New careers coordinate with new world views and exacerbating innovative technology mount. Potentials for careers in outer space challenge even the most imaginative. Homo spacialis looms on the horizon as moon villages, space towns, and Martian communities foretell a new world.

Nursing's transition from pre-science to science must be explicit if nurses are to provide knowledgeable innovative services in a space-bound world society. A new world view compatible with the most progressive knowledge available (Lauden, 1977) is a necessary prelude to studying human health and to determining modalities for its promotion both on this planet and in outer space.

As a learned profession, nursing is both a science and art. The *uniqueness of nursing*, like that of any other science, lies in the phenomenon central to its focus. Nurses' long-established concern with people and the world they live in is a natural forerunner of an organized abstract system encompassing people and their environments. The irreducible nature of individuals is different from the sum of the parts. The integralness of people and environment that coordinate with a multidimensional universe of open systems point to a new paradigm: the *identity of nursing as a science*. The purpose of nurses is to promote health and well being for all persons wherever they are. The art of nursing is the creative use of the science of nursing for human betterment.

A science is an organized abstract system. It is a synthesis of facts and ideas; a new product. Historically, the term "nursing" has been used as a verb signifying "to do." When nursing is identified as a science the term "nursing" becomes a noun signifying a "body of abstract knowledge." Theories derive from this organized body of abstract knowledge. Consequently, theories deriving from a Science of Unitary Human Beings are specific to nursing just as theories deriving from biology are specific to biological phenomena, theories deriving from sociology are specific to sociological phenomena, and theories of physics are specific to the physical world. Moreover, one must keep in mind that the study of biologists and what they do is not the study of biology. Similarly, the study of nurses and what they do is not the study of nursing.

A science has many theories. Nursing is the study of unitary, irreducible, indivisible human and environmental fields: people and their world. Complexity of investigatory methodology is not a substitute for substantive content in any field. Florence Downs (1988) noted recently ". . . our research efforts are replete with sophisticated methods applied to unsophisticated content" (p. 20). The education of nurses has identity in transmission of nursing's body of theoretical knowledge. The practice of nurses is the creative use of this knowledge in human service. Research methods are empty without substance to study. Research in nursing specifies a body of knowledge specific to nursing; research in other fields is not a substitute.

Developing nursing's abstract system demands a new world view. A language of specificity provides for precision, clarity, and communication. Replication of research becomes possible. Nursing, like other sciences, is a synthesis of facts and ideas—a new product. It is not a summation of principles and theories from other fields dealing with different phenomena and rooted in different paradigms. Nursing's focus on unitary human beings and their world as defined in this system is unique to nursing.

A universe of open systems underwrites the growing diversity of people and their environments. Furthermore, it should be emphasized that people

Table 1
Key Definitions Specific to the Science of Nursing

Energy Field:	The fundamental unit of the living and the non-living. Field is a unifying concept. Energy signifies the dynamic nature of the field; a field is in continuous motion and is infinite.
Pattern:	The distinguishing characteristic of an energy field perceived as a single wave.
Multidimensional:	A nonlinear domain without spatial or temporal attributes.
Unitary Human Beings: (Human Field)	An irreducible, indivisible, multidimensional energy field identified by pattern and manifesting characteristics that are specific to the whole and which cannot be predicted from knowledge of the parts.
Environment: (Environmental Field)	An irreducible, indivisible, multidimensional energy field identified by pattern and integral with the human field.

are energy fields. They do not *have* them. All reality is postulated to be multidimensional as defined herein. One does not become multidimensional. Rather, this is a way of perceiving reality. The use of the term "multidimensional" to replace the term "four-dimensional" does not represent any change in definition. Efforts to select words best suited to portray one's thought are difficult at best. Multidimensional provides for an infinite domain without limit.

The abstract system exists as an irreducible whole. Principles and theories derive from this irreducible whole. The nature of change finds expression in the principles of homeodynamics. New knowledge is contributing continuously to revisions of thinking. A significant change in one word in the principle of helicy occurs. Interestingly enough, the change is consistent with the abstract system and new knowledge supports it. Clarification is in order. The reader is familiar with the transition from absolutism to probability. The literature now points up that unpredictability transcends probability. Eugene Mallove (1989) writes, "To find in the late 20th century that unpredictability plays a significant role in the orderly celestial arena is not only a surprising development but a revolutionary one in the history of science" (p. 12). Peterson (1989) discusses further the unpredictability of self-organized critical systems.

The deletion of probability from the abstract system underlying the science or unitary human beings and the addition of unpredictability strengthens consistency and supports the nature of change proposed in the

Table 2
Principles of Homeodynamics

Principle of Resonancy:	Continuous change from lower to higher frequency wave patterns in human and environmental fields.
Principle of Helicy:	Continuous innovative, unpredictable, increasing diversity of human and environmental field patterns.
Principle of Integrality:	Continuous mutual human field and environmental field process.

principles of homeodynamics. The principles are now stated below in Table 2 as revised.

These principles provide fundamental guides to the practice of nursing. They continue to undergo investigation and to generate both basic and applied research in the science of nursing.

Energy fields are in continuous motion. Field pattern has been a central concept in this system from its inception over $2\frac{1}{2}$ decades ago. It is interesting to note that Ferguson (1980) wrote in her book *The Aquarian Conspiracy* that "Synthesis and pattern seeing are survival skills of the 21st century." Ferguson's comment is certainly apropos to the Science of Unitary Human Beings. Pattern within nursing's abstract system is itself an abstraction that reveals itself through its manifestations. Manifestations of patterning emerge out of the human/environmental field mutual process and are continuously innovative. The evolution of life and non-life is a dynamic, irreducible, nonlinear process characterized by increasing complexification of energy field patterning. The nature of change is unpredictable and increasingly diverse (see Table 3).

The "seems continuous" noted in Table 3 refers to a wave frequency so rapid that the observer perceives it as a single, unbroken event. Not only is field pattern diversity relative for any given individual but there is also a marked increase in diversity between individuals. The implications of this for increased individualization of nursing services is explicit.

The Science of Unitary Human Beings is equally applicable to groups as to individuals. Groups are defined as two or more individuals. The group energy field to be considered is identified: It may be a family or a social group, a crowd or some other combination. Regardless of the group identified, the group field is irreducible and indivisible to itself and integral with its own environmental field. The environmental field is unique to any given group field. The principles of homeodynamics postulate the nature of group field change just as they postulate the nature of individual field change.

Table 3
Manifestations of Field Patterning in Unitary Human Beings

The evolution of unitary human beings is a dynamic, irreducible, nonlinear process characterized by increasing diversity of energy field patterning. Manifestations of patterning emerge out of the human/environmental field mutual process and are continuously innovative. Pattern is an abstraction that reveals itself through its manifestations.

The nature of unitary field patterning is unpredictable and creative. Change is relative and increasingly diverse. Some manifestations of relative diversity in field patterning are noted below.

lesser diversity		greater diversity
longer rhythms	shorter rhythms	seems continuous
slower motion	faster motion	seems continuous
time experienced as slower	time experienced as faster	timelessness
pragmatic	imaginative	visionary
longer sleeping	longer waking	beyond waking

Questions concerning whether mother/fetus are one field or two often arise. It may be handled either way. The mother/fetus may be deemed a single indivisible field—a group field if you like. This field would be irreducible. If one determined to focus on the mother or on the fetus, these would be individual fields integral with their own unique environmental fields. Regardless of the field one chooses to study, it is essential to remember that one cannot generalize from parts to a whole. For example, studying the members of a group will not provide knowledge about the group.

The Science of Unitary Human Beings encompasses our advent into outer space. Today's astronauts are envoys to our outer space-directed future—a future that is already here. Planet Earth is integral with the larger world of human reality. The outer space future will not be how to use planetary knowledge and skills in space but rather the elaboration of a new world view in which new knowledge and new modalities raise new questions, provide new answers, and signify different evolutionary norms. Homo spacialis (Robinson & White, 1986) is proposed to transcend Homo sapiens in approximately two generations of space dwelling. Planet-bound physiological norms are already inadequate parameters for humankind in space. They are increasingly irrelevant for space travelers and to forthcoming Homo spacialis. So-called pathology on Earth today may signify health for the space bound.

Testable hypotheses derive from nursing's abstract system. Research enables one to understand the nature of human evolution and its multiple unpredictable potentialities. Description, explanation, and vision strengthen a nurse's ability to practice according to the level and scope of a given nurse's preparation and knowledge in the science of nursing. Holistic trends force new ways of thinking and spell new world views. Gould (1977) once wrote, "Facts do not speak for themselves. They are read in the light of theory" (p. 21). Unitary human health signifies an irreducible human field manifestation. It cannot be measured by the parameters of biology or physics or the social sciences and the like. The principles of homeodynamics postulate the nature of change with equal relevance for individuals and for groups, for Homo sapiens and Homo spacialis and beyond.

Education for all is undergoing considerable review. Davis (1989) has noted that "The shelf life of an education today doesn't last a working life-time" and emphasizes "a shift to a life-time of learning rather than one of knowing" (p. 16). Basic and applied research in the science of nursing is a must.

The Science of Unitary Human Beings sparks new interventive modal-ities—that evolve as life evolves from earth to space and beyond. Spin-offs from space can lead to more effective services for Homo sapiens on planet Earth. Non-invasive modalities will prevail. A positive attitude toward change is generated. Vision and imagination grow. The purpose of nurses is to promote human betterment wherever people are—on planet Earth or in outer space.

Health services are properly community based. Satellite services such as hospitals provide an orientation to pathology—not to health. As health promotion takes over, fewer and fewer people will need sick services as they currently exist. Today's world is rapidly becoming an entrepreneurial soci-ety and nurses are already into the stream of the entrepreneurial world. There is critical need for mutual respect for differences between all health personnel, between nurses, between health fields, and between fields of science.

The practice of nursing will be characterized primarily by non-invasive modalities. Research in the science of nursing is already providing support for skills deemed unscientific in the past. An excellent example is Krieger's (1979) work in therapeutic touch—relate this to the art of evening care, of back-rubs, even that cool hand on a fevered brow. There are many more examples.

As diversity grows so too does individualization of services. How do nurses best participate in enabling people to fulfill their own rhythmicities? Meditation, imagery, relaxation have undreamed of potentials. Uncondi-tional love is beginning to receive the attention it deserves. Attitudes of hope, humor, and upbeat moods are already documented to be often better therapy than drugs.

Basic research in the Science of Unitary Human Beings is increasing (Ludomirski-Kalmanson, 1985; Malinksi, 1986). Concomitantly, Senator

Clairborne Pell, in the Feburary 1988 issue of *Omni*, points out that various methods are used to prevent research that is out of the mainstream from ever getting off the ground and deplores the gearing of all research monies toward traditional disciplines of science. Nurses would do well to recognize that biomedical research is not research in nursing.

Read the chapters in this book within the context of a new world view. Examine them carefully for contradictions. Envision a future not yet here. Enjoy your forays into the unknown. Change is continuous, inevitable, and exciting.

REFERENCES

Davis, S. (1989, April). Envisioning the future. *Futurific*, 16–18.

Downs, F. (1988). Nursing research: State-of-the-art. *Journal of the New York State Nurses' Association, 19*(3), 20.

Ferguson, M. (1980). *The aquarian conspiracy: Personal and social transformation in the 1980s*. Los Angeles: J.P. Tarcher.

Gould, S.J. (1977). This view of life. *Natural History, 52*, 20–24.

Huxley, A. (1932). *Brave new world*. New York: Modern Library.

Krieger, D. (1979). *The therapeutic touch: How to use your hands to help or to heal*. Englewood Cliffs, NJ: Prentice Hall.

Lauden, L. (1977). *Progress and its problems: Toward a theory of scientific growth*. Berkeley: University of California Press.

Ludomirski-Kalmanson, B. (1985). An empirical investigation in support of M. Rogers' principle of integrality. In *Proceedings of the 10th National Research Conference* (pp. 201–204). Toronto, Ontario, Canada: University of Toronto Faculty of Nursing.

Malinski, V. (Ed.). (1986). *Explorations on Martha Rogers' science of unitary human beings*. Norwalk, CT: Appleton-Century-Crofts.

Mallove, E.T. (1989, May–June). The solar system in chaos. *The Planetary Report*, pp. 12–13.

Pell, C. (1988, February). First Word. *Omni, 14*, 32–34.

Peterson, I. (1989, July). Digging into sand. *Science News, 138*, 42.

Robinson, G.S., & White, H.M. (1986). *Envoys of mankind*. Washington, DC: Smithsonian Institute Press.

2

Changing Human Potentials and Future Visions of Nursing: A Human Field Image Perspective

John R. Phillips

The evolution of human potentials involves a lengthy history; in fact, since the beginning of humankind. Gradually, there has accumulated a large body of knowledge about human potential. However, this knowledge has emerged (for Western science) predominantly from a focus on the physical body.

Today there is an accelerated change and diversity in human potential that cannot be explained by current knowledge. As a result, conceptual models that extend our knowledge beyond the physical body and physical reality are called for. Such models exist in other disciplines—for example, Einstein's (1961) theory of relativity, Bohm's (1980) implicate order, Sheldrake's (1981) morphogenetic fields, and the current theory of Kaku (Kaku & Trainer, 1987) that the universe is made up of strings.

ROGERIAN BASIS FOR A NEW CONCEPT

The science of nursing has Rogers' (1970, 1980, 1986, 1987) model of unitary human beings that enables one to move from the world of physical facts to understand the patterns of human beings and their environments. It is from knowledge of these changing dynamic patterns that one can gain understanding of emerging human potentials and propose future visions of nursing.

A knowledge of the images of human beings and health is requisite to an understanding of these changing patterns. However, since images affect perceptions and action (Markley & Harman, 1982), both of which are involved in the emergence of human potential, a distinction must be drawn.

Generally, people hold in their minds an image of their bodies as they appear—the body image. Not only is there a physiologic aspect, but there are psychologic and social components, all of which interact to form a body image. Individual potentials are always related to some aspect of the components or their interaction. The dominant self-images persons hold are that of entities separate and independent from their environment. Such views lead to the conclusion that body image is a three-dimensional picture of the self that persons acquire in the course of their development.

It is easy to see that this understanding of body image is fragmented and out of touch with the wholeness of human beings. This is especially true since our physical awareness through the body is only a minute portion of the entirety of human awareness available. This suggests that the range of human potentials is far greater than that available from the traditional paradigm of the physical body and body image. As long as we focus on the physical body and concern ourselves with body images, the non-physical aspects of human beings will not be perceived.

The four-dimensional aspect of Rogers' model pushes the three-dimensional scales of body image from one's eyes to open up new perspectives of image. I call this perspective "human field image," which provides a four-dimensional picture of unitary human beings.

Human field image is one manifestation of the mutual process of human beings with their environments. Since it is a manifestation of the mutual process, it is also a whole that cannot be reduced to parts. Human field image is one of the innumerable manifestations of the pattern of the person that helps provide unique meaning to one's unfolding (Friedman, 1974; Richards & Richards, 1974). As one moves through the life process, there is a growing diversity of the human field image through a dynamic, ever-changing mutual process with the environmental field. Since the human field image is not confined to a static point in time, it is representative of the ever-changing relative present that synthesizes the past, present, and future. This synthesis involves all changes that have occurred in past human field images and all projected future human field images into what is known as the relative present human field image. Thus, human field image can be defined as an evolving diverse manifestation of the human field pattern that synthesizes all past and projected future images into a four-dimensional picture of human beings. As such, human field image provides a relativistic way of perceiving human field patterns. It is only when human field images are perceived that the pattern of the human field can be understood.

From these characteristics one can propose that human field image is one of the fundamental unifying principles involved in the patterning of the human energy field itself. Essentially, it is one of the matrices of the human energy field involved in the four-dimensional patterning process from which human potentials emerge. It is through human field image which involves four-dimensional patterning that one can perceive integrality with the environmental field. This perception transcends the physical body; one can move creatively beyond the boundaries of body image to experience one's wholeness. "Boundaries tend to dissolve as we find out who we really are—an extension of the unity of all life" (Global Challenges, 1982, p. 2).

From a theory–practice situation, body image and human field image provide two different views of persons with disabilities. From a body image perspective, nursing focuses primarily on the dysfunction of parts of the physical body. From a human field image perspective, nursing focuses primarily on the potentials of the person. Vash (1981) says transcendence means rising above or beyond the limits imposed by certain conditions such as disability where one must escape the mind–body trap. This view is consistent with a human field image perspective that makes it impossible to have a "trapped within the body" perception with disability that is frequently reported in the literature. As indicated by Hohmann (1981), human field image enables one to move from hating or denying one's disability toward the joyous aspects of life such as experiencing, loving, and knowing to transcend the effects of the disability.

Stephen Hawking, the world-renowned physicist, is a perfect example of how people can transcend their physical disability. He discarded a body image perspective to accept a human field image perspective. Moss (1983) points out that Hawking is concerned with life and the boundless horizon one can travel in pursuit of a greater understanding of that life.

VIEWS OF HEALTH

If human field image is to provide a new vision for nursing within a Rogerian perspective, we need to reexamine current views on health. Smith's (1981) models of health can be used to illustrate how health is viewed differently from a body image and human field image perspective, and to further delineate the distinctions between the two views of image.

The clinical model of health emphasizes that as long as people have signs and symptoms of disease they are not healthy, even though they may be productive or creative. Health is related to the disappearance of disease symptoms. The role performance model of health is related to the adequacy of performance of roles whereby sickness occurs when people are no longer able to carry out role functions. The adaptive model of health is concerned with people and their interaction with the environment, where disease occurs when people fail to adapt and cope with changes in the environment.

All such views of health emphasize a causal relationship with the environment where the person is fragmented into parts. Such views are consistent with a body image perspective composed of biologic, physiologic, psychologic, and sociologic parts or their interaction. Generally, all such models portray a problem-oriented view of health and its attainment.

On the other hand, the view consistent with a human field image perspective is a eudaemonistic model of health concerned with general well being and self-realization. In this model, health is concerned with people's actualization or realization of their potentials. Illness occurs when something impedes or prevents actualization. The goal of nursing, then, is not to cure disease, but to help people identify and realize their potentials. Certainly this is what has occurred with Stephen Hawking.

The eudaemonistic model presents an optimistic view of health and supports Martens' (1986) view that nurses need to identify strengths and resources of people and not to just diagnose problems. Winstead-Fry (1980) further defines the distinction of this type of health from a body image view of health when he states, "health transcends the merely physical domain and conveys the idea of a meaningful interaction with the environment" (p. 2). In 1970, Rogers had stated that "a field transcends its component parts. It possesses its own integrity. It acts as a whole" (p. 46). Capra (1982) also notes that fields have their own reality and can be studied without reference to material bodies.

This focus of health that moves away from a body image toward a human field image perspective is embodied in two current definitions of health in the literature. Kim and Moritz (1982) state that health is a rhythmic patterning of energy that is mutually enhancing and expresses full life potential. It is through rhythmic patterns that people can express the distinctive characteristics of their human field.

This view is similar to the more recent view of Keegan and Winstead-Fry where "health is participation in the life process by choosing and executing behaviors that lead to the [optimum] fulfillment of a person's potential" (cited in Madrid & Winstead-Fry, 1986, p. 91). Again, it is interesting to note that Rogers (1970) stated 19 years ago that nursing assists people in achieving their optimum health potentials. Others note that healing seeks to facilitate the expression of a person's greatest potential and that people should participate in their healing rather than being acted upon (Cmich, 1984; St. Aubyn, 1983).

PARANORMAL

The concepts of human field image and eudaemonistic health can be used to examine human potentials from a Rogerian perspective. One emerging phenomenon in the science of nursing related to people's participation in the life process, and that also contributes to the fulfillment of their potential, is the paranormal. Because scientists have used mainly mechanistic linear models in their decades-long attempt to explain the paranormal, they have met with little success. For example, they have not been able to explain the synchronicity of events, that is, the instantaneous perception of events that occur at long distances, where it is impossible, according to the laws of physics, for events to travel faster than the speed of light. Equally as baffling to these scientists is people's perception of future events before they occur.

Rogers' model provides a succinct explanation of the paranormal through the four-dimensional relative present that synthesizes the past, present, and future. It is reasonable to assume that one person's relative present encompasses the future of another person or one's own future. It is a person's perception of the interconnectedness between here and there, the past, present, and future that manifests in what we call paranormal. It is through the use of one's human field image that one is capable of seeing the integral patterns of the human and environmental fields.

In respect to this form of seeing, some of our current technologies (e.g., X-rays or scanners) are indicants of the paranormal potentials of human beings. Paranormal involves seeing patterns of energy fields that involve human field image rather than being confined to a physical reality and concept of body image.

Further verification of the growing potential of paranormal is given through Rogers' model where the integral human and environmental fields are also infinite with the universe. Both are four-dimensional—a nonlinear domain without spatial or temporal attributes. In such a model, energy does not have to travel from here to there since both are together simultaneously anywhere in the universe; in a dimension transcending time and space—"there isn't any there" (Ferguson, 1980, p. 192). All of this involves what Rogers calls the relative present, the infinite now. Further development of human field image will accelerate the evolution of the potentials of paranormal.

As such, paranormal is nothing more than a means by which humans seek to actualize their potentials. The paranormal is a creative thrust in the establishment of new relations with the environmental field (Ehrenwald, 1978). It signifies accelerating changes in the potentials of human beings that make other forms of communication possible that exceed those known to us today. It is significant to note that a doctoral student in the Division of Nursing at New York University is currently working on a qualitative research proposal to study nurses' experiences in caring for comatose patients with the hope of discovering what forms of nonverbal communication take place during their nursing care.

Research has shown that it is possible through the use of Kirlian photography to detect illness months before it becomes manifest in the physical body (Krippner & Rubin, 1974). Through knowledge of paranormal manifestations of human beings, nurses could make probabilistic predictions of illness before it occurs in the physical body. If so, then would it not be possible to use this knowledge to participate in the patterning process of people so they do not manifest illness? Such knowledge will make obsolete most of our nursing textbooks and schools of nursing that bow to a medical model orientation. In fact, most of the current nursing models would also be outdated. Paranormal knowledge of this kind would bring about punctuational change rather than gradual change (Lewin, 1980), especially in the health care system and in the education of health care professionals. Are we prepared for this paradigm shift?

The interconnectedness manifest in paranormal is also present in other phenomena of significance to nursing such as bonding, attachment, empathy, love, couvade, and schizophrenia. Capra (1982) points out that there is an interlocking of rhythms in the strong bond between infants and their mothers, and possibly between lovers. Schodt (1988) studied this interconnectedness by examining parent–fetal attachment and its relation to couvade from a Rogerian perspective. Again, one needs to be aware that body image and human field image provide different perspectives here. For example, Schodt states that her findings suggest there needs to be a better measurement of couvade from a Rogerian perspective rather than a physiological approach. Similarly, Bentov (1977) defines love as energy rather than an emotion since emotions are confined to physical reality, the physical body. Love from an energy field perspective "pervades the whole cosmos" (p. 92).

SCHIZOPHRENIC PATTERNING

Schizophrenia is phenomenon primarily viewed from a medical model. However, there are other views consistent with a Rogerian perspective that can be used to help schizophrenics to actualize their potentials. The eudaemonistic view of health is especially cogent when psychotic states are seen as natural paths toward health and enlightenment (Jones, 1982).

Schizophrenics, it seems, experience a reality aptly described by Rogers in her model, but do not have metaphors to deal with their experiences. Taub-Bynum (1984) believes schizophrenics experience their undivided wholeness, their interconnectedness with the environment to see past the illusion of individuality as separate selves. When they glimpse the ocean of interconnectedness they become frightened they will drown. Jones (1982) asks the question: How close is this to the absence of space and time? Isn't this reminiscent of Rogers' four-dimensionality?

Nursing can help schizophrenics create four-dimensional metaphors to understand their experiences. In this regard, it seems that metaphors of the three-dimensional world have not been overly successful. The challenge would be to use Rogers' model to create metaphors to help in the patterning of the human field so schizophrenics can actualize their potentials, expecially since schizophrenia is seen as taking the risk of evolution to the farthest point (Jones, 1982). As Rodgers (1982) stated, "you can relate to schizophrenics if you agree to meet them wherever they happen to be. They are very interesting people if you are willing to change your idea of what a relationship is" (p. 86). Nurses grounded in Rogers' model can do this.

DEVELOPMENTAL PROCESS OF DYING

The concept of human field image and a eudaemonistic view of health make it easier to understand Rogers' (1970, 1980, 1986, 1987) belief that dying is a developmental process, during which there is continued actualization of potentials. Ring (1986), who sees near-death experiences as "a generalized awakening of higher human potential" (p. 79), supports this positive view of the dying process. In fact, living/dying is a rhythmic manifestation of the life process; so much so that Hine (1982) views dying as a part of life, "the part that makes life literally whole" (p. 45).

This living/dying rhythm proposed by Rogers as diverse change in the human field is reflective of the Elizabethan philosopher Giordano Bruno who stated that "when anything 'dies,' we must believe it to be not death but change only" (cited in Croissant & Dees, 1978, p. 23). Centuries before Bruno, the Greek philosopher Apollonius questioned the process of birth and death when he said (cited in Croissant & Dees, 1978, p. 1):

> There is no death of anyone
>   but only in appearance,
> even as there is no birth of anyone,
>   save only in seeming.

The change from being to becoming
seems to be birth, and the
Change from becoming to being
seems to be death,
But in reality no one is ever born,
nor does one ever die.

The growing number of reports of people undergoing near-death experiences signifies that the dying process plays a role in helping people to actualize their potentials. Taken at face value, these experiences indicate there is continuity of life after the death of the physical body. In general, the fears of dying discussed in the literature are related to a body image perception of the physical body and one's separation from significant others through dying.

When we perceive humans as energy fields with a human field image perception of the pattern of the field, we move beyond the confines of the physical body. Rogers is correct when she proposes that dying is moving beyond the visible range of wave frequencies of the human field pattern that can be perceived by the human eye. In such a view, it is reasonable to propose that the physical body is just one of the many manifestations of the human energy field pattern. In this sense, "Death is simply a shedding of the physical body, like the butterfly coming out of a cocoon . . . and the only thing you lose is something that you don't need anymore—your physical body" (Croissant & Dees, 1978, p. 71).

Manifestations of the four-dimensional wave frequencies of human field patterning are inherent in the near-death experiences (Ring, 1980) where feelings of peace and a transcendent sense of well being that involve overwhelming joy and happiness preside. One experiences ineffable beauty with colors and music that are unforgettable and difficult to describe. One can have a moment when the whole of one's life is experienced all at once or aspects of one's life through flashforward or flashbacks. The encounter with deceased loved ones who are seen and recognized plays a significant role in the decision that one's life tasks and purposes have not been accomplished, that it is not yet time to die.

These near-death experiences play a significant role in the patterning of the human field. People who have had near-death experiences report an enhancement of self-esteem that enables them to become more assertive and accepting of others. These near-death survivors have a heightened sense of appreciation of life and a renewed sense of purpose in living with a conviction that there is a life after physical death, which inspires within them a feeling of meaningfulness (Ring, 1980).

IMPLICATIONS FOR NURSING EDUCATION

A theory-based education and practice need to take into consideration such near-death experiences to help people actualize their potentials. Nurses care for people who are having near-death experiences or paranormal experiences that can be used to enhance the quality of their lives. No doubt, in the future more schools of nursing will integrate this knowledge into their curricula, and patterning strategies will be developed to help people enhance their human field image and potentials.

A New York University doctoral student in nursing is already involved in the process of helping people visualize their dying. She plans to do a study where specific changes in participants will be looked for after they have visualized their dying. Studies of this nature can contribute to the development of individual human field image and potentials.

In a course I teach at New York University where dying as a developmental process is discussed, the following poem is distributed to all the students.

> Do not stand at my grave and weep;
> I am not there; I do not sleep;
> I am a thousand winds that blow;
> I am the diamond glints on snow;
> I am the sunlight on rippled grain;
> I am the gentle autumn rain.
> When you awaken in the morning's hush,
> I am the swift uplifting rush
> Of quiet birds in circled flight.
> I am the soft star that shines at night.
> Do not stand at my grave and cry;
> I am not there; I did not die.
>   (Author Unknown)

A student shared the poem with her dying grandmother who thought it was beautiful and requested it be read at her funeral. Members of the family were reluctant to have this done, but told the student after the funeral how much they had learned from the experience.

It is quite possible that a person's human field image can be developed at an early age. The four-dimensional aspects of Rogers' model and paranormal and near-death experiences were evident in a young child who knew he was dying of cancer. In previous interactions with the child, the nurse learned he had a dog name Jocko that had died a year before. One day while the nurse was holding the child in her lap, he looked at her and said,

"I see Jocko." The nurse smiled and asked, "Will Jocko be glad to see you?" The child nodded his head while smiling. He died later in the nurse's arms. This brief excerpt gives a glimpse of how this graduate student used Rogers' model in a theory-practice situation to enhance the potentials of the dying child. The child was able to participate knowingly in his dying since the nurse saw it as part of the living/dying rhythm of his life process. Such an approach may give rise to an interesting ethical question. Will decisions for resuscitation be based on perceptions of the human field pattern or the functioning of the physical body?

IMPLICATIONS FOR NURSING PRACTICE

Nurses currently use strategies such as meditation, imagery, visualization, and therapeutic touch where there is a primary focus on the patterning of the physical body (e.g., in manifestations such as cancer and pain). One major purpose of these strategies is to "heal" the physical body. This focus on the physical body may account for the conflicting results, both in research and practice situation. Since all manifestations, including those called illness, emerge from the mutual human field and environmental field process, these strategies should be used to help people move beyond the physical body to perceive their field patterns. This enhances the ability to participate knowingly in changing the human field pattern from which the manifestations of illness emerged. Through this patterning process people can participate actively in the actualization of their health potentials.

THE FUTURE

These changing human potentials and future visions of nursing indicate there will soon be a punctuational change in the acceptance of Rogers' model of unitary human beings. This punctuational change will affect all of nursing and the health care system. New laws and theories pertinent to the growing potentials of people will be created to give direction for the future of humankind. Rogers' model offers the framework for the evolution of this creative reality where truth will be four-dimensional (Johnston, 1984).

Human field image will serve as a window into the four-dimensional patterns of human beings enabling us to gain a greater understanding of health and illness. Of course, this human field image will only be seen through experiences in the mutual human field and environmental field process. As Dossey (1984) says, "The experienced processes of the past and the vision of an anticipated open evolution are directly grasped in a four-dimensional present" (p. 140).

The use of Rogers' model is essential since within each person's field pattern are the seeds for the images that will help people manifest their potentials. We need to nurture these seeds so they will germinate and grow (Hall, 1986). This will require the further development of such strategies as human field touch and the clear delineation of how the concept of family field image relates to the evolution of the individual's human field image. In so doing, human field image will help people to express their four-dimensional humanness as humankind moves toward a unified image of the world (Nalimov, 1982).

Nursing science can become a significant means for such advances. We need to embrace the changing potentials to give full rein to the eudaemonistic view of the health of humankind. The challenge for all of us is to continue to develop Rogers' four-dimensional vision of humankind.

REFERENCES

Bentov, I. (1977). *Stalking the wild pendulum: On the mechanics of consciousness.* New York: E.P. Dutton.

Bohm, D. (1980). *Wholeness and the implicate order.* London: Routledge & Kegan Paul.

Capra, F. (1982). *The turning point: Science, society, and the rising culture.* New York: Simon and Schuster.

Cmich, D.E. (1984). Theoretical perspectives of holistic health. *Journal of School Health, 54*(1), 30–32.

Croissant, K., & Dees, C. (1978). *Continuum: The immortality principle.* San Bernardino, CA: Franklin Press.

Dossey, L. (1984). *Beyond illness: Discovering the experience of health.* Boston: Shambhala.

Ehrenwald, J. (1978). *The ESP experience: A psychiatric validation.* New York: Basic Books.

Einstein, A. (1961). *Relativity: The special and general theory.* New York: Crown.

Ferguson, M. (1980). *The aquarian conspiracy: Personal and social transformation in the 1980s.* Los Angeles: J.P. Tarcher.

Friedman, M. (1974). *The hidden human image: A heartening answer to the dehumanizing threats of our age.* New York: Delta.

Global challenges indicate need for transcendent view. (1982, October 4), *Brain/Mind Bulletin, 7*(16), 1–2.

Hall, B.P. (1986). *The genesis effect: Personal and organizational transformations.* New York: Paulist Press.

Hine, V.H. (1982). Holistic dying: The role of the nurse clinician. *Topics in Clinical Nursing, 3*(4), 45–54.

Hohmann, G.W. (1981). Foreward. In C.L. Vash, *The psychology of disability* (pp. vii–ix). New York: Springer.

Johnston, C.M. (1984). *The creative imperative: A four-dimensional theory of human growth and planetary evolution*. Berkeley, CA: Celestial Arts.

Jones, R.S. (1982). *Physics as metaphor*. Minneapolis: University of Minnesota Press.

Kaku, M., & Trainer, J. (1987). *Beyond Einstein: The cosmic quest for the theory of the universe*. New York: Bantam.

Kim, M.J., & Moritz, D.A. (1982). *Classification of nursing diagnosis: Proceedings of the third and fourth national conferences*. New York: McGraw-Hill.

Krippner, S., & Rubin, D. (1974). *The Kirlian aura: Photographing the galaxies of life*. New York: Anchor Books.

Lewin, R. (1980). Evolutionary theory under fire. *Science, 210*, 883–887.

Madrid, M., & Winstead-Fry, P. (1986). Rogers' conceptual model. In P. Winstead-Fry (Ed.), *Case studies in nursing theory* (pp. 73–102). New York: National League for Nursing.

Markley, O.W., & Harman, W.W. (1982). *Changing images of man*. New York: Pergamon.

Martens, K. (1986). Let's diagnose strengths, not just problems. *American Journal of Nursing, 86*, 192–193.

Moss, R.L. (1983, February 27). Letters to the editor. *The New York Times Magazine*, p. 86.

Nalimov, V.V. (1982). *Realms of the unconscious: The enchanted frontier*. Philadelphia: ISI Press.

Richards, F., & Richards, A.C. (1974). The whole person: The embodied and disembodied images. *Journal of Humanistic Psychology, 14*(3), 21–27.

Ring, K. (1980). *Life at death: A scientific investigation of the near-death experience*. New York: Coward, McCann, & Geoghegan.

Ring, K. (1986). Near-death experiences: Implications for human evolution and planetary transformation. *ReVision, 8*(2), 75–85.

Rodgers, J.E. (1982, July/August). Roots of madness: The schizophrenic's reality is not ours. *Science*, 84–91.

Rogers, M.E. (1970). *An introduction to the theoretical basis of nursing*. Philadelphia: F.A. Davis.

Rogers, M.E. (1980). Nursing: A science of unitary man. In J.P. Riehl & C. Roy (Eds.), *Conceptual models for nursing practice* (2nd ed.) (pp. 329–337). New York: Appleton-Century-Crofts.

Rogers, M.E. (1986). Science of unitary human beings. In V.M. Malinski (Ed.), *Explorations on Martha Rogers' science of unitary human beings* (pp. 3–8). Norwalk, CT: Appleton-Century-Crofts.

Rogers, M.E. (1987). Rogers' science of unitary human beings. In R.R. Parse (Ed.), *Nursing science: Major paradigms, theories, and critiques* (pp. 139–146). Philadelphia: W.B. Saunders.

St. Aubyn, L. (1983). *Healing*. North Pomfret, VT: David & Charles.

Schodt, C.M. (1988). *Patterns of parent-fetus attachment and the couvade syndrome: An application of human-environment integrality as postulated in the science of unitary hu-*

man beings. Unpublished doctoral dissertation, New York University, New York.

Sheldrake, R. (1981). *A new science of life: The hypothesis of formative causation.* Los Angeles: J.P. Tarcher.

Smith, J.A. (1981). The idea of health: A philosophical inquiry. *Advances in Nursing Science, 3*(3), 43–50.

Taub-Bynum, E.B. (1984). *The family unconscious: "An invisible bond."* Wheaton, IL: The Theosophical Publishing House.

Vash, C.L. (1981). *The psychology of disability.* New York: Springer.

Winstead-Fry, P. (1980). The scientific method and its impact on holistic health. *Advances in Nursing Science, 2*(4), 1–7.

Unit II
Visions of Rogers' Science-Based Practice

Nursing's concern is with people—all people. Its commitment is to promoting human health and welfare through knowledgeable nursing services.

Martha E. Rogers

3

Rogers' Science-Based Nursing Practice

Elizabeth Ann Manhart Barrett

Nursing's story is a magnificent epic of service to mankind. It is about people: How they are born, and live and die; in health and in sickness; in joy and in sorrow. Its mission is the translation of knowledge into human service.

Nursing is compassionate concern for human beings. It is the heart that understands and the hand that soothes. It is the intellect that synthesizes many learnings into meaningful ministrations.

For students of nursing the future is a rich repository of far-flung opportunities—around this Planet and toward the further reaches of man's explorations of new worlds and new ideas. Theirs is the promise of deep satisfaction in a field long dedicated to serving the health needs of people.

Martha E. Rogers, 1966

Florence Nightingale (1860/1969) initiated pre-science in nursing with her directive to nurse the person, not the disease. Today nurse scientists are defining distinctive knowledge for "nursing the person." "Science-based practice is the use of substantive nursing knowledge, developed through logical analysis and quantitative and qualitative modes of inquiry" (Barrett, 1988, p. 50). According to Rogers (1988), what is unique about nursing is its concern with unitary, irreducible human beings and their respective environments.

Rogers' Science of Unitary Human Beings provides a structure whereby one can view and understand the world (Moccia, 1986). It includes, like the structure of other conceptual models of nursing, basic assumptions about human beings, the definition of nursing, the purpose of nursing, the view of health and illness, as well as key concepts and major implications for research (Waltz, Strickland, & Lenz, 1984). Use of a conceptual model to guide nursing practice is a hallmark of success in practice (Fawcett & Carino, 1989). Use of a conceptual model also helps to distinguish between the practice of nursing and the practice of other disciplines and facilitates identification of nursing-specific client health issues.

PROMOTING HEALTH AND WELL BEING

"The purpose of nursing is to promote human health and well being" (Rogers, 1988, p. 100). Health promotion is a cornerstone of Rogerian science-based nursing practice. "Nursing exists to serve people" (Rogers, 1970, p. 112). "The arenas of nursing's services extend to all areas where there are people: at home, at school, at work, at play, in hospital, nursing home, and clinic, on this planet and now moving into outer space" (p. 86).

Rogers' science-based practice is theory and research-based. The four concepts (energy fields, openness, pattern, four-dimensionality) and three principles (resonancy, helicy, integrality) provide the abstract framework that is now being further fleshed out through theory development and research and translated into practice through knowledgeable caring for clients. Rogerian science presents a different way of looking at nursing phenomena based on its substantive knowledge.

Rogers' major writings cited in the Reading List in Appendix B of this volume provide the theoretical basis for Rogerian science-based practice. There is no substitute for these primary sources. Additionally, Fawcett's (1989) presentation of Rogers' work provides an accurate and clear overview of major tenets of this science. Contributors to Malinski's (1986) *Explorations on Martha Rogers' Science of Unitary Human Beings* provided a beginning research basis for Rogerian nursing practice. Writings contributed to this book represent a further effort to underwrite nursing practice with substantive knowledge.

There is still only minimal basic nursing research that focuses on understanding human health (Pender, 1987). "The primary focus of nursing research has been on the care of people in illness" (p. 460). Bender (1985) indicated the need for case studies of individuals who exhibit high levels of health behaviors over a sustained time. Additional research knowledge about unitary humans and their health generating interchange with the environment will give further practice direction (Pender, 1987).

Both health and sickness are expressions of the life process; they are not dichotomous, discrete entities (Rogers, 1970). Both health and sickness are value terms. Rogers maintains that manifestations of human and environmental field pattern considered to have high value are labeled wellness by society, and those considered to have low value are labeled illness (Rogers, 1980). In the Science of Unitary Human Beings, health is ultimately defined by individuals for themselves.

In Rogerian science health can be viewed as a process of actualizing potentials for well being by knowing participation in change. Health patterning is assisting clients with their knowing participation in change (Barrett, 1988). Health patterning enhances clients' capacity to transform themselves in creative mutual process with their environments. In nursing practice the nurse uses substantive nursing knowledge to facilitate patterning the health of humankind. Keegan and Winstead-Fry defined health as "participation in the life process by choosing and executing behaviors that lead to the maximum fulfillment of a person's potential" (cited in Madrid & Winstead-Fry, 1986, p. 91). Malinski (1988) defined well being as optimal patterning for a particular person.

ROGERIAN PRACTICE METHODOLOGY

The Rogerian practice methodology (Barrett, 1988) calls for (1) pattern manifestation appraisal and (2) deliberative mutual patterning. The nurse and client (individual, family, or other group) work together to facilitate well being throughout the life process.

> Pattern manifestational appraisal is the continuous process of identifying manifestations of the human and environmental fields that relate to current health events. Deliberative mutual patterning is the continuous process whereby the nurse with the client patterns the environmental field to promote harmony related to the health events. (p. 50)

See Cowling's chapters in this volume for further discussion of practice methodology.

Pattern Manifestation Appraisal

In practice the nurse identifies manifestations of pattern of both the client's human field and environmental field, recognizing their integral nature. "Each environmental field is specific to its given human field. Both change continuously, mutually, and creatively" (Rogers, 1986, p. 5). Energy field is "a means of perceiving people and their respective environments as irreducible wholes" (p. 4).

In the first phase of the Rogerian practice methodology, pattern manifestation appraisal, various health assessment tools can be employed (Clark, 1986; Dossey, Keegan, Guzzetta, & Kolkmeier, 1988; Pender, 1987). Such tools are useful only to the extent that they facilitate appraisal of pattern manifestations of four-dimensional irreducible human and environmental fields. Pattern manifestation appraisal may include lifestyle parameters of human health such as nutrition, work and play, exercise, substance use, sleep/wake cycles, safety, decelerated/accelerated field rhythms, space—time shifts, interpersonal networks, and professional health care access and use.

Deliberative Mutual Patterning

In the second phase of the Rogerian practice methodology, deliberative mutual patterning, the nurse facilitates the client's actualization of potentials for health and well being. Well being is choosing to be well. Practice modalities are options that can be used by clients to pursue a way of living, to assist in lifestyle change, to increase awareness of opportunities to be well, and to provide information that may be helpful in making health-related choices.

Many modalities can promote power enhancement whereby clients use their capacity to participate knowingly in change to actualize certain potentials. Health education and wellness counseling will be the practice modalities of choice if actualization is inhibited by lack of information or its use. Considerable health information literature is available although it may not be research based. However, providing information is seldom adequate since its use rather than its procurement often creates difficulty. In some cases where clients are better informed than the nurse—they may have become familiar with the literature during their process of attempting change—they still may experience difficulty in actualizing such informed choices. In this light, power enhancement often requires additional practice modalities in order for clients to experience comfort, hope, healing, well being, and health.

At times the deliberative mutual patterning process itself is the healing modality. This is the case when human therapeutic contact is deemed essential to enhancing the health of the person. Meaningful presence, usually though not necessarily accompanied by dialogue, is the medium for expression. As the song tells us, people need people. After assessing more than 37,000 people on the effects of isolation (few or weak social ties) over periods of up to 12 years, Goleman (1988) found that being cut off from friendships and one's family doubles a person's chances of sickness or death.

Moccia (1988) commented on the power of authentic dialogue between the nurse and client:

[it has the] power to change the lived experiences of both patient and nurse, to change the situation, to change the world. . . . The person who really listens to what we are saying, who really tries to understand our lived experiences of the world and who asks the same from us. When found, it brings the same exhilarating feeling of self-affirmation and the comforting feeling of well being. (p. iv)

Indeed, the importance of meaningful dialogue as a health patterning modality is not to be minimized.

It is important to note that, strictly speaking, there is no such thing as a nurse–client relationship or therapeutic use of self from the Rogerian perspective. In this system one person can't interact with another. There are just the two fields, human and environmental, and they are in continuous mutual process. The nurse is in continuous mutual process with her or his unique environment; the client is in the nurse's environment. This is true for all human fields (individual, family, group). Therefore, the client is in mutual process with his or her unique environment; the nurse is in the client's environment (Madrid, 1988). Regardless of the practice modality being used, the nurse's objective is to pattern the client's environment to promote health and well being.

Unitary Human Field Practice Modalities

Increasingly, as new practice modalities are generated by Rogerian science, the need to develop and test them will rise (Rogers, 1989). Such practice modalities will evolve from basic research on the parameters of unitary human health and the increasing complexity of human life (Rogers, 1989). In Rogerian science, practice modalities concern human life patterning and reflect the wholeness of the unitary person in continuous innovative change with the universe. Currently, in order to select appropriate practice modalities from the full range of choices available, it is necessary to examine the nature and knowledge claims of various strategies as openly and critically as possible. For example, a meta-analysis of relaxation approaches used to treat conditions such as nausea, vomiting, headache, insomnia, and pain was conducted for the purpose of synthesizing findings from 48 experimental studies of non-mechanically assisted relaxation approaches. All treatments included in the analysis except Benson's relaxation technique demonstrated evidence of effectiveness, especially for non-surgical samples with chronic health conditions (Hyman, Feldman, Harris, Levin, & Malloy, 1989).

Studies testing the effectiveness of relaxation as well as other unitary human field practice modalities used alone or in combinations will be needed to assess the usefulness of these approaches for Rogerian science-based practice. For example, considerable research has been conducted on the effectiveness of therapeutic touch as a healing modality (Kreiger, 1987; Meehan, 1988). However, Meehan's work demonstrates both theory development and practice of therapeutic touch from a Rogerian science perspective.

In addition to scientific research evidence of effectiveness and "goodness of fit" with the Rogerian system, a modality also requires "goodness of fit" with an individual client. For example, imagery and affirmations are powerful practice modalities. Not all clients are able to tolerate the intensity of emotion they may evoke. Based on an understanding of what may be useful for a particular client, the nurse selects a combination of modalities. These modalities allow the client's health patterns to develop, evolve, or change in ways that foster healing. The nurse does not attempt to change anyone to conform to arbitrary health ideals. Rather, nursing care enhances the client's efforts to actualize health potentials from his or her point of view. The nurse helps create an environment where healing conditions are optimal and invites clients to heal themselves as they participate in various modalities used in deliberative mutual patterning.

Unitary human field practice modalities based on motion, sound, light, and color are especially useful in Rogers' science-based practice (Rogers, 1989), including: movement/dance/imposed motion, rest/activity, and music. Other modalities that may be indicated include imagery, meditation, humor, relaxation, nutrition, affirmations (expressions of intentionality), therapeutic touch, bibliotherapy (selected readings prescribed as therapeutic treatment), and journal keeping. Esthetic experiences of art and nature may be useful (Moch, 1989). Haiku, a form of poetry, may be composed by the nurse for the client to convey unique healing messages (Rapacz, 1989). Centering is central to many of the modalities (Krieger, 1987). Often the nurse and the client center themselves at the beginning of a particular encounter. Centering is a necessary aspect of therapeutic touch for the healer and may also be useful for the client. Centering facilitates the use of imagery as well.

The Science of Unitary Human Beings provides a perspective for conceptualizing scientific information evolved from other frameworks. Rawnsley (1985) illustrated the process of translating available techniques into healing modalities appropriate for unitary humans. According to Rawnsley, "The assumption is made that there are many therapeutic activities currently implemented from a three-dimensional framework that could be designed so that the meaning is logically consistent with the four-dimensional reality set forth in the concepts and principles of the Science of Unitary Human Beings" (p. 25).

Rawnsley (1985) used the term "conceptual motion" to describe changing focus from a three-dimensional to a four-dimensional view of events. Knowledge emerging from this paradigm shift from a three-dimensional to a four-dimensional view, when used creatively to promote health, constitutes the practice dimension of nursing science. A different paradigm requires a different interpretation of data. Terms and concepts from three-dimensional models must be examined for their "goodness of fit" with Rogerian science. For example, Rawnsley pointed out that the term "intervention" is defined by Webster as "to come in or between, by way of hindrance or modification" and is, therefore, logically inconsistent with integrality of fields in mutual process.

According to Rawnsley (1985), "Healing patterns refer to non-repeating rhythmicities or behaviors that facilitate motion toward health" (p. 26). Rawnsley used the acronym H-E-A-L-T-H to demonstrate some of the healing behaviors that express the unique field patterning of the nurse. She translated the behaviors from their three-dimensional definitions to four-dimensional interpretation. These healing behaviors were humor (H), empathy (E), altruism (A), language (L), transcendence (T), and harmony (H). For example, transcendence in the Rogerian world view is free from three-dimensional restrictions of time and space. Rather, it is characterized by timelessness where time neither moves slowly nor quickly. Instead time is perceived as an "expanded relative present, a dilated time-window through which events that have already occurred and those not yet manifest in temporal reality are experienced as 'now'. Transcendence is the human field moving through the process level of events to a synthesis of thought, feeling and action experienced as wholeness or harmony of fields" (p. 27).

The conceptual motion shift from three- to four-dimensionality provides a model for translation of other non-invasive healing approaches to unitary human field practice modalities. These modalities are specific examples of how deliberative mutual patterning can be used to promote health. Knowledge and healing modalities from other new world views are more likely to yield a "goodness of fit" and thus be appropriate for reconceptualization from a Rogerian science view than knowledge based on old world views.

For Rawnsley (1985), the purpose of healing in Rogerian science is "to tune into that basic harmony of a specific human experience relative to a larger contextual pattern of environmental change" (p. 27). Healing is motion and "the intent of healing is to facilitate motion toward harmony of human and environmental fields" (p. 27).

Malinski, in her chapter in this book, conceptualizes therapeutic touch, imagery, and meditation from a four-dimensional Rogerian science world view. Her description of these modalities also serve as eloquent examples for describing other practice modalities for use in Rogerian science-based practice.

Also in this volume, Boguslawski provides a clear and detailed discussion of human field practice modalities that she uses in her private practice. Relaxation and knowing, imagery, therapeutic touch, affirmations, and nutrition along with the modality of deliberate use of oneself are vividly described through case study illustrations. Other authors in this book discuss these as well as other modalities that they use in practice. There is need for development of unique Rogerian nursing science modalities.

In summary, the two phases of the Rogerian practice methodology are neither linear nor necessarily sequential (Barrett, 1988). Unitary human field practice modalities need to be further defined, developed, and scientifically tested. Other modalities that demonstrate "goodness of fit" with Rogerian science are also appropriate for use, particularly if they have evolved from new world views. Three-dimensional approaches, if appropriate for use, require reconceptualization from a four-dimensional Rogerian world view as demonstrated by Rawnsley (1985) and other authors in this book. Unitary human field practice modalities allow for change; they don't require it. Health-related change priorities are decided by the client. The process of assisting clients with their knowing participation in change is called health patterning. One uniquely Rogerian unitary human field practice modality is called "power enhancement." Power is the capacity to participate knowingly in the nature of change characterizing the continuous patterning of the human and environmental fields (Barrett, 1986). Power is the avenue whereby humans participate in creating their own reality by actualizing some potentials for change rather than others.

It is likely that many of these practice modalities will become an important aspect of all of our lives in the 1990s. They reflect a new way of thinking that is woven into the fabric of the quiet revolution that has been brewing for some time.

THE MILIEU FOR SCIENCE-BASED NURSING PRACTICE IN THE 1990s

In 1970, Rogers warned that "economically, educationally, and socially deprived groups struggle for opportunity and recognition while vested interests endeavor to maintain an obsolete hierarchical control" (p. 119). In 1989, Maraldo proposed that the health care system is close to a state of collapse; "we have a huge medical industrial complex that is no longer suited to respond to people's health needs or socioeconomic imperatives" (1989b, p. 302).

Maraldo also reported that the National League for Nursing is developing a nursing-sponsored national health plan that centers around home care and provides access to nursing care for all Americans. The plan would include "prevention as an overarching priority," nurse-managed care proposals that can compete for contracts with employers or public sponsors, restructuring of long-term care, and payment for nursing services (1989a, p. 2).

Health problems of the 1990s will be those that require nursing knowledge (Moccia, 1989). An increasingly sick citizenry denoting the deteriorating public health of the nation will increase the demand for graduate education for direct care providers. Poverty, drug abuse, acquired immune deficiency syndrome (AIDS), homelessness, the elderly, and chronic illness present health problems that the current sickness system cannot solve. Nursing leadership and nursing knowledge allow for creative approaches to designing a nursing care delivery system relevant to the health needs of our society. Increasingly, people cannot afford to be sick and when they are sick, they cannot access the care that is available. The care that is available often is not the care required or suitable care does not exist. Baccalaureate and higher degree nurses can develop various types of entrepreneurial and/or corporate arrangements so that nursing care can be delivered in the manner in which it is designed and so that nurses can practice as they have been prepared. Nurse-owned and nurse-operated corporations will increasingly contract with hospitals to provide services. This may prove to be beneficial in terms of assuring what services will be provided and in assuring the quality of work life. "As more of the nursing enterprise moves outside hospital walls, community health nursing would once again expand in scope instead of, as today, constricting toward simply transplanting what is done in hospitals to some other site" (Milio, 1986, p. 47). Creative avenues for delivering nursing services are needed.

Moccia (1989) noted the "ever quickening decline of acute-care empires" and warned of "hostile takeovers and the expropriation of nursing knowledge" by medicine (p. 16). Andrews (1986) also proposed that with the surplus of physicians in the 1990s physicians may attempt to take over nursing activities. This is an opportunity for nursing and medicine to clarify turf issues, thereby fostering expert nursing medical services, in a manner that will benefit society. Lines of demarcation based on knowledge domains will dictate practice territories. It is likely that physicians will reclaim "medical activities which previously had to be abandoned owing to a shortage of physicians" (Andrews, 1986, p. 52). While there is some commonality in service provided, it is appropriate for physicians to practice medicine and for nurses to practice nursing. Differences require clarification particularly if Lewis Thomas is correct that "we are on the verge of a disease-free society" (quoted in Bezold, Carlson, & Peck, 1986).

To avoid physicians' claim of nursing activities, nurses will need to clearly articulate the knowledge domain of nursing science that underlies the art of nursing practice. The profession will also need to be prepared to defend nursing territory both in terms of practice activities and practice settings. For example, the director of practice activities for the American College of Obstetricians and Gynecologists has stated, "We are opposed to non-physicians in private practice" (Andrews, 1986, p. 52). Nurse midwives who have established independent birthing centers have seen the impact of those words as efforts to restrict where nurses practice. Is this another way to sustain the inferior status of nurses, similar to attempts to curtail unversity-based professional education for nurses? Meanwhile, Moccia (1989) noted that reforms in medical education are beginning to sound like what nurse educators have been teaching and what nurses have been doing throughout our history, such as holistic approaches to histories, care plans that respect cultural and social differences, and talking to clients. Similarly, it has been suggested that clients will soon be able to select between "high-tech medicine or high-therapeutic touch medicine" (Bezold, Carlson, & Peck, 1986, p. 100). Detmer (1986) also noted that with the increasing supply of physicians, "some will want to provide nursing care instead of medical care" (p. 20). The explosive growth of wellness programs in hospitals and industry that are offered without nursing input provide further evidence that competitive forces are moving into nursing's territory. Also, a variety of types of corporations are marketing programs to promote health and some are being franchised (Bezold, Carlson, & Peck, 1986).

Defining nursing as a body of unique knowledge is a declaration of nursing independence. In order to stake out claims to a legitimate nursing territory, the profession will need to make a solid argument for its capabilities to consumers, legislators, the business community, and insurance companies (Andrews, 1986). These potential allies of nursing need to be educated as to how nursing can improve the health status of citizens of this country.

"Consumers are the key force driving the systems of the future" (Detmer, 1986, p. 20). Not only will they demand a say in the health care they want, they will also become a strong voice in designing the delivery system through the choices they make in the marketplace. If we shift our focus to increased excellence in a nursing knowledge-based practice of promoting well being in health and sickness, nurses will be highly visible and respected as a professional force in health care. The alternative is for nurses to return to their handmaiden status and "become even more task-oriented, responding to someone else's orders, including unions, management, and medical staff" (p. 22). What will the professional, technical, and vocational nurse be doing in the year 2000? What will nursing have become?

Various and vast efforts to design cost-effective medical care have failed to reduce health care costs. Numerous demonstration projects have proved the economic value of nursing services. Maraldo (1989b) notes that the research of Brooten and colleagues indicates that nurse specialists can provide effective care for low birth weight infants at home safely at a savings of $2,000 per day. Similarly, a New York City study demonstrated that the Visiting Nurse Service can provide care for clients with AIDS for $800 a day at home whereas hospital care is now $3,000 a day (Maraldo, 1989b). The nursing profession needs to raise the consciousness of the American public as to the cost-effectiveness of nursing services.

The winds of change are blowing strongly. New modes of delivery and modalities of care are imperative. Knowledge claims in practice are rooted in the science of the discipline. As the profession demonstrates that nursing makes a difference through designing and implementing cost-effective programs to enhance health, nursing will have a stronger claim on limited resources.

The power of the emerging information society is working to create a health care system in which millions of consumers are reshaping both consumer demands and health care practices (LeRoy, 1986). The passive client has become an active consumer. Evidence of the change is the personal health enhancement market. It was recognized as an independent part of the economy in 1977 and is the fastest growing part of the health care industry (Andrews, 1986). Since nursing's purpose is to promote health (Rogers, 1988) and this is what many consumers want, nursing has entered a period of unprecedented opportunity. Much more sophisticated knowledge will be increasingly understood and used by clients. No one owns knowledge; it is not a commodity to be bought and sold by health professionals, nor do health professionals maintain a monopoly over the unique knowledge that distinguishes them as a profession.

As hospitals become intensive care units and recovery continues elsewhere, the movement of clients to various kinds of homes requires a new organization of nursing services. Perhaps each family needs its own "family nurse." A baccalaureate-prepared family nurse generalist could function as an education and information resource for all family members on a continuous basis. With increasing concern and accountability by clients for their own health and illness management, effective negotiation of the health delivery system could be coordinated by the family nurse. Appropriate referrals to nurse specialists and other health professions would be expedited.

One major role of the family nurse would center around teaching related to informational, instructive, and monitoring requirements for self-care. Knowledgeable caring with continuity of concern and advocacy would be inherent in the role. Increasing health awareness and patterning the environment to enhance healing would be important. The Rogerian practice methodology would focus on pattern manifestation appraisal for the family as a unit and deliberative mutual patterning would require use of unitary human field practice modalities to assist the family as a unit. Depending on particular health priorities, at times the individual, rather than the family as a whole, would be the primary focus for patterning the environment. Nurses would involve clients in designing their care plans; they would provide options and facilitate clients' use of options based on informed choices. Advocacy would be based on the paradox, "You alone do it, but you don't do it alone" (Pilch, 1981, p. 18).

In summary, nursing doesn't change in a vacuum. The limits of medicine are slowly being recognized and this recognition is reshaping the delivery of health care (Bezold, Carlson, & Peck, 1986). Likewise, there are mutual "changes in consumers including increased knowledge of and participation in their own health care, decreased trust in organizations and governments, questioning of health costs and health care delivery, and interest in health behavior and promotion" (Bezold & Carlson, 1986, p. 69). Nurses can align themselves with consumers to enhance the power of both groups for betterment of health care.

We cannot assume progress. What the future will bring is not "out there" waiting to happen; nor is it "in there" in a black box known as a computer (Milio, 1986). "Rather, the future will emerge from the choices made yesterday, now, and in the decades ahead. . . . Nonetheless, the future is open, and its shape is limited only by the most inventive of all systems: People acting in concert" (Milio, 1986, p. 49).

Nursing practice, like the life process, is alive with the dance of change. The usefulness of Rogerian science-based nursing practice will speak for itself, and this voice will echo more loudly and clearly as the science evolves. Rogers' vision challenges the nursing imagination to previously unfathomable horizons of scientific humanitarianism.

REFERENCES

Andrews, L.B. (1986). Health care providers: The future marketplace and regulations. *Journal of Professional Nursing, 2,* 51–63.

Barrett, E.A.M. (1986). The relationship of human field motion and power. In V. Malinski (Ed.), *Explorations on Martha Rogers' science of unitary human beings* (pp. 173–184). Norwalk, CT: Appleton-Century-Crofts.

Barrett, E.A.M. (1988). Using the science of unitary human beings in nursing practice. *Nursing Science Quarterly, 1,* 50–51.

Bender, R.C. (1985). Health definition and health behavior of well adults. Unpublished master's thesis, Texas Women's University, Denton, TX.

Bezold, C. & Carlson, R. (1986). Nursing in the 21st century. *Journal of Professional Nursing, 2,* 69–71.

Bezold, C., Carlson, R., & Peck, J. (1986). *The future of work and health.* Dover, MA: Auburn House.

Clark, C.C. (1986). *Wellness nursing: Concepts, theory, research, and practice.* New York: Springer.

Detmer, S.S. (1986). The future of health care delivery systems and settings. *Journal of Professional Nursing, 2,* 20–27.

Dossey, B.M., Keegan, L., Guzzetta, C.E., & Kolkmeier, L.G. (1988). *Holistic nursing: A handbook for practice.* Rockville, MD: Aspen.

Fawcett, J. (1989). Rogers' science of unitary human beings. In J. Fawcett, *Analysis and evaluation of conceptual models of nursing* (2nd ed.) (pp. 263–305). Philadelphia: F.A. Davis.

Fawcett, J., & Carino, C. (1989). Hallmarks of success in nursing practice. *Advances in Nursing Science, 11*(4), 1–8.

Goleman, D. (1988, August 4). Researchers add sounds of silence to the growing list of health risks. *The New York Times,* B7.

Hyman, R., Feldman, H., Harris, R., Levin, R., & Malloy, G. (1989). The effects of relaxation training on clinical symptoms: A meta-analysis. *Nursing Research, 38,* 216–220.

Krieger, D. (1987). *Living the therapeutic touch.* New York: Dodd, Mead & Company.

LeRoy, L. (1986). Continuity in change: Power and gender in nursing. *Journal of Professional Nursing, 2,* 28–38.

Madrid, M. (Speaker). (1988). *Small group discussion of Rogers' science of unitary human beings* (Cassette recording). New York: Third Rogerian Conference.

Madrid, M. & Winstead-Fry, P. (1986). Rogers' conceptual model. In P. Winstead-Fry (Ed.), *Case studies in nursing theory* (pp. 73–102). New York: National League for Nursing.

Malinski, V. (Ed.) (1986). *Explorations on Martha Rogers' science of unitary human beings.* Norwalk, CT: Appleton-Century-Crofts.

Malinski, V. (Speaker). (1988). *Small group discussion of Rogers' science of unitary human beings* (Cassette recording). New York: Third Rogerian Conference.

Maraldo, P.J. (1989a, Summer). As the pendulum swings nursing can triumph. *National League for Nursing Executive Director Wire,* pp. 1–2.

Maraldo, P.J. (1989b). Home care should be the heart of a nursing-sponsored national health plan. *Nursing and Health Care, 10,* 301–304.

Meehan, T.C. (1988, October). Theory development. *Rogerian Nursing Science News,* 4–8.

Milio, N. (1986). Telematics in the future of health care delivery: Implications for nursing. *Journal of Professional Nursing, 2,* 39–50.

Moccia, P. (Ed.). (1986). The theory–practice dialectic. In P. Moccia (Ed.), *New approaches to theory development* (pp. 23–38). New York: National League for Nursing.

Moccia, P. (1988). Preface. In J. Paterson & L. Zderad. *Humanistic nursing.* New York: National League for Nursing. (Original work published 1976.)

Moccia, P. (1989). 1989: Shaping a human agenda for the nineties: Trends that demand our attention as managed care prevails. *Nursing & Health Care, 10*, 15–17.

Moch, S.D. (1989). Health within illness: Conceptual evolution and practice possibilities. *Advances in Nursing Science, 11*(4), 23–31.

Nightingale, F. (1969). *Notes on nursing: What it is and what it is not.* New York: Dover Publication. (Original work published 1860.)

Pender, N.J. (1987). *Health promotion in nursing practice* (2nd ed.). Norwalk, CT: Appleton & Lange.

Pilch, J. (1981). *Wellness: Your invitation to a full life.* Minneapolis, MN: Winston Press.

Rapacz, K. (1989, June 21). Personal communication.

Rawnsley, M.M. (1985). H-E-A-L-T-H: A Rogerian perspective. *Journal of Holistic Nursing, 3*(1), 25–28.

Rogers, M.E. (1966, June). Nursing's story. *The Education Violet.* New York: New York University.

Rogers, M.E. (1970). *An introduction to the theoretical basis of nursing.* Philadelphia: PA: F.A. Davis.

Rogers, M.E. (1986). Science of unitary human beings. In V. Malinski (Ed.), *Explorations on Martha Rogers' science of unitary human beings* (pp. 3–8). Norwalk, CT: Appleton-Century-Crofts.

Rogers, M.E. (1988). Nursing science and art: A prospective. *Nursing Science Quarterly, 1*, 99–102.

Rogers, M.E. (1989). *Nursing in space* (Cassette Recording No. W4-491-89). Seattle, WA: National League for Nursing Convention.

Waltz, C.F., Strickland, O.L., & Lenz, E.R. (1984). Nursing theories, measurement resources, and methods for data collection in nursing. In C. Waltz, O. Strickland, & E. Lenz (Eds.), *Measurement in nursing research* (pp. 341–383). Philadelphia: F.A. Davis.

4

A Template for Unitary
Pattern-Based Nursing Practice

W. Richard Cowling, III

Rogers (1970, 1980) has advocated that nursing science is the basis of creative nursing practice, or the art of nursing. Furthermore, nursing science is identified as a body of knowledge specified in an abstract system of concepts (Rogers, 1988). Science is defined as "an organized body of abstract knowledge arrived at by scientific research and logical analysis" (p. 100). The creative use of this body of abstract knowledge defines the art of nursing.

Recently, Barrett (1988) and Huch (1988) have addressed the issue of integration of theory into practice which they respectively described as science- and theory-based practice. Barrett has defined science-based practice as "the use of substantive nursing knowledge, developed through logical analysis and quantitative and qualitative modes of inquiry, to care for people in their worlds" (p. 50). The mode of establishing science-based practice advocated by Barrett is to use a conceptual model to provide the structure for organizing nursing knowledge and delivering care based on that knowledge. Barrett offers an example of science-based practice using the conceptual system of the Science of Unitary Human Beings.

Huch's (1988) attention to theory-based practice for structuring nursing care is more generic. She makes the case that all nursing practice is implemented through some frame of reference, but the idea of theory-based practice is relatively new. Huch states, "Theory-based practice is nursing care guided by propositions from a nursing theory or framework" (p. 6). Consequently, the practice of nursing is directed by the theoretical structure. More specifically, according to Huch, nursing practice methodologies, concrete modes of action, emerge from frameworks or theories. Use of theory-based nursing practice is a means of pragmatically testing nursing theories. Evaluation methodologies are developed and used to test outcomes of modes of action.

The purpose of this chapter is to present considerations for developing nursing practice based on Rogers' Science of Unitary Human Beings (Rogers, 1970, 1980, 1986, 1988). Emphasis is placed on clarifying some of the conceptual issues in using the system as a guide for practice. A unitary pattern-based practice model is proposed that is consistent with the major tenets of the conceptual system. This model is offered as a template in the form of constituents which might be considered to guide development of nursing practice. It should be noted that other ways of developing and evolving practice based on this conceptual system may be relevant as well.

CONCEPTUAL SYSTEM

The conceptual system proposed by Rogers (1970, 1980) which has been further explicated in recent works (Rogers, 1986, 1987, 1988) specifies the focus of nursing as unitary human beings in mutual process with their environment. Human beings and environments are described as open systems and energy fields. Energy fields are identified by pattern perceived as a single wave. However, Rogers (1988) notes that "one perceives manifestations of field pattern, but one does not perceive field pattern itself" (p. 100). Unitary human beings are irreducible and manifest "characteristics which are specific to the whole and that cannot be predicted from knowledge of the parts" (p. 100). The human and environmental energy fields are four-dimensional and integral with one another.

Rogers (1986) delineates four critical elements or building blocks for this conceptual system: energy fields, open systems, pattern, and four-dimensionality. Because energy provides a sense of the dynamic nature of humans and field implies unity, energy fields typify dynamic unities. They are infinite, open systems that, by definition, contradict the concepts of homeostasis, equilibrium, adaptation, and steady state. Pattern is the distinguishing feature of each energy field and consequently the source of its uniqueness. All reality is viewed as four-dimensional, nonlinear, and without spatial or temporal attributes.

Rogers has proposed three principles of homeodynamics, derived from the conceptual system, that help to describe, explain, and predict the nature of human and environmental change. These principles are stated as:

Principle of Resonancy: The continuous change from lower to higher frequency wave patterns in human and environmental fields.

Principle of Helicy: The continuous, innovative, probabilistic, increasing diversity of human and environmental field patterns characterized by nonrepeating rhythmicities.

Principle of Integrality: The continuous, mutual human field and environmental field process.

It is important to note that change, according to Rogers (1980), is relative and specific to the particular human energy field. It is always in the direction of increasing heterogeneity, differentiation, diversity, and complexity of pattern. Furthermore, the nature of change is probabilistic. "The goal of nurses is to participate in the process of change so that people may benefit" (Rogers, 1988, p. 101). "The purpose of nursing is to promote human health and well being" (p. 100).

CONCEPTUAL FEATURES: CLARIFICATION FOR PRACTICE

The major conceptual features of the Science of Unitary Human Beings (Rogers, 1970, 1980, 1986, 1987, 1988) are outlined as follows:

1. Humans are unitary, irreducible, four-dimensional energy fields.
2. Energy fields are distinguishable by patterns which are not perceived directly but through manifestations.
3. "Each human field pattern is unique and is integral with its own unique environmental field" (Rogers, 1987, p. 143).
4. Consequently, "characteristics and manifestations of unitary human beings are specific to the whole" (Rogers, 1988, p. 101), encompassing human energy field and environmental energy field.
5. Energy field pattern change is continuous, innovative, probabilistic, increasingly diverse, from lower to higher frequency, and characterized by nonrepeating rhythmicities.
6. Human and environmental fields are integral and in mutual process.
7. Individuals have "the capacity to participate knowingly and probabilistically in the process of change" (Rogers, 1987, p. 141).

Elaboration of the implications of these conceptual features for nursing practice provides the basis for the template of a unitary theory-based practice model. Conceptualizing the person as a unitary, irreducible energy field implies that parts are nonexistent. Consequently, one who is attending to a person conceptualized as an "irreducible whole" cannot distinguish parts. What we describe as psychological phenomena, physiological phenomena, spiritual phenomena, emotional phenomena, and the like are manifestations of the whole (encompassing integral human and environmental energy fields) which cannot be reduced to parts. These labels have been used in prior conceptualizations from other disciplines. The issue is not whether such phenomena exist; rather the issue is how they are conceptualized in congruence with the system. They can be described through experience, but to define them as manifestations of parts is to acknowledge the existence of reducible parts. This logical realization has not been identified previously in writing on this conceptualization.

This is a central point: All phenomena have relevance because all phenomena are manifestations of the whole. This is an inclusive, rather than exclusive stance concerning what one considers as relevant in practice. The difference between the unitary perspective and a psychological perspective is that the phenomena we label as psychological are relevant in the context of unitary human beings rather than in the context of some theoretical entity labeled psychological man or the psychological part of the human being, which has no relevance in a unitary conceptualization. Likewise, other phenomena labeled in particular terms conceptually have relevance to unitary human assessment. However, as I will discuss later, the ability to observe, be aware of, and know these phenomena is through processes different from those associated with the theories underlying the conceptualization of these phenomena in particular terms.

The distinction between phenomena as percepts and the labeling of them for meaning as concepts may be useful here. This distinction, posed by LeShan and Margenau (1982), involves the movement from encountering a phenomena to labeling it as a concept. Percept refers to "deliverances of our senses," the main property being a certain spontaneity, a "giveness"; "their occurrence is somehow independent of our volition—we do not feel responsible for the fact we see a tree" (p. 46). Generally, percept is viewed as encompassing that which is conveyed by the senses (perceptions, sensations). However, LeShan and Margenau widen percept to include introspective insights and intuitive apprehensions because they share the spontaneity characteristic of percepts. "A sudden unexpected recollection, the coming of a pain, the incidence of a mood—all these are given in a sense very similar to sensations" (p. 47).

The notion of concepts, on the other hand, as described by LeShan and Margenau (1982), "are products of thought, imagination, and memory" (p. 46). Concepts are abstract ideas associated with a class of all phenomena labeled the same conceptually. The concept "tree" is an abstract idea associated with a class of all trees. In other words, "a concept is related to a percept as a set is related to one of its members" (p. 47). However, LeShan and Margenau note a major difficulty with this analogy in that some concepts can never be a collection of perceptible entities or happenings. "Nobody has ever seen, heard, or smelled an electron—electrons are much too small to display these sensory attributes—yet the concept 'electron' is important to the current theory of atoms" (pp. 47–48). This idea will be revisited in the later discussion of human energy field pattern. LeShan and Margenau describe these experiences of perceiving and conceptualizing as cognitive processes. From the perspective of the Science of Unitary Human Beings, they would be unitary processes.

The idea that energy fields are four-dimensional is consistent with unitary thinking as described by Koplowitz (1984). Time and space are a four-dimensional continuum; they do not exist independently as one temporal dimension and three spatial dimensions, a common interpretation of four-dimensionality. The division of experience into spatial and temporal dimensions is an action like the division of a map into north and south taken by a knower. Unitary thinking postulates four-dimensionality as an intrinsic aspect of reality. "Time and space are both seen as constructs, artifacts of the knower's attempt to make sense of his/her experience, rather than as intrinsic aspects of reality" (p. 287). Rogers describes logically that fields are four-dimensional and in mutual process of change. This is logical since two events or objects, such as fields, would be considered adjacent to each other [in mutual process] if no space or time separated them. "All things are interconnected" (Toben, 1975, p. 134). More specifically, this implies that a practice intervention might go beyond the perceived boundaries of the system from which the problem occurs (Koplowitz, 1984, p. 288).

Three significant implications of the four-dimensional perspective are:

1. The developmental perspective of linearity is inconsistent so that chronological age as a referent for development is inappropriate.

2. Experiences that a person would describe as extremely similar to a past experience or the feeling of connectedness to a person or object that is not in one's three-dimensional space could be explained as four-dimensional phenomena.

3. Since events and objects are mutually connected, regardless of space and time, an event or object from another space or time may participate in immediate experiences. This could be useful in understanding how "past" experiences relate to "current" problems.

Since energy fields are identified by pattern and pattern cannot be perceived directly, manifestations of field pattern are extremely important assessment devices in nursing practice. Rogers (1986) has postulated correlates or indices of patterning delineated in Malinski's text. These are described as in the direction of higher frequency, shorter rhythms, and faster motion toward what seems continuous. Additionally, correlates or indices are sleeping/waking experiences toward beyond waking, temporal experience toward timelessness, greater diversity, and from pragmatic to imaginative to visionary.

The next three conceptual features have relevance to understanding the implications of manifestations for practice:

1. Each human field pattern is unique.
2. Manifestations are specific to the whole.
3. Pattern change is continuous and probabilistic.

Taken together, these three imply, as Rogers (1986) has noted, that change is continual and relative to that particular field with varying forms of manifestations that are somewhat predictable.

For practice this means a consideration of the manifestations relative to the individual in developing practice aims. Using the manifestations for practice means putting them into the context of the individual who is the focus of care, rather than using them as normative indices of development. The capturing of manifestations that are in continual change requires techniques of assessment that focus on the relative present, yet do not ignore the relative past and future. However, from a four-dimensional perspective, manifestations have relevance regardless of linear time and three-dimensional space.

The theoretical feature of the conceptual system that human and environmental fields are integral and in mutual process means that assessment of the human field pattern captures environmental field assessment as well. In other words, pattern reflects the human-environmental process, and thus, it is not clear whether the environmental assessment can be extracted from the general pattern manifestations.

The previous argument for the relevance of phenomena labeled in conceptual terms in other frameworks as psychological, physiological, spiritual, and so forth has significance here. These phenomena, conceptualized as unitary field pattern manifestations, provide clues to the nature of the pattern. What needs particular attention is the validity of physiological changes as human field pattern manifestations. Since humans cannot be separated into parts, or reduced to parts, what is the significance of data we specify as physiological in the assessment of pattern? Perhaps this data is useful, but not central. Nonetheless, the use of this data in assessment is advocated on the grounds that all phenomena are unitary. The assessment would involve placing this data, as well as other data, into a unitary context. The wide array of phenomenal features in human experience would be considered relevant in this frame of reference. These phenomena provide clues to human field pattern. In Wilber's (1982) words, "you get the footprints, but never the beast itself" (p. 92).

In the Science of Unitary Human Beings the most important conceptual feature for practice is the capacity of the person to participate knowingly and probabilistically in the process of change. Herein lies the potential for a meaningful intervention aimed at knowing participation. However, the capacity for participation by the nurse in another's unitary human field pattern is unclear. Unlike other practice models that advocate the centrality of nurse–patient/client interaction, the nurse, in this conceptualization, cannot be extracted from the whole of human-environmental process. Additionally, to what extent may one human field "know" another human field? This point is particularly relevent to assessment. Two avenues for nurse involvement in knowing change of another's human field pattern are possible. One might be to create ways in which the client might become more aware of his or her field and collaborate with the nurse in proposing and using patterning strategies. Another might be that the nurse could knowingly participate in human field patterning through his or her interconnectedness to the client, possible in a four-dimensional universe of open fields. The nurse might have the capacity through various modes to participate in change. For instance, it has been suggested that a human to human field process operates in therapeutic touch through the mode of commitment of intentionality on the part of the nurse (Krieger, 1981).

Barrett (1986) has conceptualized power as "the capacity to participate knowingly in the process of change characterizing the continuous patterning of human and environmental fields" (p. 50). In 1986, she developed and implemented research based on this conceptualization of power and offered two years later a practice model with a clinical example. In this model health patterning is defined as assisting clients with their knowing participation in change. Nursing practice methodology involves two phases, pattern manifestation appraisal and deliberative mutual patterning. Appraisal of pattern manifestations focuses on "identifying manifestations of human and environmental fields that relate to current health events" (Barrett, 1988, p. 50). Deliberative mutual patterning is "the continuous process whereby the nurse with the client patterns the environmental field to promote harmony related to the health events" (p. 50). The goal is substantive change in health dynamics and change in the direction of health as defined by the client. Client participation is an essential element to both appraisal and patterning.

PATTERN-BASED PRACTICE: A TEMPLATE

Here I will propose a model that serves as a guide for developing nursing practice strategies consistent with the theoretical perspective of the Science of Unitary Human Beings. In some ways this model is an extension of what Barrett (1988) has proposed. By way of this model I can address the scope of phenomenal elements and features considered in pattern appraisal and suggest a reconceptualization of deliberative mutual patterning. Additional proposals for constituents of a pattern-based practice follow:

Constituent 1. The basic referent of nursing practice is human energy field pattern. The human energy field pattern emerging from human and environmental field mutual process is the central focus for considering nursing strategies. The development of nursing interventions derives from knowledge of the individual pattern. Another way to state this is that nursing is pattern-appropriate rather than, for instance, age-appropriate, disease-appropriate, or gender-appropriate.

Constituent 2. Human field pattern is appraised through manifestations of the pattern in the form of experience, perception, and expressions. The person is able to experience pattern manifestations that form a wide variety of phenomena. Experience is meant in the broadest sense, and not merely sensory experience which is often the limiting conception of experience. Wilber (1982) describes it as covering all modes of awareness:

> For instance, there is a sense in which I experience not only my own sensations and perceptions (sensibilia) but also my own ideas, thoughts, and concepts (intelligibilia)—I see with the mind's eye, I experience my train of thoughts, my personal ideals, my imaginative displays.
>
> These are subtler experiences than a clunk on the head, but they are nonetheless experiential, or directly and immediately perceived by the mind's eye. Likewise, there is a sense in which I can experience spirit—with the eye of contemplation or gnosis, I directly and immediately apprehend and experience spirit as spirit, the realm of transcendelia. (pp. 81–82)

The experience of pattern manifestations is accompanied by perception. Perception means that the person has the capacity to be aware to some degree of pattern manifestations. Without this capacity, knowing participation could not exist. Perception is the basis for sharing something of the pattern manifestation with another.

Pattern manifestations are expressed in a variety of forms that range from very subtle to direct. Examples of direct expressions might be a verbal response of a feeling or the response on an instrument designed to capture human field manifestations. Subtle expressions are less obvious—I will discuss several examples later in a clinical context. The importance of expression in "geist sciences," those dealing with all realms of experience, not merely physical or empirical, has been noted by Wilber (1982). "Expression is required because the underlying spiritual structure is grasped only in and through its external expressions" (p. 100). Translated in unitary terms, expression is required because the underlying pattern is grasped only in and through its expressions.

Constituent 3. Pattern appraisal requires an inclusive perspective of what counts as pattern information. LeShan and Margenau (1982) embrace the notion of experience to include all strands of meaning as defined by William James as "any item or ingredient within our stream of consciousness" (cited in LeShan & Margenau, p. 44). It is this type of inclusivity that is necessary for pattern appraisal. However, LeShan and Margenau draw some distinctions between two categories of experience: cognitive and noncognitive. Cognitive experiences are those that lead to knowledge or understanding. Feelings, values, beauty, friendship, love, esthetic enjoyment are not cognitive. To provide an example that illuminates this distinction further, LeShan and Margenau discuss the human dwelling: the house. While a house conveys an architectural structure, a home conveys a feeling. The former is cognitive, the latter is noncognitive.

A unitary perspective is one that does not embrace such distinctions. For instance, the conveyance of feeling and the accompanying thought are equally valid sources of pattern information. Pattern appraisal attends to sensory information, thoughts, feelings, awareness, imagination, memory, introspective insights, intuitive apprehensions, and more. Major recurring themes and issues that pervade a person's life are also rich sources of pattern information. The distinctions between experiences as internal or external, cognitive and noncognitive, subjective and objective, and past, present, and future have little or no meaning within the unitary perspective of pattern appraisal.

Furthermore, pattern appraisal includes information expressed in the form of language, mainly metaphors, and visualizations or images described by the person or represented in pictorial format. These expressions of unitary pattern information, which are not often considered in other conceptual models of practice, provide clues to features of pattern experience and perception.

Constituent 4. Knowledge derived from pattern information involves multiple modes of awareness by the nurse. The nurse is informed of pattern by way of experience, perception, and expressions of the individual client.

Expressions include physical sensations reported by the client as well as physically represented entities (gait, position, activity level, posture, sleeping behaviors, etc.) observed by the nurse. Typically, assessment of appraisal is based on observing, noticing, monitoring, and listening. These are essential elements in ascertaining pattern information as well. However, knowledge of pattern involves more than these modes of awareness.

The ways in which nurses come to know the pattern of a client is a critical issue because it is through pattern knowledge that the nurse comes to decisions about intervening. The issue of pattern recognition in the holistic assessment of human beings has been addressed by several authors. Newman (1986) has been most explicit about the concept of pattern recognition. Through her work in the arena of nursing diagnosis she has elaborated pattern recognition generally and specifically. She describes pattern recognition as a general "going into ourselves and getting in touch with our own pattern and through it in touch with the pattern of the person or persons with whom we are interacting" (p. 72). Furthermore, Newman elaborates that pattern recognition is more a function of "reading" one's own pattern than collecting information "external" to oneself. The process of focusing is advocated as a first step in awareness of one's own pattern. More specifically, however, Newman delineates a pattern assessment framework based on unitary pattern manifestations of a person, namely, exchanging, communicating, relating, valuing, choosing, moving, perceiving, feeling, and knowing. Each of these pattern manifestations is operationalized in brief definitions.

Others have focused more generally on what is needed for pattern recognition or viewing the person as a whole. Phillips (1988) recently addressed the need for facilitating pattern recognition in nursing research, and this perspective also has relevance for practice. From his perspective uncovering human-environment patterns of wholeness requires methodologies that provide a "wedding of observable and unobservable manifestations" embodying both concreteness and abstractness (p. 96).

Smith (1988) suggests three potential approaches to viewing the person as a whole. One is the particular or zoom lens which focuses on a summation of parts. Another, the interrelationship or wide-angle lens, goes beyond the additive view focusing on identifying manifestations of the whole from a person-environment interrelationship perspective. Another approach is suggested because it can be argued, according to Smith, that neither of the other two really address wholeness as unitary. Unitary implies that the person is inextricably tied to the environment in a dynamic (flowing) web of interconnections. The focus is on the person-environment process as it unfolds. This perspective requires a motion lens approach which has not yet been formulated. However, Smith does say that the lens approach would involve "a creative leap to identify configurations of the rhythmical flow in the person-environment process" (p. 94).

Recently, Agan (1987) reported an inquiry into perceptions of the phenomena of holistic nursing held by nurses describing themselves as holistic. A key theme that emerged was "a feeling or sensing level of knowing, described as intuitive, psychic, subconscious, or instinctual" (p. 63). The role of intuition in effective nursing intervention has been argued by several researchers other than Agan (Benner & Tanner, 1987; Rew & Barrow, 1987; Schraeder & Fischer, 1986). Benner (1984) has also identified intuition as a characteristic associated with expertness in nursing. "It allows a gestalt of holistic understanding that bypasses building the situation up element by element and then grouping or synthesizing the elements into a conclusion or whole picture" (p. 295).

Rew (1986) did a concept analysis of intuition as a group phenomenon involving an extensive review of the literature. This researcher ascertained the following attributes of intuition:

1. knowledge of a fact or truth, as a whole;
2. immediate possession of knowledge; and
3. knowledge independent of the reasoning process. (p. 23)

Rew cited a study (Cosier & Aplin, 1982) in which intuition is described as allowing "the mind of the individual or group to perceive 'wholes' rather than 'bits and pieces' characteristic of the linear reasoning process" (p. 23).

An additional point here has relevance for a unitary perspective on knowing and modes of awareness. Koplowitz (1984) has formulated a theory of unitary thinking that has some striking similarities, as well as some distinctive differences, to concepts posed by Rogers. This is a cognitive theory about the possibilities of thinking in a unitary way. Of relevance is a notion of unitary knowing that distinguishes it from formal operations and general systems thinking. This notion is "that objects are constructed by the knower to make sense of perceptual data and that objects are not an aspect of reality waiting, as it were, to be noticed by an observer" (p. 290). This, perhaps, may be the fundamental grounds for participative knowing by the nurse with the client. This also implies that the nurse's encounter with pattern information involves construction as part of that participation. LeShan and Margenau (1982) describe construction as "a passage from the data of perception to the realm of concepts and ideas" (p. 49). This aspect of knowing participation on the part of the nurse represents a critical juncture in pattern appraisal. Constituent 5, therefore, is aimed at addressing the way in which information is constructed to be consistent with the unitary perspective.

Constituent 5. Pattern information has meaning for pattern appraisal only when constructed within a unitary context. The act of constructing information within a unitary context involves considering the conceptual features of the unitary perspective. Four features considered relevant are:

1. Data or information from the client is unitary, and not particular.
2. Inclusion of information expressed from a temporal dimension is understood as four-dimensional.
3. Pattern information does not exist separately in reality.
4. Human and environmental fields are in constant mutual process; thus being inseparable, any use of boundaries is constructed.
5. Pattern information is specific to the individual client.

The idea that phenomena arising from experience, perception, and expressions represent unitary manifestations has been emphasized previously in the nature of knowing the human field pattern. It is worth reiterating that information does not have meaning out of the context of a unitary perspective. For instance, the sensation of pain can be considered a physical manifestation from a particular perspective that suggests a physical change. The sensation of pain cast in a unitary context could be an indicator of pattern change. The first connotation would lead one to consider, appropriately, physical measures of relief. Pain viewed as a unitary pattern phenomenon has different implications. The experience of pain derives from something more basic, the human field pattern. Thus, additional information about the pain may lead to a configuration forming an impression about the pattern. This is not to negate the value of using a physically based rather than a unitary perspective. The point is that the sensation of pain has different implications for knowing and intervening in practice from these different perspectives.

Information that is presented from a temporal dimension to the nurse from the client has relevance from a four-dimensional perspective. Thus, if a client experiences an event similar to that of an earlier point in time with accompanying perceptions and behavioral expressions, this is relevant as pattern information in the relative present. Clients may similarly project through images fear of the future. Another way in which pattern information is reflected is through major recurrent life themes and dominant issues in a person's life. This information seems to fit a linear perspective, but in a unitary, four-dimensional perspective it cannot be separated from the current moment. From the unitary perspective it provides information about the pattern of that particular individual.

Any pattern information does not exist separately from other pattern information. According to Koplowitz (1984), a unitary view incorporates the consideration of an essential unity among variables. Another way to state this idea might be that pattern information viewed configuratively has value in understanding human field pattern, rather than isolating information or accumulating it additively. Smith (1988) alludes to this in describing a lens for viewing information from a unitary perspective. She describes the lens as requiring "a creative leap to identify the configurations of rhythmical flow in person-environment process as a starting point for inquiry" (p. 94). Benner and Tanner (1987) characterize pattern recognition as recognizing configurations and relationships without prespecifying the components of the situation. "Context-free criteria or lists are never adequate to capture either the essential relationships or subtle variations in the pattern" (p. 24).

Since human and environmental fields are integral, and pattern arises from their mutual process, the human field pattern information is really information about both. The point is that there is no apparent validity in segregating information into human field pattern information and environmental field pattern information. Appraisal of human-environmental mutual process and environmental field pattern is simultaneous since human and environmental fields are integral.

Pattern information is specific to the individual pattern being appraised. The generalizability of pattern information for appraisal is questionable, although there may be some similarities in pattern characteristics. Allport (1960) has addressed this issue by way of making a distinction between the general and unique in psychological science which also has pertinence to the uniqueness of unitary fields. Allport made the case that it is not appropriate to argue that an individual system is unique and then that it is only the general laws of system functioning that lead to comprehension. "The human system, unlike all others, possesses a degree of openness to the world, a degree of foresight and self-awareness, a flexibility and binding of functions and goals that present a unique structural challenge far more insistent than that presented by any other living system" (pp. 406–407).

Two forms of information may lead to predictions: dimensional and morphogenic. Prediction based on dimensional information is derived from the commonalities that run through all individuals. Prediction based on morphogenic information is derived from the unique world and experience of the particular individual. The latter form of prediction is sometimes referred to as clinical prediction. This is a useful idea for practitioners since pattern information is relevant to the pattern of that individual even though there are commonalities or trends in human and environmental pattern across individuals that are postulated in the principles of homeo-dynamics. Pattern manifestations of the same kind may have different im-plications for pattern appraisal in different individuals because they need to be considered in context, the context of that unique human field pattern and its accompanying multiple manifestations.

Constituent 6. Variant formats for presenting and conveying pattern ap-praisal are applicative to the unitary perspective. The pattern information configured to provide a pattern appraisal may be presented in varying for-mats because the appraisal will have individual meaning for the nurse and client and may be used for different goals and purposes. In other words, there is no one format prescribed for all pattern appraisals.

One potential format might be a single word or phrase that captures the essence of the pattern based on the information ascertained. This could be a function of clarity of the information as it conforms in the appraisal by the nurse; that is, the information might bombard the nurse's senses in a way that the essence of the pattern is clearly evident. A single word or short phrase might capture this essence.

Another format might be a pattern profile that incorporates pattern properties, features, or qualities that emerge from the pattern information. This format would be a description of the pattern profile based on distinc-tive properties or qualities. Since the pattern profile is inferred from the pattern information reflected in the client's experience, perception, and ex-pressions, the pattern information and inferred profile would be included. The profile might be presented in a listing, diagrammatic, or narrative form.

The central purpose of the pattern appraisal is to provide a focus from which to consider nursing intervention. Since this is accomplished in a reciprocal way with the client, the most important consideration in deter-mining a pattern appraisal format is the degree to which it captures and conveys the experience, perception, and expressions of the client. Thus, the client's opinions and impressions about the format are important in the decision. Pictorial and diagrammatic representations of the pattern ap-praisal may best convey the pattern profile or the essence of the pattern. Using the subject's own words and phrases in validating pattern observa-tions is another potential approach. The value of this approach was affirmed in a recent pilot study (Cowling, 1986) in which pattern information was reflected back to subjects who reported that it was a meaningful representa-tion of capturing life themes and issues. Likewise in clinical practice, the use of the client's own words and phrases might be the optimum mode of conveying pattern appraisal.

Constituent 7. The primary source for validating pattern appraisal is the client. From this perspective, self-knowledge represents another form of pattern information and is valued in the process of validating the pattern information and the inferred pattern appraisal. Validating pattern appraisal is also an important phase in the practice model because it provides the direction for setting specific goals and considering intervention strategies. It can be structured in a way that deliberative mutual patterning (see the discussion of constituent 8) is launched.

Validating pattern appraisal is consistent with knowing participation in change. The major aim of validating the pattern appraisal is to ascertain from the client's perspective the degree to which the presented format of the pattern appraisal represents his or her experience, perceptions, and expressions. This is why the format needs to be structured in a way that is meaningful to the client. It also provides an opportunity for further reflection which might lead to additional pattern information.

Many clients understand the notion of an underlying pattern while others do not. An effective way to express the intent of the pattern appraisal is to describe it in terms of experiences and perceptions related to life and health. Observations of expressed pattern information such as sensations and physical information are incorporated and related to other pattern information in a complete profile. For those who understand the notion of an underlying pattern, the synthesized pattern profile can be validated readily.

For some clients the validation focuses more on the pattern information and the degree to which it represents the experience, perceptions, and expressions of the client. In this case the pattern appraisal itself (word, phrase, narrative statement, diagram, or profile) is presented as a synthesis of the information and the client is asked whether this is a good summation of the information.

The validation process might also lead to alterations in the pattern appraisal based upon additional information or corrected impressions or inferences. The alterations are made at the time in an attempt to have the best description of pattern available from which to develop intervention strategies. It is possible to identify goals at this point.

Constituent 8. The basic foundation for intervention is knowing participation in change. Barrett (1988) defines health patterning as "assisting clients with their knowing participation in change" (p. 50). Furthermore, power is viewed as essential in health patterning. Power is operationalized by indicators of awareness, choices, freedom to act intentionally, and involvement in creating changes. This is a highly useful conceptualization of power as participating knowingly in change. Strategies can be oriented to these particular power dimensions. Some strategies employed by Barrett with an actual client included facilitating family communication, exploring options for cancer treatment openly, and acknowledging the client's intentions to act freely.

Developing meaningful interventions involves going from knowledge gained from the pattern appraisal to identifying changes that might be implemented to facilitate health patterning goals. Barrett (1988) defines deliberative mutual patterning as involving environmental patterning to promote harmony.

The term "deliberative mutual patterning" does capture the nature of the process, and from the perspective outlined here it would focus on human field patterning which is integral with environmental field patterning. The process would be comprised of sharing knowledge gained from pattern appraisal from the client's perspective and the nurse's perspective, collective reflecting on the meaning of the pattern knowledge for the client's health goals, and formulating intervention strategies that reflect the nature of change desired by the client. The role of the nurse would be one of suggesting and reflecting on alternatives for facilitating healthful changes. In a sense, the nature of the nurse–client mutual process is as co-clinicians.

Intervention strategies arise from the creative use of pattern knowledge to promote health and well being. Introduction of potential strategies is in the context of exploration rather than imposition. Clients are asked to appraise how the strategy fits for them in terms of their experience and perceptions.

Nursing intervention embraces a wide array of potential strategies specific to the individual situation. At this point in the development of the Science of Unitary Human Beings it seems unwarranted to limit the potential strategies that might be employed. As in any other practice model, strategies must be responsibly designed within the scope of ethical and legal practice of nursing. The most evident criteria for intervention selection would be: (1) its probability of healthful patterning change; (2) its capacity to offer knowing participation in change; and (3) its consistency with pattern appraisal.

Although many potential strategies consistent with the Science of Unitary Human Beings have been suggested by Rogers (1980, 1986, 1987, 1988) and others (Barrett, 1988; Malinski, 1986), the listing of strategies here would be inappropriate taken out of the context of the individual pattern appraisal. However, it is noteworthy that many of the strategies employed in health patterning efforts go beyond the general bounds of traditional clinical practice. Some that are often associated with the unitary perspective involve a wider range of human potentials such as imagery, meditation, movement, psychic abilities, and incorporate environmental elements such as music, light, and color.

Additionally, there are those outside of nursing who are using strategies derived from other perspectives consistent with unitary pattern-based nursing practice. Examples of these include the rebirthing and loving relationship training developed by Ray (1976) and Mandell (1986), the energy techniques utilized by Moss (1981), the healing methods of Hay (1984), and the visualization/imagery work of Siegel (1986). All of these practices are built on an idea that there is an underlying and enduring process that accounts for the health problems and issues faced by individuals. Each involves getting in touch with this underlying process through awareness techniques. There is a deemphasis on analysis and a heavier focus on exploring alternative ways of viewing things for greater consistency with health. Imagination, imagery, affirming oneself, letting go of past thoughts, accepting feelings, using natural processes like breathing, music, and body work in a broader context are advocated in these practices.

Constituent 9. Evaluation methodologies are focused on continual pattern appraisal and confirmation of alterations with the client. Evaluation requires a return to the original appraisal format after monitoring and collecting additional pattern information as it unfolds during the implementation of nursing intervention strategies. The pattern information is considered in the context of continually emerging health patterning goals affirmed by the client. The client may use a journal or some other form to record experiences, perceptions, and expressions of pattern information to be considered in the pattern reappraisal. Individual clients are involved in identifying where they are and where they would like to go from that point. It is possible that at the time of pattern reappraisal, new intervention strategies, or modifications in suggested intervention strategies, might be introduced. The same forms of pattern information are used in the continuous pattern appraisal as were considered in the original appraisal. The evaluation process is ongoing and not necessarily as sequential as presented for explanatory purposes.

A CLINICAL EXAMPLE OF THE TEMPLATE

Mr. Jones was a 54-year-old man who came to my practice in health promotion asking for assistance with phantom limb pain. He had tried multiple treatment modalities including a large number of medically prescribed analgesics and psychotherapy. While doing a pattern appraisal, I asked him a number of questions about the pain, the circumstances of losing the arm, his choices, his life in general, and what he wanted to achieve in working with me. His goal was very specific; he wanted to be able to manage the phantom limb pain. His wife made the office visit with him and talked freely about their life and their relationship. A strong sense of real support for each other was evident.

What he described was a life in which he had been very productive and useful. He owned his own business—a hardware store. Everything he did in his life demonstrated responsibility. He also loved motorcycles and it was while riding one that he had an accident in which his arm was left paralyzed. He described the weight of the arm as incredibly heavy and how difficult life had been trying to work and deal with the paralyzed arm. A surgeon recommended that he have the arm amputated and he decided this was the best course under the circumstances. Following the amputation, he had severe burning sensations in the arm. The sensations subsided, but would return intermittently without warning. He was extremely afraid of the pain, not knowing when it might strike him. His wife described the physical reaction when the pain hit as extremely severe. It could happen almost any time of the day or night with no regular pattern. Other than this pain he described himself as happy and healthy.

I noted that Mr. Jones was extremely organized and systematic about things. He described how his hardware store was organized with detailed labeling and an efficient arrangement of the stock. His wife remarked about his neatness and orderliness in regard to his garage and workshop.

This man was extremely ambivalent about the decision to amputate the limb, yet everything else in his life was clear. He referred to the decision to amputate the limb as based on its uselessness, and its effect on his ability to function proficiently. He had control of everything in his life but the pain.

Apparent to me was a major theme of pattern information concerning control and order. Life was good when he had control and when things were in order. The loss of the limb was an asymmetry in his physical body according to his perception. However, he was open to the possibility of change. His pattern profile, when placed in the context of experience, perceptions, and expressions, was:

> Experience: anticipatory fear of pain, disrupted order in life and health, loss of control
>
> Perceptions: ambivalence about limb and amputation, guilt about motorcycle accident and amputation, uncertainty about potential for pain relief, openness to possibilities
>
> Expressions: physical signs of pain, vivid and explicit description of pain sensation, metaphorical representations of pain used, such as hot as coals, uneasiness, and discomfort from loss of control.

These elements were used to offer a pattern appraisal of fear, ambivalence, guilt, disorder, and asymmetry as major themes of pattern manifestations.

The client was offered an opportunity to describe to me how he would change the pain if he could do this visually. This was done purposely to give him a sense of control and clarity. He was asking for control, but in actuality he was gaining involvement in his mutual process through knowing participation. Since he liked to fish, he said the ultimate relief would be imagining that the limb was soaking in a cool stream. I guided him through a visualization using his own images and taught him how to use guided imagery for himself. This was done to facilitate pattern change in the direction of health which was very specific in regard to pain relief. Additionally, I offered him the opportunity to explore the relationship of fear and searching for ultimate control. Over a number of weeks he experienced relief of pain at his will on several occasions using guided imagery. He began to incorporate a change in thinking about letting go of control and experiencing life more fully in his own terms. The strategies were evaluated based on the accomplishment of his one goal of pain relief and on the grounds of his own sense of growth and satisfaction with his life situation. Dialogue, reflection, and exploration were the features of our interactions.

SUMMARY

Unitary pattern-based practice is one creative approach to nursing intervention based on the conceptual and theoretical perspective of the Science of Unitary Human Beings. Considerations for practice were derived from the major concepts and theoretical tenets of the framework. Continued clarification and operationalization of the conceptual features in practice is warranted. A template for nursing practice with specified constituents provides a mechanism for implementing practice strategies. Processes of pattern appraisal, deliberative mutual patterning, health patterning, and evaluation were elaborated for the consideration of clinical scholars. Debate and dialogue on these issues is anticipated to further explicate the practice potential of this conceptual system.

REFERENCES

Agan, R.D. (1987). Intuitive knowing as a dimension of nursing. *Advances in Nursing Science, 10*(1), 63–70.

Allport, G. (1960). The general and unique in psychological science. *Journal of Personality, 30*, 405–422.

Barrett, E.A.M. (1986). Investigation of the principle of helicy: The relationship of human field motion and power. In V.M. Malinski (Ed.), *Explorations on Mar-*

tha Rogers' science of unitary human beings (pp. 173–184). Norwalk, CT: Appleton-Century-Crofts.

Barrett, E.A.M. (1988). Using Rogers' science of unitary human beings in nursing practice. *Nursing Science Quarterly, 1*, 50–51.

Benner, P. (1984). *From novice to expert*. Menlo Park, CA: Addison-Wesley.

Benner, P., & Tanner, C. (1987). How expert nurses use intuition. *American Journal of Nursing, 87*, 23–31.

Cosier, R.A., & Aplin, J.C. (1982). Intuition and decision making: Some empirical evidence. *Psychological Reports, 5*, 275–281.

Cowling, W.R. (1986). *Proposal for pattern study*. Unpublished manuscript.

Hay, L. (1984). *You can heal your life*. Santa Monica, CA: Hay House.

Huch, M.H. (1988). Theory-based practice: Structuring nursing care. *Nursing Science Quarterly, 1*, 6–7.

Koplowitz, H. (1984). A projection beyond Piaget's formal-operations stage: A general system stage and a unitary stage. In M.L. Commons, F.A. Richards, & C. Armon (Eds.), *Beyond formal operations* (pp. 272–295). New York: Praeger.

Krieger, D. (1981). The creative nurse: A holistic perspective. In D. Krieger (Ed.), *Foundations for holistic health nursing practices: The renaissance nurse* (pp. 137–148). Philadephia: Lippincott.

LeShan, L., & Margenau, H. (1982). *Einstein's space and Van Gogh's sky: Physical reality and beyond*. New York: Macmillan.

Malinski, V. (1986). Nursing practice within the science of unitary human beings. In V. Malinski (Ed.), *Explorations on Martha Rogers' science of unitary human beings* (pp. 25–32). Norwalk, CT: Appleton-Century-Crofts.

Mandell, B. (1986). *Two hearts are better than one*. Milbrae, CA: Celestial Arts.

Moss, R. (1981). *The I that is we*. Milbrae, CA: Celestial Arts.

Newman, M. (1984). Nursing diagnosis: Looking at the whole. *American Journal of Nursing, 84*, 1496–1499.

Newman, M. (1986). *Health as expanding consciousness*. St. Louis: C.V. Mosby.

Phillips, J.R. (1988). The looking glass of nursing research. *Nursing Science Quarterly, 1*, 96.

Ray, S. (1976). *I deserve love*. Berkeley, CA: Celestial Arts.

Rew, L. (1986). Intuition: Concept analysis of a group phenomenon. *Advances in Nursing Science, 8*(2), 21–28.

Rew, L., & Barrow, E.M. (1987). Intuition: A neglected hallmark of nursing knowledge. *Advances in Nursing Science, 10*(1), 49–62.

Rogers, M.E. (1970). *An introduction to the theoretical basis of nursing*. Philadephia: Davis.

Rogers, M.E. (1980). Nursing: A science of unitary man. In J. Riehl & C. Roy (Eds.), *Conceptual models for nursing practice* (2nd ed.) (pp. 329–337). New York: Appleton-Century-Crofts.

Rogers, M.E. (1986). Science of unitary human beings. In V. Malinski (Ed.), *Explorations on Martha Rogers' science of unitary human beings* (pp. 4–23). Norwalk, CT: Appleton-Century-Crofts.

Rogers, M.E. (1987). Rogers' science of unitary human beings. In R.R. Parse (Ed.), *Nursing science: Major paradigms, theories, and critiques* (pp. 139–146). Philadelphia: W.B. Saunders.

Rogers, M.E. (1988). Nursing science and art: A prospective. *Nursing Science Quarterly, 1*, 99–102.

Schraeder, B.D., & Fischer, D.K. (1986). Using intuitive knowledge to make clinical decisions. *Maternal Child Nursing Journal, 11*, 161–162.

Siegel, B. (1986). *Love, medicine, and miracles.* New York: Harper and Row.

Smith, M.J. (1988). Perspectives of wholeness: The lens makes a difference. *Nursing Science Quarterly, 1*, 94–95.

Toben, B. (1975). *Space, time, and beyond.* New York: E.P. Dutton.

Wilber, K. (1982). The problem of proof. *ReVision: A Journal of Consciousness and Change, 5*(1), 80–100.

5

The Science of Unitary Human Beings and Theory-Based Practice: Therapeutic Touch

Thérèse C. Meehan

In the world of contemporary health care with its emphasis on specific diseases, complex technology, and cost containment, the importance of a nurturing relationship between nurse and patient and between the whole environment and the patient is often overshadowed. Responsibility for ensuring this relationship is a fundamental aspect of professional nursing, for to nurse is to nurture in the professional sense of fostering human growth and development and tending the flow of human life in ways that promote wholeness and health. The Science of Unitary Human Beings (Rogers, 1986; Malinski, 1986) provides a broad perspective within which to conceptualize the nature of this nurse–patient, environmental–patient relationship. It can give renewed theoretical impetus to the use of long standing (and all too often long forgotten) methods of practice such as the back rub, and supports the development of innovative new methods of practice such as therapeutic touch. Figure 1 provides a schematic example of the conceptual-theoretical-practice levels of the Science of Unitary Human Beings with emphasis on the focus of this paper.

In this chapter the use of therapeutic touch as a nursing intervention will be described in detail and its conceptual and research basis will be reviewed. Suggestions will be made for learning therapeutic touch and for integrating it into nursing practice.

Figure 1
An Example of Conceptual-Theoretical-Practice Levels
of The Science of Unitary Human Beings

		Science of Unitary Human Beings	
		Resonancy-Integrality-Helicy	

Conceptual View (Deduction)

Theory-linked Hypotheses

Imposed rocking motion will improve quality of sleep and perceived restedness

Therapeutic touch will decrease anxiety and pain and promote comfort

A back-rub procedure administered by a nurse who is centered will increase feeling of calmness in both patient and nurse

Unconscious patients experience a level of awareness which allows them to knowingly participate in change

Testing Hypotheses

Gueldner (1984)

Quinn (1984)
Meehan (1985)
Quinn (1989)

Not tested

Not tested

Theory-based Practice

Rocking elderly patients in a rocking chair to promote rest and sleep

Treating patients with therapeutic touch to decrease anxiety and pain and promote comfort

Restructure the back rub to include centering by the nurse

Knowing that "unconscious" patients can be aware of activity in their environment

Conceptual View (Induction)

Experience in Practice

e.g. Intuition, Meditation, Therapeutic Touch

THERAPEUTIC TOUCH: A NURSING INTERVENTION

The practice of therapeutic touch involves direct subjective experience of energy field patterning and is not easily described to those who are not familiar with it. Except for the work of Lionberger (1985), few detailed descriptions of the practice appear in the nursing literature. Also, in many situations, especially those dominated by the medical model, therapeutic touch is considered unconventional and nurses are unsure of how to introduce the treatment to patients. The following practice example, described in detail in the first person, is presented to help illustrate the nature of the practice and the kind of situation in which it can be offered to a patient.

"Can't you do *something* to help me," the man asked in a tense, weary voice. Holding himself guardedly, he sat on a stool in an examining room of the inpatient ambulatory care section of a large medical center. His tired eyes held the eyes of his nurse as she sat across from him considering his situation.

Mr. Cullen had been admitted three days previously for reassessment and possible further treatment for metastatic cancer, and for pain management. Despite the chemotherapy, the cancer seemed to be spreading. But his most immediate problem was pain: persistent, aching, and at times excruciatingly sharp pain in his back and abdomen. His analgesic medication had been increased to morphine 8 mgs by subcutaneous injection every 3 hours PRN and methadone 10 mgs every 8 hours. It was 1½ hours since his last injection of morphine and 1½ hours until he could have another. The pain persisted, although its sharp edge had been dulled. Mr. Cullen was by nature a stoic man but the pain was beginning to wear him down.

"Well," the nurse said, "there is one thing you could try. It's a bit different from the kinds of treatment you've been having but patients often say that it helps them to feel better. It's a nursing treatment called therapeutic touch. I learned it in my college courses in nursing. It doesn't involve actual physical touch. It's different in that it's based on the idea that you extend beyond your skin and that the nurse can use her hands, a few inches away from your body, to smooth what's considered an energy flow around you. It's a bit like the Eastern idea of acupuncture. With acupuncture needles are used to unblock and balance energy as it flows through the body. With therapeutic touch the nurse uses her hands to unblock and balance energy as it flows around the body."

An expression of surprise momentarily replaced the tiredness in Mr. Cullen's eyes. "It sounds ridiculous," he said. "I don't believe in those kind of things." Mr. Cullen had for many years taught high school mathematics and had no time for what he called "unknown quantities."

"Well," the nurse continued, "there have been some studies done which indicated that it can help patients relax and may help relieve pain. Many nurses believe it helps relieve pain. It may or it may not help relieve your pain. If you'd like, I could give you a treatment now and you could try it."

"But—Oh, I don't know." The pain and weariness seemed to overwhelm him. "I don't think it'll help, but I guess you could try it. I just want to get rid of this pain."

Mr. Cullen remained seated on the examining room stool while the nurse administered therapeutic touch. Before beginning, she explained in simple terms what she would do. "I'm going to be moving my hands, in gentle, sweeping downward movements, from your head to your feet, at a distance of 2 to 4 inches from your body. I'll be working sometimes at the back of you and sometimes at the front of you. I'll be focusing my attention on my hands and probably won't be talking much, but if you want to talk or have any questions, just say. It'll take about 10 minutes, but if at any time you want me to stop, just say."

Before beginning, the nurse assumed a meditative state of awareness called "centering." This meditative state is of central importance in the practice of therapeutic touch and is maintained throughout the intervention. The nurse centered herself by shifting her awareness from a direct focus on her environment to a focus on, and attunement with, the center of her own being. Through centering she was able to put aside any personal concerns, achieve a sense of calm and balance within herself, and experience herself as a unitary whole. Although she was still very aware of her environment, it had merged into the background. Her attention was specifically focused on Mr. Cullen as a unitary whole, not on his body systems, and not on the disease or the distress it engendered in him. It was from this meditative state of awareness that she made the specific intent to therapeutically assist Mr. Cullen. This meditative awareness enabled her to attend to him with a sense of balance and compassion, yet without personal attachment to his need to be helped or her need to help him. It also helped quicken her intuitive sense of him and made it easier for her to become aware of sensory cues in her hands as she carried out the intervention.

Her assessment of Mr. Cullen actually occurred continuously throughout the intervention but was particularly focused on at the beginning. Her assessment was carried out on two levels. On one level she took into consideration everything she knew about him from nursing and medical records and from her general observation. This included knowledge of such factors as his usual daily activities, his attitudes toward different aspects of his life, his relationship with family members, the tone of his voice, and how he held himself as he sat on the stool. From her meditative state of awareness, knowledge derived from this level of assessment formed an overall perception of Mr. Cullen as a unitary whole and formed the context within which she carried out the second level of assessment: that of the energy field pattern.

To begin the energy field assessment she stood behind Mr. Cullen and moved her hands gently and symmetrically, about 3 inches from his body, in a downward motion through the energy flow from his head to his lower back. As she did this she was able to determine the pattern of the energy flow by perceiving qualitative differences in extremely subtle sensory cues, similar to changes in temperature or pressure, in her hands. These cues gave rise to images through which she conceptualized the pattern of the energy flow. She recognized that the energy flow did not have an open or symmetrical quality but instead felt "slightly heavy" or "tight" in places giving, in metaphoric language, the impression of thin, elastic strings and scattered knots. She then stood in front of him and continued the assessment, perceiving similar sensory cues as she moved her hands over his chest and abdomen. As she moved her hands over his legs the sensory cues changed, giving the impression of "emptiness" and lack of energy flow.

For most patients, after completing the initial assessment, the nurse would have stopped for a minute to tell the patient, in general terms, her perception of the energy flow, and review with the patient her plan for the treatment. However, since Mr. Cullen was quite skeptical, and weary from the pain, she continued directly on. In treating Mr. Cullen, she kept her awareness of him and of herself as unitary wholes constantly at the forefront of her attention. This enabled her to stay centered and to project to him her own sense of balance and calm. It also enabled her to be constantly aware that he had, beyond the overriding dissonance and distress of the disease, a source of vitality continuously flowing forth which was characterized by order, balance, and health. It was her specific and constant intent to facilitate this flow of vitality; in effect, to facilitate Mr. Cullen's own natural healing potential. The nurse did this by being aware of the vitality which constantly flowed forth within herself; a vitality which she shared with all life in the universe. Because she was centered she perceived this vitality as flowing through the center of calm and unity in herself and as separate from her own personal energy. By staying centered she was able to ensure that it was the vitality flowing through the center of calm and unity in herself that was flowing to Mr. Cullen during the treatment and not her own personal energy. At the same time, she used her hands in sweeping motions through the energy field to smooth and balance the energy flow, to remove areas of tension and congestion, and to facilitate as open and balanced an energy flow as possible. She did this by conceptualizing the quality of her intent in images and directing them to Mr. Cullen using her hands as focal points. For example, where the quality of the energy field gave the impression of "tightness" and "scattered knots," she directed the image of a gentle waterfall flowing through the area loosening the tension, dissipating the knots and smoothing the energy flow. Where the quality of the energy field gave the impression of "emptiness" and a lack of energy flow, she directed the image of rivulets of water gently falling through a barrier and streaming into the earth.

The nurse worked this way for about 10 minutes. A couple of times she said to Mr. Cullen, "How are you feeling?"

He said, "I'm O.K." but otherwise did not say anything and did not seem discomforted by the method of therapeutic touch.

As the nurse worked, her perception of the pattern of the energy flow changed continuously. For example, over one side of his lower back the quality of the energy flow changed to give the impression of "warmth." As she moved her hands over this area she directed the image of a gentle, cool mountain breeze with the intent that the quality of this image would flush out the imbalance signified by the impression of warmth. After she had worked for about 10 minutes, and even though the energy flow still had a disrupted, tentative, and nonsymmetrical quality, she felt that, for a first treatment, this was long enough. If this treatment helped him and if he wanted another, she could treat him again later in the day. To complete the treatment she knelt to one side of him and placed one hand in front of him, just above his waist, and her other hand directly opposite over his back. She held her hands this way for about 2 minutes, being especially aware of the source of vitality continuously flowing forth within herself and directing her image of the source of this vitality to her left hand with the intent of making this energy available to him to use in whichever way he needed. Again, her intent was motivated by compassion, but detached from personal involvement. As she did this the quality of the sensory cues in her hands gave the impression of a concentrated flow of energy between her hands and Mr. Cullen.

"I've finished the treatment now," she said, standing aside from him. "How do you feel?"

Mr. Cullen continued to sit, still somewhat guardedly, on the stool. "I don't really feel any different," he said. "I don't think it made any difference to the pain."

"Well," the nurse said, "I'm sorry it didn't help. It doesn't always help, but at least you tried it. I'll try to think of something else that might help and I'll talk to the physicians again about changing or increasing your pain medication. Come back in an hour and I'll be able to give you another injection."

Mr. Cullen went off, still appearing tense and weary. He had an appointment to attend a group class in the patient education center. The nurse went on working with her other patients.

Two hours went by before the nurse noticed that Mr. Cullen had not returned for his injection. At about the same time a nurse from the education center stopped to ask her about the "treatment with her hands" that she had done for Mr. Cullen. She explained that Mr. Cullen had attended his class and reported that he had begun to feel better. He had told the group that his nurse had "done something with her hands" and that even though he still had the pain, it didn't bother him any more. After the class he had gone to his room to rest for a while.

An hour later Mr. Cullen returned to see his nurse. The pain was beginning to increase again and he wanted another injection of morphine. Six hours had passed since his last injection, the longest period of time he had gone without an injection of morphine in several days. He sat again, somewhat less guardedly, on the examining room stool while the nurse administered the injection.

"I don't know what you did," he said, "but it did help after a while—at least I think it did. It was odd how the pain was still there but it didn't bother me anymore." Though he was still weary, and somewhat puzzled, his voice held a hint of hope.

"If you'd like, I could give you a treatment again this afternoon," the nurse said.

"Yes," he said. "Yes, I think I'd like to try it again—if you've got time? I know you're very busy."

"I will have time," the nurse said, thinking to herself that whatever else happened, she or one of the other nurses would make time.

For the remainder of his stay at the medical center, Mr. Cullen received a therapeutic touch treatment twice a day. He continued to receive the morphine, but at less frequent intervals: about every 6 to 8 hours. He began to sleep for longer periods and to feel more relaxed generally. One of Mr. Cullen's sons became interested in learning therapeutic touch. The nurse taught him to do it, and he continued the treatments for his father after he returned home.

CONCEPTUAL BASIS FOR PRACTICE

Consideration of therapeutic touch brings into sharp focus the difference between nursing and medical models for practice. Although nurses who are responsible for the care of patients receiving medical treatment must have a working knowledge of the medical model, only a nursing model can direct nursing practice. It is immediately clear that therapeutic touch is quite different from the medical model. Because the medical model is based primarily on the mechanistic, physical-sensory world view, it allows for touch only as direct contact and does not allow for the source of touch to have any relevance to its effect other than its quantitive sensory impact (Weber, in press). Most nursing models are based primarily on the psychological-humanistic world view espoused in existential philosophy. From this view they allow for touch as a purposive way of reaching out and communicating feelings, such as empathy or compassion, between self-conscious and imaginative human beings. The Science of Unitary Human Beings is based entirely on a field world view and allows for touch as an energy field process which can include but does not require physical contact. When nursing values, such as nurturance and compassion, are incorporated with the Science of Unitary Human Beings model of human-environmental energy field process, the use of therapeutic touch as a nursing intervention can be logically proposed and explained.

It is important to note that from the perspective of the Science of Unitary Human Beings, therapeutic touch is not viewed in quite the same way as when it was first introduced into nursing (Krieger, 1975; Krieger, Peper, & Ancoli, 1979). For example, therapeutic touch is not viewed as being derived from the laying-on of hands. Instead, the nurse is viewed as being integral with the patient's environmental energy field patterning, and therapeutic touch treatment is viewed as a purposive patterning of energy field mutual process in which the nurse uses his or her hands as a mediating focus in the continuing patterning of the mutual patient-environmental energy field process. Also, change in a patient-energy field patterning is not viewed as being mediated by a flow of *prana*, a human energy field concept from Eastern philosophy. Instead, it is viewed as change which occurs in the human-environmental energy field patterning as the nurse assumes a meditative state of awareness, recognizes his or her own unitary nature and integrality with the environmental field, and focuses his or her intent to help the patient.

In considering Mr. Cullen, his nurse was using the Science of Unitary Human Beings as a perspective for viewing him and her relationship to him, and from which to gain insight into his experience and determine how she might best be able to treat his responses to the metastatic cancer. Because she was using this model her perspective held that energy fields were the fundamental units of herself, Mr. Cullen, and their respective environments. She, Mr. Cullen, and their respective environments were interconnected, unitary wholes in a continuous mutual process of motion and change, and simultaneously giving rise to their own unique patterns of characteristics. From this perspective, the nurse viewed Mr. Cullen's experiences of pain and weariness as rising from his unitary nature wherein his mental and physical aspects were inseparable. The nurse felt confident in using the model as a basis for her practice because she had studied its basic concepts and was familiar with the support for the energy field view provided by contemporary scientists and scholars (Bohm, 1973; Cushing & McMullin, 1989; Prigogine, 1980; Weber, 1986).

Thus, Mr. Cullen's nurse perceived that she and Mr. Cullen extended beyond their bodies, each being an energy field pattern in the other's environment. She assumed, based on the experiences of a large number of nurses familiar with the practice of therapeutic touch, that in a state of health the energy field as it extended beyond Mr. Cullen's body would move in an open and symmetrical flow from head to feet. She also assumed that she could, through the natural sensitivity of her hands, perceive the pattern of the energy flow as subtle sensory cues in her hands. Moreover, she assumed that the pain and weariness that Mr. Cullen was experiencing would be reflected in the energy field pattern as it extended beyond his body. As she did the field assessment of Mr. Cullen, she perceived that the pattern of the energy field as it extended beyond him was not flowing freely and symmetrically. In treating him, her intent was to continuously direct the patterning of the field to facilitate a more open and symmetrical patterning which in turn would enhance his own healing potential. The nurse knew from experience that she would have an intuitive sense of when to end the treatment; of the right "dose" of the treatment in relation to the needs of the particular patient. From the perspective of the Science of Unitary Human Beings, therapeutic touch is one example of how "Professional practice in nursing seeks to . . . strengthen the coherence and integrity of the human and environmental fields, and to knowingly participate in patterning of the human and environmental fields for realization of maximum well-being" (Rogers, 1988).

RESEARCH BASIS FOR PRACTICE

The nurse's decision to suggest therapeutic touch to Mr. Cullen was based on her experience with using it and her knowledge of clinical research studies which have tested hypotheses about the effects of therapeutic touch on anxiety and pain. Heidt (1981), in an early study, found that hospitalized cardiovascular patients who received therapeutic touch had a significant decrease in situationally induced anxiety compared with patients who received casual touch or no touch. In a constructive replication of Heidt's study, Quinn (1984) found that patients who received therapeutic touch had a significantly greater decrease in anxiety compared with patients who received a mimic treatment. Fedoruk (1984) found that hospitalized premature infants had a significant decrease in physiological indicators of stress when they received therapeutic touch compared with when they received a mimic treatment or only the presence of a nurse. However, Parks (1985) found no significant difference in anxiety levels in elderly hospitalized patients who received therapeutic touch compared with those who received a mimic treatment or no study treatment. In a recent study which replicated and extended her previous work, Quinn (1989) found no significant difference in preoperative anxiety levels in patients who received therapeutic touch compared with patients who received a mimic treatment or standard nursing care. Two studies on the effect of therapeutic touch on pain have also been reported. Meehan (1985) reported that therapeutic touch had no significant effect in decreasing postoperative pain compared with mimic treatment or standard narcotic analgesia. However, a secondary analysis of the therapeutic touch and mimic treatment data alone indicates that therapeutic touch is significantly effective in decreasing postoperative pain and that patients who received therapeutic touch wait a significantly longer period of time before requesting more analgesia (Meehan, 1986). Keller and Bzdek (1986) found that individuals with tension headache pain who received therapeutic touch had a significant and sustained reduction in headache pain compared with those who received a mimic treatment.

The scientific investigation of therapeutic touch is still in its early stages, and only the Quinn and Meehan studies, noted above, specifically identified the Science of Unitary Human Beings as the theoretical rationale. Although study findings so far are mixed, there is evidence that it does have potential for therapeutic effect (see Figure 1). As the findings of studies accumulate, they can be used to make decisions about using therapeutic touch to treat patients. For example, the nurse treating Mr. Cullen knew that it could decrease anxiety in hospitalized patients, and Mr. Cullen was quite anxious. She also knew that therapeutic touch could be moderately effective in decreasing pain and that patients tend to wait a longer period of time between requests for analgesic medication.

LEARNING THERAPEUTIC TOUCH

Learning therapeutic touch is sometimes thought of as being quite simple but it is, in fact, a very complex process. While traditionally nurses have used their hands as a focus for communicating therapeutic intent to patients, the practice of therapeutic touch demands that the nurse become more consciously aware of the dynamics of such interaction. In treating a patient with therapeutic touch the nurse is consciously using him or herself as a therapeutic tool. Therefore, the nurse must develop insight into his or her motivation for using self in this way so that the nurse can move beyond his or her own needs and better meet the needs of the patient. Learning and understanding the concepts of the field world view and the principles of the Science of Unitary Human Beings and learning to use these as a basis for practice requires disciplined attention and serious study. Although centering is not difficult to learn, to use it effectively requires disciplined practice. Also, it is likely to take some period of time to come to terms with the experience of being able to perceive the subtle feeling of the energy flow; of being able to tactilely perceive something that is not physical. At the same time, the practice of therapeutic touch brings the nurse face to face with the essence of professional nursing: the nurturing of human life through specialized nurse–patient interaction. In turn, this experience provides the opportunity for the nurse to learn more about nursing and about him or herself as a nurse.

Meditation and centering may be new and intimidating concepts to some nurses. However, centering is a fairly simple form of meditation and is easily learned and incorporated into daily activity. Kunz (1988) suggests that a short meditation or centering exercise, for about 5 minutes, at the beginning of each day will help the nurses to develop awareness of their inner center of unity and peace. This enables them to establish a sense of quiet and calmness that will become part of their daily activity and upon which they can draw in times of stress.

Nurses who are curious about the experience of using one's hands to perceive an energy flow could do a hand exercise developed by Krieger (1979) and adapted here as follows: (1) Sit comfortably with both feet flat on the floor, loosen any tight clothing, and take a couple of deep breaths in and out to help loosen any tension in your body. (2) Hold your elbows away from your body and your hands in a free and comfortable position in front of you at about the level of your waist. (3) Extend your fingers so that the palms of your hands are flat and facing one another but are at the same time relatively relaxed, and hold your hands in this way throughout the exercise. (4) Bring the palms of your hands as closely together as possible without actually touching, then move the palms of your hands slowly and steadily apart about two inches. (5) Continuing in a slow, steady motion, bring the palms of your hands as close as possible together again without actually touching, then move them apart again about four inches. (6) Repeat step 5 twice, the first time moving your hands six inches apart and the second time moving your hands eight inches apart. As you do this be aware of any perceptions or sensations which you may feel in the palms of your hands or fingers or in the space between your hands. (7) Continue to move the palms of your hands together and apart in the same slow and steady motion, continuing to be aware of any perceptions or sensations for about a minute. Some nurses, when they first do this exercise, are not able to feel anything. Others do feel different kinds of perceptions and sensations that are similar to those felt when using therapeutic touch. Books by Macrae (1988), Krieger (1979), and Borelli and Heidt (1981) provide information guidelines for beginning learners.

It is recommended that nurses who want to learn therapeutic touch do so within a nursing context such as an undergraduate or graduate nursing program, or in a continuing education program in a school of nursing or health care agency department of nursing. The initial learning of therapeutic touch should take place over a time period of at least 6 months. Learning should include regular, daily practice of centering and at least 60 hours of instruction in the theory and practice of therapeutic touch. At the end of the initial learning period nurses should: (1) have a basic understanding of the Science of Unitary Human Beings; (2) have confidence in their ability to use therapeutic touch in the nursing care of selected patients; (3) have read and be able to discuss the books noted above and all of the literature on therapeutic touch published in peer-reviewed journals; (4) have an in-depth knowledge of the arguments both for and against the use of therapeutic touch as a nursing intervention; (5) be able to discuss therapeutic touch in terms that can be understood by fellow nurses, other health professionals, and patients who are not familiar with therapeutic touch; and (6) have as much supervised experience in practice on relatively healthy individuals as is necessary to develop skill in energy field assessment and treatment and self-confidence in the ability to practice.

In learning therapeutic touch nurses are encouraged to be open to new ideas but, at the same time, discriminating and questioning with regard to presentations of philosophical bases and logic underlying the ideas. Care should be taken not to accept sweeping generalizations about the effects of therapeutic touch that are not carefully documented in the professional literature. Nurses are encouraged to avoid the use of "new age" jargon such as "healee" instead of patient or client. They are also encouraged to avoid the use of Eastern terms such as "prana" or "chakra" as these terms are not necessary to the practice of therapeutic touch and are often poorly understood and misinterpreted in Western culture.

INTEGRATION INTO PRACTICE

There are two ways in which therapeutic touch can be integrated into practice. It can be added to the skills that a nurse already has as is demonstrated in the example of the nurse caring for Mr. Cullen, or concepts inherent in the practice of therapeutic touch can be integrated into other nursing activities.

Nurses in private practice can easily integrate therapeutic touch into practice. Nurses who practice in an organization such as a community health agency, hospital, or medical center will need to lay a foundation for using the Science of Unitary Human Beings and interventions such as therapeutic touch. The concepts and principles of the model and advantages of practice based on the model should be discussed with colleagues, especially head nurses and nursing administrators, to gain their support. While it is obviously not appropriate for physicians to prescribe nursing interventions for patients, interventions that are new and different should be discussed with physicians responsible for patients' medical care so that they understand what it is and how it can help patients. Because the medical model is dominant in most health care organizations, therapeutic touch is often viewed, at least initially, with skepticism and caution. However, when it is clearly explained, most nurses and other health professionals accept the possibility that it can help patients. The nurse should expect to be asked about "the literature" on therapeutic touch, and should have at hand copies of articles and research reports from peer-reviewed professional journals and be ready to discuss them. Then, when a patient situation arises in which therapeutic touch is indicated, the nurse will feel confident in offering therapeutic touch to the patient.

The concepts of centering and focused intent to help, inherent in the practice of therapeutic touch, can be integrated into all aspects of traditional nursing practice from assessing a patient to administering medication or giving a back rub. In caring for a patient from a centered perspective the nurse is able to perceive the patient as a unitary whole, is better able to recognize the patient's individuality, and be receptive to the patient's experience in the moment. Thus, the nurse is better attuned to the patient and better able to communicate receptivity, compassion, and intent to help. Patients often seem to recoginze this, and it is probable that this kind of attuning to the patient is, in itself, therapeutic. The regular practice of centering can also lead to deeper insight into the many levels of human awareness and to the complex and profound role intuition can play in nurse–patient interaction.

Centering also helps nurses protect themselves against burnout. Kunz (1989) explains that in ordinary nursing practice nurses, in wanting to help and care for patients, will open themselves up to the suffering and anxiety ill patients often experience. The patients, being depleted of energy due to illness, will naturally draw upon and drain the nurses' personal energy. If this process continues, nurses become exhausted or burned out and tend to leave nursing practice. However, if nurses center themselves, their receptivity to and intent to help patients will be focused through a center of unity and calm in themselves. Through this center they are detached from a personal relationship with patients and instead experience a universal feeling of compassion toward patients. This kind of interaction with patients is intensely humanitarian but at the same time non-personal. Nurses can then direct the energy that continuously flows through this center to assist patients, promote their comfort, and facilitate their healing. Nurses who practice from a centered perspective find that they feel invigorated by their practice rather than drained or burned out.

Thus, this overview of therapeutic touch illustrates one example of the innovative, enriched nature of nursing practice using the Science of Unitary Human Beings. The use of interventions such as therapeutic touch provide the opportunity to gain greater insight into the nature of nursing and to promote professional development and self-awareness. Through practice generated by the Science of Unitary Human Beings, nurses can renew their commitment to nursing and to their fulfillment of the profession's mandate to nurture human life in ways that promote unity, peacefulness, and well being.

REFERENCES

Bohm, D. (1973). Quantum theory as an indication of a new order in physical law. *Foundation of Physics*, *3*, 144–156.

Borelli, M.D., & Heidt, P. (Eds.). (1981). *Therapeutic touch*. New York: Springer.

Cushing, J.T., & McMullin, E. (Eds.). (1989). *Philosophical consequences of quantum theory*. Notre Dame: University of Notre Dame.

Fedoruk, R.B. (1984). *Transfer of the relaxation response: Therapeutic touch as a method of reduction of stress in premature neonates.* Unpublished doctoral dissertation, University of Maryland.

Gueldner, S.H. (1983). *A study of the relationship between imposed motion and human field motion in elderly individuals living in nursing homes.* Unpublished doctoral dissertation, University of Alabama, Birmingham.

Heidt, P. (1981). Effect of therapeutic touch on anxiety of hospitalized patients. *Nursing Research, 30*, 32–37.

Keller, E., & Bzdek, V. (1986). Effects of therapeutic touch on tension headache pain. *Nursing Research, 35*, 101–105.

Krieger, D. (1975). Therapeutic touch: The imprimatur of nursing. *American Journal of Nursing, 75*, 784–787.

Krieger, D. (1979). *The therapeutic touch*. Englewood Cliffs, NJ: Prentice Hall, Inc.

Krieger, D., Peper, E., & Ancoli, S. (1979). Therapeutic touch: Searching for evidence of physiological change. *American Journal of Nursing 79*, 660–662.

Kunz, D. (1988). Nursing practice colloquium. Department of Nursing, New York University Medical Center, New York.

Kunz, D. (1989). Seventeenth annual invitational workshop on therapeutic touch, The Pumpkin Hollow Foundation, Craryville, New York.

Lionberger, H. (1985). *An interpretive study of nurses' practice of therapeutic touch.* Unpublished doctoral dissertation, University of California, San Francisco.

Macrae, J. (1988). *Therapeutic touch: A practical guide.* New York: Alfred A. Knopf.

Malinski, V. (1986). *Explorations on Martha Rogers' science of unitary human beings.* Norwalk, CT: Appleton-Century-Crofts.

Meehan, M.T.C. (1985). *The effect of therapeutic touch on the experience of acute pain in postoperative patients.* Unpublished doctoral dissertation, New York University.

Meehan, T.C. (1986). *The effect of therapeutic touch on acute pain: Secondary analysis.* Unpublished report, Department of Nursing, New York University Medical Center, New York.

Parks, B. (1985). *Therapeutic touch as an intervention to reduce anxiety in elderly hospitalized patients.* Unpublished doctoral dissertation, University of Texas, Austin.

Prigogine, I. (1980). *From being to becoming.* San Francisco: W.H. Freeman & Co.

Quinn, J. (1984). Therapeutic touch as energy exchange: Testing the theory. *Advances in nursing science, 6,* 42–49.

Quinn, J. (1989). Therapeutic touch as energy exchange: Replication and extension. *Nursing Science Quarterly, 2,* 79–87.

Rogers, M. (1986). Science of unitary human beings. In V. Malinksi (Ed.), *Explorations on Martha Rogers' science of unitary human beings* (pp. 3–8). Norwalk, CT: Appleton-Century-Crofts.

Rogers, M. (1988). Personal communication.

Weber, R. (Ed.). (1986). *Dialogues with scientists and sages: The search for unity in science and mysticism.* London: Routledge & Kegan Paul, Ltd.

Weber, R. (In press). Philosophical perspectives on touch. In T.B. Brazelton & K. Barnard (Eds.), *Touch: The foundation of experience.* National Center for Clinical Infant Programs Clinical Infant Report Series, Madison, WI: International University Press.

6

Unitary Human Field Practice Modalities

Marie Boguslawski

The Science of Unitary Human Beings (Rogers, 1970, 1986) provides a basis for the nurse's use of unitary human field practice modalities. Rogerian science is concerned with change (Madrid & Fry, 1986). Releasing, transforming, and transcending one's present energy field pattern are changes that portend new manifestations of health. With clarity of goal, patience, and perseverance, everyone can participate in creating desired changes in their life. For some, creating this change seems relatively easy; for others, it is one of the most difficult tasks they have ever attempted to accomplish. Regardless of whether it is easy or difficult, releasing old familiar pattern manifestations and developing new, yet unknown, characteristics is a challenging endeavor requiring courage and trust that the process will be in the service of well being and worth the effort. Trust is essential here because the process has its moments of provoking disruptive and painful emotions before the person feels its releasing and enriching qualities. To enhance this change the nurse, working in the Rogerian mode, has various unitary human field modalities to use. All such modalities, when used together, create a power for change that surpasses any one modality used alone. In Barrett's (1983) view, "Power is the capacity to participate knowingly in the nature of change characterizing the continuous patterning of the human and environmental fields."

NUTRITION

One modality the nurse uses to assist people in creating change relates most directly to the "physical" energies which are manifestations of the field. Diet, vitamins, minerals, and herbs give nourishment to the basic complex of energies we call the "physical" body. Nourishment harmonizes the energy field pattern and, thereby, strengthens the basic organization through which power for change is created. Nutrition, as an energy source, can enhance the momentum toward health and probabilistic goal attainment. Health and probabilistic goal attainment refer to goals as defined by the individual seeking assistance.

ACTIVITY AND REST

Another aspect of the human field pattern that requires attention by the nurse is the appropriate balance between activity and rest. Activity harmonizes the energy field pattern and, by its very nature, creates more energy for change. On the other hand, if too much activity is engaged, instead of creating power for change, it can actually be depleting and, subsequently, interfere with goal attainment. The same is true for rest. A proper amount can enhance healing whereas too much can deplete one's energies. Tuning in to the rhythm of one's own pattern provides the best clue to that proper, power inducing, balance. Tuning in is a skill that can be learned. Once learned, the person is able to perceive the subtle messages of the human field pattern and to participate in directing change quickly at critical moments to sustain the momentum of probabilistic goal attainment.

RELAXATION AND KNOWING

Tuning in to hear one's own messages is greatly enhanced through the art of relaxation. Relaxation is an activity that promotes changes in the human field pattern to allow a quietness to occur so the subtle nature of the messages can be discerned with clarity. Often, however, when these messages are really heard, one discovers that they are counter to one's desired goals. All energy has its opposite. So too it is with human beings. The unaware sabotage of well being is, ironically enough, a well-developed skill in many people. When the opposing aspect of one's energies is discovered, acknowledged, and accepted, the person can begin to change so that human field patterning flows predominantly in the direction of probabilistic goal attainment and health promotion. After these messages are acknowledged and accepted, then the most productive way to begin creating change is to explore their nature and source.

These messages frequently evolve out of early childhood/family energy field patterns. However, while pattern manifestations that the child developed in mutual process with his or her family were health promoting then, they may not be productive when used in adult contexts now. Through the exploration of these previously acquired behaviors, knowledge is gained to release them and to transform field patterning toward attainment of personal goals. This transformation can be realized quite rapidly or, as is more often the case, emerge gradually over time. Once these new and desirable patterns begin to emerge, it is essential that the person creates the power to strengthen them. Of course, this power is enhanced greatly by the innate healing potential of the human field, that momentum toward health that exists in all of us, often manifested through the art of relaxation. Even though we all possess this natural momentum toward health, certain characteristics of the human field pattern can interfere with its manifestation. When this healing power of the human field is impaired, a different energy flow exists and disease often begins to manifest in specific patterns. The continuing practice of relaxation is a key to allowing healing power to manifest.

In addition to tuning in to one's unique human field pattern, relaxation also allows the freedom to perceive and interpret environmental activity so that a health promoting mutual process becomes a way of life. Being relaxed and centered, the person is better able to be aware of multiple perceptions of self and environment. This heightened awareness gives the person a more accurate perception with which to act and a greater mastery of human encounters. In addition, relaxation is a key element in the facilitation of imagery. Both relaxation and imagery are unitary human field modalities used by the nurse practicing within the perspective of Rogerian science.

IMAGERY

Imagery is the process of (1) allowing spontaneous images to manifest and exploring the nature of these images experientially to provide information about oneself, (2) using images to create the power to change disharmony—disease—into harmony, and (3) utilizing images to experience the attainment of goals in the relative present and, thereby, increase the potential of attaining those goals.

Imagery is a powerful tool available to discern and change previous patterns, focus energies on the attainment of health goals, and enhance one's own healing power. Imagery promotes four-dimensional awareness and is not space or time bound. Experiences from the relative past can be brought to the relative present. The adult is now able to speed up the evolution of childhood patterns by releasing their energy through a deliberate relinquishing of emotions in these patterns and directing that energy into health promoting adult patterns. Confidence, patience, and perseverance are necessary in this effort. Energy is in constant motion and will flow in the direction of deliberately held health promoting goals that have been designed by the person. It is a process with a high probability of success. In addition, during this process it is helpful to remember that energy is a wave form, with valleys and plateaus. What may appear to be a low point or continuing plateau is only an aspect of the life process. A crest will come. When this process is viewed from a broader and somewhat more distant vantage, it can be observed that movement continues in a steadily forward direction toward the fulfillment of individual goals.

During this process of identifying, exploring, releasing, and changing obstacles toward health, the focus gradually shifts from self to environment. By reason of mutual process with the environment, as the person participates knowingly in health promoting patterns focused on the environment, flow patterns within the person are changed and goal attaining health patterns are enhanced. As the sluggishness, weakness, tautness, and solidity of flow patterns in the person are changed through mutual process (Boguslawski, 1979), healing manifests in the human and environmental fields.

If the person has the intention of knowing the disruptive aspects of life patterns but is not yet ready to fully experience them, they will frequently manifest in imagery through symbolism in much the same way as dreams. The person then must interpret the symbolism to realize its intended message. Often there is a rhythm in imagery between symbolism and actual memory as the process unfolds.

AFFIRMATIONS

Affirmations are succinct, declarative statements encompassing all of one's desired life goals and are repeated verbally or subvocally while experiencing the goals as already attained in one's imagination.

Affirmations grant important assistance to the person in creating change toward probabilistic goal attainment. They help to focus on what is really desired and provide a direction and organization for the energy. However, it is sometimes easier to know what is not wanted than to know what is wanted out of life. By focusing on affirmations, the person begins to change pattern manifestations in opposition to them. This change makes it easier to discover defeating pattern manifestations along with their nature and origin.

THERAPEUTIC TOUCH

Therapeutic touch is an intentional interaction between a nurse's energy field and that of another to potentiate that person's natural self-healing abilities by enhancing universal, orderly, harmonious healing energy (Boguslawski, 1979, 1980, 1983).

Therapeutic touch is a powerful unitary human field modality that the nurse uses to enhance relaxation, imagery, and the entire healing process. Pertaining to the nurse, it encompasses an aware intent to help another, relaxation, centering, confidence, perceptive skills of subtle energy patterns of the human field, intuition, and imagery. The person receiving therapeutic touch realizes a greater facility in relaxation, centering, confidence, imagery, knowing, creating power, healing, and goal attainment.

Therapeutic touch is an assistance to the person participating in creating change toward health and well being. This person has the responsibility to participate knowingly and deliberately in the process of attaining health. Therapeutic touch patterns the person's energies so that they are readily available to use in creating the necessary momentum toward health as defined by that person. While the person is receiving therapeutic touch, therefore, greater energy transformation can usually be realized than when the person is working alone.

ONESELF

An important unitary human field modality possessed by the nurse is something that is quite elusive and intangible but very powerful—oneself (Boguslawski, 1983). Its power comes frequently through such things as a simple gesture, a word, a facial expression, posture, or environmental changes by which the nurse intentionally gives support to another. The application of knowledge from the Science of Unitary Human Beings enhances this power. Those who experience this mutual process know that it is something other than three-dimensional energy that is primarily responsible. When people who have successively emerged from a hardship are asked what had been most helpful to them, they will frequently answer by naming the presence of some other person. The nature of this mutual process is a powerful presence in a person's "will to live," the energy available to support that "will to live," and the confidence, patience, and perseverance necessary to achieve an optimal, healthy lifestyle. Because of its power, this is a modality about which a nurse can become very excited. It seems so simple and easy to use. However, as the nurse develops and manifests the deliberate use of this modality into a process of mutual awareness, its complexity can seem overwhelming. Apparent too is an educational and ethical issue. Because of the nature of mutual process, what responsibility does the nurse have for self-development? For example, if a nurse is not feeling well on a particular day, what implications does this have for mutual process with the people for whom he or she is caring?

PRACTICE NOTES

What follows are examples of how the nurse, using unitary field practice modalities within the perspective of Rogerian science, cares for a person who has received a medical diagnosis. The person comes to the first session with a diet summary and a listing of the vitamins and drugs that he or she is taking. An extensive health history is begun. From this information comes an assessment of the person's human field pattern manifestations and a beginning mutual plan of action to achieve desired health goals. Nutrition, vitamins, and herbs for optimal nourishment in relation to the person's lifestyle are discussed. Decision making remains the person's prerogative. Changing dietary, vitamin, and herb intake to promote health within the context of one's lifestyle often is the first decision and challenge confronted. Some make the change quickly and with apparent ease. Others find it difficult and make the change more slowly over time while affirming that they are "eating only nourishing food for their system and have perfect digestion and metabolism." A change in diet can mean a significant change in how one interacts with food and with others. Sustaining a change in diet may require a strong conviction that it is the right thing to do and a strong sense of self in relation to others. The nature of the nurse's support and guidance provides the foundation for a nurturing mutual process that enhances success. Incorporating appropriate activity, rest, and relaxation into one's lifestyle is usually more easily accomplished. Generally, it does not require as much change in lifestyle or in one's sense of self in relation to others that a diet change requires.

One man with a medical diagnosis of cancer, having difficulty accepting his unique pattern manifestations, could never bring himself to order different foods than his colleagues during business luncheons and dinners. He was the president of a firm and these luncheons and dinners were frequent. He was having marital problems. His wife did not believe in his changed diet and she would not cook the kind of meals that he perceived would be most helpful to him. Also, after more than a year, he still needed to listen to relaxation and imagery tapes since he had not developed the ability to do imagery and affirmations on his own. He had sought help from various practitioners offering "alternative care" throughout the United States and Canada. His pursuit of help was out of a distrust of the medical model of care and not from a conviction that "alternative care" was of value in getting well. He wanted to get well without the disruptions of a change in lifestyle. During the admission interview, his pattern manifestations indicated that the cancer was progressing. Increasing the probability of attaining one's goals for new manifestations of health requires a deliberative participation in change and courage (to be different, to deal with marital problems), perseverance (doing imagery and affirmations), and trust in the process (valuing one's choice). To ensure the highest probability of success with a decision, one must participate fully and self-confidently in that decision.

In another situation, one's lifestyle and sense of self readily became a focus of attention for a person with a medical diagnosis of acquired immune deficiency syndrome (AIDS). Death became real. Relationships with others were changing rapidly. The illness brought into awareness a very deep pain and sorrow about this person's relative present.

Through counseling, imagery, and therapeutic touch, the healing process proceeded. Using imagery to explore the dynamics of his feelings began with the acceptance of his unique identity and common humanity. With acceptance came a basis for the development of strength. This person became so comfortable and confident that he attended an important function with such panache that no one dared inquire about several large blisters on his face from having had Kaposi's sarcomas removed. Acceptance at work was not as easily gained. It took several months before his partners and staff fully involved him in the business of the firm. It was as if they did not want to include him in planning out of fear that he would not be there to complete the projects, and they would have to deal with loss. He did not feel fully accepted until a business crisis occurred that everyone wanted to avoid. He handled it with ease and expertise. Within 6 months after his initial visit, his confidence had evolved to the degree that one session was spent on his plans for retirement some 30 years hence. Healing requires an aware investment in life. Feeling a strong desire to live with an enthusiasm to accomplish particular life and career goals is a powerful mobilizer of healing energy.

The mobilization of healing energy and strength can be seen in the person's imagery. Initially, it may be difficult to imagine a favorite place that is all one's own: a place that is very private and nourishing. Beginning favorite places may be of childhood experiences or of public places. As the person develops power, favorite places frequently become beautiful private gardens and beaches. Favorite places may change and have visitors in accordance with specific personal and lifestyle issues to be addressed. Healing evolves as the person learns to deal with the challenges of these spontaneously changing images. These images offer information, direction, and encouragement to the person who is working toward health.

Disease is not an isolated event. It is a manifestation of the whole. Getting well entails resolving the issues that are present in all aspects of one's life. First comes an awareness of these issues. Then the process of healing in relation to these issues begins. Healing evolves through mutual process in weekly or twice weekly sessions with the nurse over an extended period of time. Lifestyle patterns emanating frequently from childhood typically are not resolved quickly. It is usually too disruptive of one's being, and it is more likely that the person might instinctively reject the change rather than incorporate it. As the person becomes more intuitively aware of self, it is not uncommon to discover a subtle, but strong, resistance to getting well. The nurse supports and educates about the dynamics of change so that the person can continue to focus on health goals with patience and perseverance. This is a critical aspect of mutual process, especially if desired health goals are slow in manifesting. It is a sign that the probability for manifesting desired health goals and general well being has increased when the person begins to participate more deliberatively in mutual process with the environmental energy field. In the continuing sessions, disease is frequently not even mentioned as the person focuses on career, social, and life goals.

Focus can also be centered on the immediacy of the disease process itself. Four sessions with another person with advanced AIDS resulted in the decision that death was permissible. For him, the elusiveness of success did not warrant the effort required. Shortly thereafter, he entered the hospital for the last time.

Another person with a medical diagnosis of rectal/pelvic cancer died, probably not from the cancerous process, but because he felt that life with colostomy and urinary bags did not seem worth living. He discerned that he was having difficulty in swallowing and was avoiding food because he did not want to have any stool. He was experiencing traumatic issues around stool and urine that he had experienced as a child. In addition, he was now in direct competition with a much younger wife for whom he had been a mentor. In discussions about death, he was reassured that death was a permissible option even though, with effort, he probably could live for an indefinite length of time.

CONCLUSION

Attaining health, defined in each instance by the individual, is a complex process. It requires consideration of all life experiences free from spatial and temporal boundaries. In the Science of Unitary Human Beings the past, present, and future are not separate. They are one. That oneness informs our experiences. In mutual process, the nurse is aware of the fullness of that oneness, the manifestations of wholeness relative to irreducible human and environmental fields, and uses the information to assist people in attaining their health goals.

REFERENCES

Barrett, E.A.M. (1983). An empirical investigation of Martha E. Rogers' principle of helicy: The relationship of human field motion and power. *Dissertation Abstracts International, 45.* (University Microfilms, No. 84-06-278)

Boguslawski, M. (1979). The use of therapeutic touch in nursing. *The Journal of Continuing Education in Nursing, 10,* 9–15.

Boguslawski, M. (1980). Therapeutic touch: A facilitator of pain relief. *Topics in Clinical Nursing, 2,* 27–37.

Boguslawski, M. (1983). Use of self in intervention strategies, including therapeutic touch and imagery. In P. Ashwanden (Ed.), *Interventions in Pain Management* (pp. 15–22). New York: Columbia University Comprehensive Cancer Center.

Madrid, M., & Winstead-Fry, P. (1986). Rogers' conceptual model. In P. Winstead-Fry (Ed.), *Case studies in nursing theory* (pp. 73–102). New York: National League for Nursing.

Rogers, M.E. (1970). *An introduction to the theoretical basis of nursing.* Philadelphia: F.A. Davis Company.

Rogers, M.E. (1986). Science of unitary human beings. In V.M. Malinski (Ed.), *Explorations on Martha Rogers' science of unitary human beings* (pp. 3–8). Norwalk, CT: Appleton-Century-Crofts.

BIBLIOGRAPHY

Advances. Quarterly Journal of the Institute for The Advancement of Health. New York, NY.

Barrett, E.A.M. (1986). Investigation of the principle of helicy: The relationship of human field motion and power. In V.M. Malinski (Ed.), *Explorations on Martha Rogers' science of unitary human beings.* Norwalk, CT: Appleton-Century-Crofts.

Hannah, B. (1981). *Encounters of the soul: Active imagination as developed by C.G. Jung.* Santa Monica, CA: Sigo Press.

Holistic Medicine. Bimonthly Newsletter of the American Holistic Medical Association and the Holistic Medical Foundation. Seattle, WA.

Holos' Practice Report. Monthly Publication of the Holos Institute of Health. Springfield, MI.

Klinger, E.K. (1981). *Imagery.* Vol. 2, Concepts, results and applications. New York: Plenum Press.

Korn, E.R., & Johnson, K. (1983). *Visualization: The uses of imagery in the health professions.* Homewood, IL: Dow Jones-Irwin.

Noetic Sciences Review. Quarterly Publication of the Institute of Noetic Sciences. Sausalito, CA.

Rossman, M.L., & Bresler, D.E. (1984). *Guided imagery. An intensive training program for clinicians* (2nd ed.). Workbook. Pacific Palisades, CA.

Sheikh, A.A. (1984). *Imagination and healing.* Farmingdale, NY: Baywood Publishing Company.

Sheikh, A.A. (1986). *Anthology of imagery techniques.* Milwaukee, WI: American Imagery Institute.

Sheikh, A.A., & Pachuta, D.M. *Guided imagery. Workshop training manual.* Milwaukee, WI: American Imagery Institute.

Shorr, J.E. (1983). *Psychotherapy through imagery.* New York: Thieme-Stratton.

7

The Participating Process of Human Field Patterning in an Acute-Care Environment

Mary Madrid

It was the evening of Christmas day. I had just received my private duty assignment: a patient with a medical diagnosis of acquired immune deficiency syndrome (AIDS) and gastrointestinal bleeding. The assignment was disturbing and disappointing, but I did not refuse it because I believe it inappropriate to reject any assignment if I have the skills and knowledge necessary to carry it out.

Intellectually, I rationalized that calendar days or patient diagnosis should not make a difference as far as nursing and human values are concerned. It was my choice to work this Christmas and not for the first time would I care for a patient with this medical diagnosis.

Realistically, though, I did not want the assignment. I felt guilty, and I was concerned that the patient would sense my feelings. I did not want my behavioral manifestations to reflect any hesitation or value judgments in relation to patient care. I had not resolved these issues as I entered the room but I was determined to find a way to view the patient, whose name was Roger, as a unitary human being and not a person with AIDS and gastrointestinal bleeding.

Roger was 30 years old and had been in the hospial for an extended time. The room had the distinct look of his being "settled in." Colorful posters decorated the wall. The tape, yellow with age, that was holding them in place showed that they were not new. A collage of multiple faces, pictures of friends, had been cut out and arranged in a design. Since Roger was confined to his bed, the collage had been strategically placed upside down on the opposite wall so that he could view it without effort. The windowsill was covered with plants and flowers, some crisp and fresh, others wilted. A commode, no longer in use, was in a corner of the room piled high with linen and Chux. The nightstand by his bed was covered with supplies needed for his care. A round bedside table held a radio, a tape deck, and a small Christmas tree with colorful lights. Cards with expressions of love from family and friends stood upright on his overbed stand. The wastebaskets were stuffed with discarded Christmas wrappings, and a cot against the wall held neatly stacked boxes of already-opened gifts. Roger's bed was in the middle of the room and it appeared too big for his small body. His friend, Gary, was sitting by the bed holding his hand and making light conversation.

Roger looked frail and tired, as if he were depleted of energy. He was lying on multiple layers of eggcrate mattresses. His body was emaciated and covered with lesions of Kaposi's sarcoma. Bony prominences, sharp and distinct, stood out against the white linen. A drainage bag covered the insertion site of a leaky gastrostomy tube that had recently been removed. The skin surrounding the area was shiny, weeping, and had an angry red color. Roger winced in pain when I touched his skin to assess his abdomen. It was firm and distended. An NG tube was draining coffee-ground material and a tube feeding was infusing through a jejunostomy tube. The rigid, tense position of his body expressed discomfort. He seemed afraid to move.

Roger had recently received chemotherapy. A towel, placed over his pillow, was covered with hair and as he turned his head from side to side, more would profusely fall out. He coughed, then expectorated into a tissue, making no attempt to wipe the residual from his mouth. It seemed to be a strenuous effort for him to even manage these body mechanics. They left him exhausted.

Gary reached over, gently wiped his mouth, and continued talking to him, small talk about sports and movies he had recently seen that Roger might like. Roger kept his eyes closed and was not an active participant in the conversation. When Gary directed questions to him, his replies were laconic and the tone unreflective. There were long periods of silence. Gary left a short time after I arrived.

It was not difficult to see that Roger was very sick and in a great deal of pain. If I were going to make a difference and promote even a small change in the human-environmental process that might ease his situation, I had to stop thinking of him only as "an AIDS patient who is a gastrointestinal bleeder."

I began talking to Roger, asking him about the things he liked to do and what life was like before he became ill. His answers were brief. He told me he worked as a research pharmacologist and had grown up in the country. He referred to the good times he had had with his brothers and the long walks he had taken, accompanied by their family dog. As he presented the information, I used imagery to transpose it into scenes that were alive and real. Although he only offered a few words, I was able to achieve an elaboration of the material through the process of imagination and imagery. A holistic picture, rich in detail and dynamic in nature, was available to me. I was able to view Roger's human field pattern at a time when he had strength and vigor and in a place where there was joy and beauty. I pictured him running with his brothers over a beautiful countryside, the dog, excited and enthusiastic, following along. I saw him as a scholar, diligently solving problems at his desk, conducting experiments in the laboratory, and enjoying the conviviality associated with college life. The pattern manifestations of his human and environmental energy fields were so alive and real that they gave me an entirely different perception of him as a person. I saw him as a holistic being, an interesting person that I would enjoy knowing. When I moved beyond the terms of pathology and diagnosis, I was able to see that Roger was a unique individual who experienced the environment in his own special way. I wanted my participation in this experience to be as pleasant for him as possible.

I offered to give him a back rub and assist him with relaxation exercises that might promote comfort. Roger responded that nothing seemed to help. Medication for pain was ineffective and only made him nauseous. Stabbing pain reverberated through every muscle when he moved. The sheets against his skin felt like a blanket of fire. I put medicated cream on the weeping areas of his side and abdomen, but he requested that I not turn or move him. I explained the concept of therapeutic touch and its usefulness in this situation. As long as he did not have to move, he was willing to give it a try.

After 30 minutes of therapeutic touch, I noted an observable change in his human field pattern. He took on a new appearance. The squint around his closed eyes disappeared and his facial expression became serene and peaceful. His chest gently rose with each restful respiration. I saw the tense muscles of his body slacken and become relaxed. When I thought he was asleep, I quietly sat down. The silence was interrupted. "I'm not asleep," he said. "Whatever you did, it feels great!" We were both delighted.

There was less skepticism now in Roger's willingness to have me reposition him, rub his back, and change the linen on his bed. As I worked, I talked him through relaxation techniques and they helped. Roger deliberately became aware of the pattern manifestation of his muscles and how he could control their degree of relaxation. By focusing on feelings of warmth and weightlessness he was able to maintain a sense of relaxation.

After a long interval of sleep, he awoke refreshed and began to talk about his life process. He spoke of meaningful events, some recent and others that had occurred at a much earlier point in time. His voice and mannerisms reflected the joy and enthusiasm he was experiencing as he recalled special family gatherings during his childhood and social events from his college years. He expressed pride in the accomplishments he made within his profession and described the exuberant feelings experienced when he finally solved a problem after hours of study, pondering, and experimentation. He verbalized his sadness about his present state of health, the long days during which he would lie in bed with time dragging, the feelings he experienced from social rejection. Roger's speech was free flowing and filled with emotion. There was no hesitation in his delivery as different phases of his life process unfolded. He was sincere and honest in his comments regarding his successes and failures, his joys and disappointments. He spoke; I listened and shared his world.

He talked at great length and then stopped suddenly. His body became rigid and tense and he made whimpering sounds of pain. His hands shook as he put the urinal in place. Straining his abdominal muscles, he forced short bursts of urine into the urinal. My comments about relaxing were forgotten as he spoke of losing control when he felt the urge to void. The rhythmic spasms of his bladder were painful and prohibited him from passing urine normally. The only way he found relief was to strain and push, urinating small amounts at a time until his bladder was emptied. The painful process consumed his whole being.

Placing my hands over his pelvis, I centered and concentrated on transferring and increasing energy to this area. I asked Roger to take deep breaths and relax his abdominal muscles. At first, he could not change the pattern of his rapid, shallow respirations. The tremor in his hands increased and prevented him from holding the urinal. He kept repeating that he could not stop the tremors or change his rapid breathing pattern. His general expressions of movement demonstrated a pattern of agitation and frustration. I held the urinal and continued to direct energy to the pelvic area. I asked Roger to focus his attention on my breathing pattern. He began to synchronize his breathing pattern with mine. Gradually, his respiratory rate decreased and a regular, deep inspiratory rhythm was established. I then turned attention toward his relaxing the abdominal and pelvic muscles and suppressing the urge to strain. He became engrossed in my suggestions to enhance relaxation, concentrating on one muscle at a time until he was completely relaxed. When he released a gentle stream of urine that seemed endless, Roger was relieved and thankful. We reviewed how he could use deep breathing and relaxation techniques. He proudly gave me a demonstration of his ability to use them.

Roger was beginning to take an interest in activities that would promote health patterning goals and I wanted to encourage that interest. I noted that his hair was matted and dull and had not been washed for some time. My offer to give him a shampoo was received apologetically. He knew "it was a mess" and was "falling out like crazy," and said there probably wouldn't be much left when I got through shampooing. I padded the bed and filled the wash basin. As I shampooed, his hair did come out in large clumps, but when I finished the sparse hair remaining was soft and shiny.

Roger felt great! His whole expression changed. He rubbed his head with his hands, commenting on how good it was to "feel the air on his scalp." He asked that I help to sit him up and position the mirror on the nightstand so he could see himself. Intently, he looked in the mirror and commented on his appearance. Looking pensive, he stroked his chin, smoothed his mustache, and turned his head from side to side so that he could see his face from different views. He pushed the mirror away and began to list articles—shaving equipment, scissors, and other items—he needed to groom himself. I assembled what was available and watched him shave and trim his mustache. As I recalled the manifestations of his human field pattern when I first began the shift, his lack of energy and how different and unimportant it was for him to perform a simple task such as wiping his mouth, I was gratified to observe the changes. Patterning the environment was continued.

I suggested a rearrangement of the flowers on the windowsill so that he could see them easily from his bed. He had a grand time orchestrating the task. He pulled dead leaves off plants and instructed me as to which flowers should be discarded and where others were to be placed. I had to move them numerous times until "the right spot" for each one was found. A satisfied grin lit up his face when I finished.

Shortly after, Roger's friend, Tom, came to visit, bringing a large bouquet of flowers, long-stemmed lilies and birds of paradise. He placed them on the floor, cut the stems, and began to arrange them in a vase. Roger repeatedly asked him to move the vase so he could see it. Each time, Tom placed the vase elsewhere, but Roger was not content with its location. He began to manifest a pattern of restlessness. I saw that Tom did not grasp the full meaning of Roger's request. Roger did not want to miss seeing the evolving pattern of the arrangement as each flower was added. I asked Tom to stand where Roger could see every move he made. There was silence as Roger intently watched the arrangement take form. His facial expression was like that of someone completely absorbed in hearing a beautiful piece of music. When the last flower was in place, he chose a spot on the windowsill for the arrangement.

Tom enjoyed his visit and conversation with Roger. He remarked on how amazed he was to see the changes in Roger's attitude and his interest in the environment. He laughed when referring to Roger as "a little tyrant about his flowers."

Roger slept after Tom left. Upon awakening, he listened to his favorite selection of soft music on the tape deck, and he was content to immerse himself in the experience of integrating the musical wave patterns into his field pattern. I explained how he could concentrate on the expression of the music, striving to capture its peaceful, harmonious rhythm, blending it into the wave frequency of his energy field to create a sense of wholeness with the universe. Although the melody was familiar, he listened from a new frame of reference and heard as he never had before. Roger described his experience as being multidimensional and boundless in nature. He felt as if he had lost all physical, spatial attributes and was infinite with the universe. Although he experienced his presence on the earth, he also experienced it elsewhere at the same time. The experience was unique to himself. He wanted to share it with me through expression but could not find the words. I used a quote from *Thoughts* by Blaise Pascal as an analogy to best exemplify what I thought he had experienced. Referring to the universe, the French mathematician and philosopher said, "It is an infinite sphere whose center is everywhere, it's circumference nowhere." Roger was satisfied that I had achieved a degree of understanding.

Through a mutual process, Roger and I had established a trusting relationship. There were times during the rest of the evening when Roger reached out to draw strength from my presence. On two separate occasions he hurriedly requested the bedpan, crying out in fright when he filled it to capacity with blood. It was necessary for him to immediately transfer the flow to another bedpan, and he was distressed at seeing so much blood being expelled. He wept as I cleaned him. When I finished, I sat with him and held his hand. We both knew the seriousness of what had taken place. There were no medical orders to initiate when this information was reported to the staff. Neither of us spoke but there was communication through feeling and touch. By my being there, he received a measure of comfort.

Roger sadly began to speak of his belief that he would never again be able to spend an evening on the beach. He had spent many evenings there alone, reading a book, hearing the ocean, and watching a beautiful sunset. He explained that this was a time when he could clear his thoughts and work out his problems. The beauty and tranquility were refreshing. His mind would wander and it seemed that after he viewed the sunset, there was real peace within himself.

I knew that Roger could live that experience again through imagery. I explained to him that his human energy field did not have to be confined to a spatial dimension. Time and space were relative and it was possible for him to see the sunset on the beach, and yet, not physically leave the room. Roger easily grasped what I was saying, relating it to the experience he had earlier when listening to the music. He participated in the process of being guided through visualization and imagery in order to capture an evening similar to those he had enjoyed so many times before. Once again, Roger sat on the beach and enjoyed the sunset. He was deeply moved by the experience.

I was sorry to see the evening come to a close when my shift was over. Caring for Roger had been a rich, rewarding experience. He asked that I return the next day to care for him. I told him that I would be off the next day and though my work schedule did not permit me to accept the case the following day, I would enjoy stopping by for a visit.

The next afternoon, I stopped for my visit with Roger. I was excited and looked forward to seeing how he was doing with the imagery and relaxation exercises he had learned. When I reached his room, I found a new patient in it. Roger had died the morning of December 26th.

Once again, I found myself having mixed feelings about Roger. I was happy that he had been able to be at peace with himself and privileged to have been able to be involved in the participating process of guiding him to use a measure of his infinite potential. From this, he was able to enter meaningful experiences that held no limitations. I was also very sad that he was gone.

It was not sophisticated technology that made such a difference that evening. It was the art of nursing, based on the science of nursing, that Roger would have remembered, the caring and application of knowledge to human betterment. This knowledge was generated from the principles of resonancy, helicy, and integrality which are set forth within the conceptual system of the Rogerian model. Continuous change is inherent in each principle. The Rogerian practice methodology described by Barrett (1988) that I used consisted of pattern manifestation appraisal and deliberative mutual patterning.

Human energy fields are characterized by their own unique pattern (Rogers, 1986). Barrett defines pattern manifestation appraisal as the "continuous process of identifying manifestations of the human and environmental fields that relate to current health events" (p. 50). Although this may refer to a mutual process involving nurse and client, I believe that pattern manifestation appraisal may also be directed toward oneself.

Humans have the capacity for thought, sensation, and emotion, and these qualities underline the humaneness of unitary beings (Rogers, 1970). One of the ways in which we demonstrate our humaneness is by our ability to experience both self and environment. Feelings and thoughts are characteristics of human behavioral patterns. They are unique in relation to the individual and to the environment. When I learned of my assignment of Christmas day, I was in mutual process with the environmental field and I was experiencing the feeling manifestations of my energy field. The experience was unpleasant. Self-appraisal of pattern manifestations was important if my presence in the human environmental process was to be of benefit. I had to look within myself, honestly examine my intentions and motivations, recognize my fears and weakness, and accept what I found without illusion (Quinn, 1981).

In that relative present I did not want the assignment. I felt regret over choosing to work that day, concern for self-safety, and guilt for having these thoughts and feelings. There was also concern for the patient because I was afraid that he might perceive how I felt. I knew that "one cannot not communicate" (Watzlawick, Helmick-Beavin, & Jackson, 1967, p. 51) and that "the process between human and environmental fields is continuous and mutual" (Rogers, 1983, p. 4). It was not my nature to view a patient in terms of pathology. Unitary human beings cannot be compartmentalized and reduced to being viewed in terms of a diagnosis, but that was what I was doing. I believed my feelings and perception of the situation were inappropriate. My desire to use my knowledge and technical skills to promote harmony and well being took precedence over all else. I wanted to find a way to change my perception of Roger so that I would view him as a person, an irreducible whole, more than and different from the sum of his parts.

Self-appraisal of pattern manifestations allowed me to face the situation as it was. By bringing those uncomfortable feelings out into the open, I was able to recognize them for what they were. I could then knowingly pattern my energy field so that I would experience the situation differently and to Roger's benefit.

The use of imagery gave me the opportunity to be in mutual process with Roger at a different time and place. Since space and time are four-dimensional and nonlinear, my human energy field was not tied to conventional reality and I could enter another domain. There was an undivided wholeness of our energy fields in a different dimension and from a different frame of reference. This allowed me to experience Roger's energy field in the relative past and to bring this reality to the relative present. Reality was an imaged representation of the physical and behavioral manifestations of Roger's human energy field. This reality gave me a different perspective so that I was able to set aside my fears and concerns and participate with Roger in the patterning process that evolved.

When I entered Roger's room, I directed pattern manifestation appraisal toward Roger's human and environmental energy fields. The pattern of his environmental field reflected the pattern manifestations of those closely involved with Roger. The love, thoughtfulness, and caring of Roger's relatives and friends were evidenced by the tree, cards, gifts, cot, and personal items that one needed to stay in the hospital for extended periods. The plants that had lost their beauty and the posters left hanging for long periods of time may not seem important when ranked with Roger's other issues and concerns. However, Roger was continually in mutual process with his environment, which was coextensive with the universe. His family and friends were a unit or system and their pattern manifestations could not be viewed as a separate issue. Their perception of Roger and his illness would constantly be reflected in his human self-image which was continuously evolving. Viewing Roger as a holistic being involved my looking through a "motion lens" at the rhythmic flow of the human and environmental mutual process and the "dynamic web of interconnections" (Smith, 1988, p. 94). I attempted to observe and appraise patterns in an all-inclusive manner. At times, the appraisal was made intuitively.

The hospital had been Roger's home for many months and he had experienced many personal myths. These myths were part of his identity and gave meaning and organization to his illness and hospital experiences (Madrid & Winstead-Fry, 1986). He knew the exuberance and joy of anticipated recovery associated with trials of new modalities for treatment, but was also familiar with the disappointments of failure as one after another method of treatment was rejected. His family and friends had attempted to bring the world to his room with tangible items, bits of news and verbal descriptions of their experiences, but a vicarious experience of the world had a different flavor. From the time he had first entered the hospital, the outward appearance associated with his human energy field had been continuously changing, manifesting new and different pattern manifestations. His human self-image was also in continual flux. Pattern changes in his energy field were continually occurring ranging from faster to slower rhythms, from time racing to time dragging, from feelings of hopefulness to feelings of hopelessness. There was a time when he had the strength to shave and shower, the satisfaction of admiring a newly donned wardrobe. Now, in the relative present, even though it was Christmas, he expressed no interest in participating in the mutual process with his environment. It was too much of an effort. His strength was minimal. He was concentrating on keeping his body as immobile as possible, avoiding any movement that would inflict pain. Roger was aware of his environment and his mutuality with it but his human field rhythm was in a range of low frequency. Time was dragging. Roger validated this pattern manifestation appraisal of the human and environmental fields as we spoke later that evening.

The appraisal that was the first phase of the Rogerian practice methodology described by Barrett (1988) would provide the direction for the next phase: deliberative mutual patterning.

Roger's goal was to be relieved of the pain that consumed him. His energy was focused on pain and he was not able to use the healing powers that were within his capacity. Using therapeutic touch, I assessed the rhythm and energy flow of his human field and found that it was in a range of low frequency. By means of therapeutic touch, I was able to focus and direct energy to his human field. A new pattern emerged as changes in his energy field took place. His human field manifested a higher wave frequency and his physiological parameters served as indices of change in his energy field. McDonald (1986) posits that the concept of pain is a "rhythmic phenomenon having wavelike characteristics" (p. 121). It was evident from an appraisal of the manifestations of his field that Roger was experiencing a harmonious, rhythmic flow of energy. As I rubbed his back and changed his bed, he was able to maintain that state of comfort by drawing upon his own resources.

The changes that took place in Roger's human field pattern that evening were changes that came from within himself. He had power and the capacity to knowingly participate in the process of change (Barrett, 1988; Rogers, 1970). My role was not to direct, but rather to open doors to reveal new horizons. Therapeutic touch, deep breathing, relaxation techniques, and imagery were choices that he was made aware of and could participate in for the purpose of health patterning. I was there to be of assistance, but it was Roger who consciously chose to actualize his well being and pattern his human and environmental field. The process was not passive.

Therapeutic modalities do not necessarily have to be complex. Something as simple as a shampoo facilitated a change in human self-image. Roger felt good after the shampoo but he also recognized the difference it made in his appearance. A familiar pattern of behavior was emerging—his desire to be well groomed and his concern about his appearance. His intention was to actively participate in his hygiene and he directed me toward the fulfillment of this goal.

Healing also took place through empathy, which is defined as a feeling attribute emerging from the human and environmental mutual process (Raile, 1982). Continuous motion and evolving patterns were associated with both of our human energy fields. Empathy encompassed the totality of this process. I understood and experienced Roger's world through an interconnectedness of our human energy fields. These fields resonated together, sharing feeling patterns to the end that there was a mutuality of feeling and a comprehension of the "shared experience of the four-dimensional integral self" (Rawnsley, 1985, p. 27). Roger knew that I cared and he was not hesitant to reveal his inner self to me. Through open expression, he had the opportunity to sort out and resolve feelings and experiences that troubled him. He found it invigorating to engage in the process of reminiscence. I listened as he brought experiences from the relative past into the relative present so that he could enjoy them from a new and different perspective. When he was frightened, he knew that he would not be abandoned.

It is important to note that the process of empathy does not imply that Roger's energy field was in mutual process with my energy field. This trust and confidence evolved through the mutual process of his human and environmental energy fields. Environmental energy fields are coextensive with the universe and my energy field could not be separated out from this universal whole. This point is made not to minimize my role as a nurse in the patterning process of his human energy field toward health-related goals but to recognize that my contribution blended in and was integral to all that surrounded Roger.

Roger experienced those 8 hours as if he were living rather than dying. He lived them to the fullest, appreciating and capturing the beauty of music and flowers, integrating their presence into his energy field so that its pattern reflected an accelerated frequency that seemed continuous. His awareness was heightened as he reached out to synthesize the experiences of his life process, drawing new meaning and personal fulfillment from them. The wave patterns of Roger's human energy field resonated with those of the universe, becoming harmonious and synchronous. The perceptual features of his field pattern were diverse and visionary.

I don't believe that Roger was sad or afraid when he died. He was content to let go of the life in which his energy field was associated with physical manifestations and move on to a more diverse existence. It was my privilege to have been able to have shared a portion of this transformation with him.

REFERENCES

Barrett, E.A.M. (1988). Using Rogers' science of unitary human beings in nursing practice. *Nursing Science Quarterly, 1*, 50–51.

Madrid, M., & Winstead-Fry, P. (1986) In P. Winstead-Fry (Ed.), *Case studies in nursing theory* (pp. 73–102). New York: National League of Nursing.

McDonald, S. (1986). The relationship between visible lightwaves and the experience of pain. In V. Malinski (Ed.), *Explorations on Martha Rogers' science of unitary human beings* (pp. 119–127). Norwalk, CT: Appleton-Century-Crofts.

Pascal, B. (1931). *Thoughts*, as cited in Walsh, W. *The international encyclopedia of prose and poetical quotations* (p. 706). Philadelphia: Winston.

Quinn, J. (1981). Client care and nurse involvement in a holistic framework. In D. Krieger, *Foundations for holistic health nursing practices: The renaissance nurse* (pp. 197–210). Philadelphia: J.P. Lippincott Co.

Raile, M. (1982). *The relationships of creativity, actualization, and empathy in unitary human development*. Unpublished doctoral dissertation, New York University, New York.

Rawnsley, M. (1985). Health: A Rogerian perspective. *Journal of Holistic Nursing, 3*(1), 25–29.

Rogers, M.E. (1970). *An introduction to the theoretical basis of nursing*. Philadelphia: F.A. Davis.

Rogers, M.E. (1983). *Science of unitary human beings: A paradigm for nursing.* Unpublished manuscript.

Rogers, M.E. (1986). Science of unitary human beings. In V. Malinski (Ed.), *Explorations of Martha Rogers' science of unitary human beings* (pp. 3–8). Norwalk, CT: Appleton-Century-Crofts.

Smith, M.J. (1988). Perspectives of wholeness: The lens makes a difference. *Nursing Science Quarterly, 1*(3), 94–95.

Watzlawick, P., Helmick-Beavin, J., & Jackson, D. (1967). *Pragmatics of human communication*. New York: Norton & Co.

8

Health Patterning with Clients in a Private Practice Environment

Elizabeth Ann Manhart Barrett

Science-based nursing practice is the use of substantive nursing knowledge to facilitate patterning human health. This chapter provides a glimpse of how science-based practice is implemented in one private nursing practice. In this practice the Science of Unitary Human Beings (Rogers, 1970, 1983, 1986) is linked to knowledgeable caring for clients. The theoretical matrix creates a unique experiential involvement in the human-environmental mutual process of life's innovative emergence.

HEALTH PATTERNING

Assisting clients with their knowing participation in change defines the process of health patterning, a nursing science alternative to psychotherapy. Even holistic modes of psychotherapy focus on the mind as a "part" of a whole human being. However, operating in the Rogerian mode, I do not think of clients as having "psychological" or "physical" problems since I am not treating minds or bodies in and of themselves; rather,my concern is with manifestations of whole human beings.

Clients are health seekers concerned with the quality of their lives. Often, they are searching for more meaning and ways to make changes. The focus of health patterning is to assist clients with lifestyle changes and resolution of difficulties in living and dying. In the health patterning process, people are helped to become aware of feelings, thoughts, and attitudes within a special environmental context that involves deliberate use of theory and associated unitary human field practice modalities. This interface of science and art is designed to facilitate participation in changing particular field manifestations that the client decides to attempt to change. Individual decision is crucial in this regard as compliance is antithetical to the Rogerian system.

Health patterning involves the two major phases of the Rogerian practice methodology. First, there is pattern manifestation appraisal, "the continuous process of identifying manifestations of the human and environmental fields that relate to current health events" (Barrett, 1988, p. 50). Second, there is deliberative mutual patterning, "the process whereby the nurse with the client patterns the environmental field to promote harmony related to the health events" (p. 50). In these two phases, pattern manifestation appraisal and deliberative mutual patterning, clients are assisted to knowingly participate in health decisions related to their experience of themselves and others, work and play, nutrition, substance use, sleep/wake cycles, safety, decelerated/accelerated field rhythms, space time shifts, and professional health care. In addition to wellness counseling and health education, unitary human field practice modalities include meditation, innovative imagery (content derived from Rogerian science, e.g., imagery reflecting the Rogerian power theory), laughter, affirmations as expressions of intentionality, imposed motion/movement/dance, breathing/rest/relaxation approaches, descriptive dream experience, therapeutic touch, poetry, drawing, as well as use of color, light, and sound.

The scientific basis for health patterning practice is diagrammed in Figure 1 (Barrett, 1989). Rogers (1986) maintains that nursing's phenomenon of concern is people and their world. According to the Science of Unitary Human Beings, people and their world are four-dimensional energy fields which means that reality is a nonlinear domain without spatial or temporal attributes. Unitary human beings are irreducible wholes; they are more than and different from the sum of their parts. The uniqueness of each human and environmental energy field is defined by pattern which is ever changing. There is no causality or regression in this reality of openness (Barrett, 1988).

Consistent with the building blocks of energy fields, pattern, openness, and four-dimensionality, the power theory that I developed in previous work (Barrett, 1983, 1986) was derived from Rogers' (1983) principle of helicy which describes the continuous, innovative, probabilistic, increasing diversity of human and environmental field patterns characterized by non-repeating rhythmicities. The operational indicators of power, that is,

Figure 1
Derivation of the Power Model for Practice

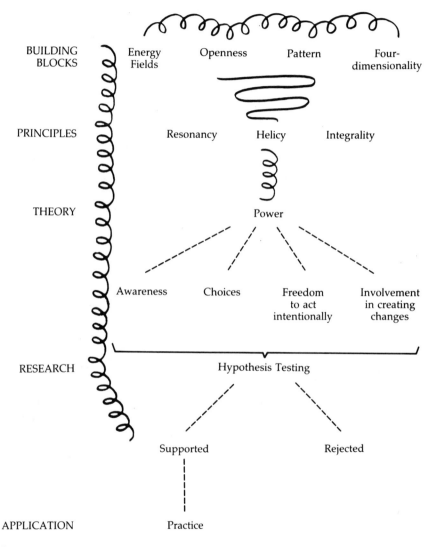

BUILDING BLOCKS — Energy Fields Openness Pattern Four-dimensionality

PRINCIPLES — Resonancy Helicy Integrality

THEORY — Power

Awareness Choices Freedom to act intentionally Involvement in creating changes

RESEARCH — Hypothesis Testing

Supported Rejected

APPLICATION — Practice

From "A Nursing Theory of Power for Nursing Practice" by E.A.M. Barrett, 1989. In J. Riehl-Sisca (Ed.), *Conceptual models for nursing practice*, 3rd ed. (p. 209). Norwalk, CT: Appleton & Lange. Used with permission of the publisher.

awareness, choices, freedom to act intentionally, and involvement in creating changes allowed for testing the hypothesis that power was related to human field motion, an index of unitary human change (Barrett, 1983, 1986, 1989). Human field motion is a perceptual experience of motion that manifests the continuously moving position and flow of the human field pattern (Barrett, 1983). Support of the hypothesis provided a beginning scientific basis for implementing the theory in practice (Barrett, 1983, 1986, in press).

Nursing care in this system is concerned with patterning the environmental field. The nurse, together with the client, patterns the environment to promote healing and comfort. The goal is change in the client's health dynamics with a principal focus on process.

In both phases of the Rogerian practice methodology I use the power theory, previously tested in research (Barrett, 1983, 1986), to assist clients with their knowing participation in change. Health patterning evolves as clients participate more knowingly in the changes occurring in their lives, including health care decision making. Health patterning is a dynamic process that enhances power and other avenues for actualizing human potentials for change.

"Power" is defined as the capacity to participate knowingly in the nature of change characterizing the continuous patterning of the human and environmental fields as manifest by awareness, choices, freedom to act intentionally, and involvement in creating change (Barrett, 1983, 1986, 1989). Power, a continuous theme in life experiences, dynamically describes the way human beings interact with their environment to actualize some potentials for change rather than others and, thereby, share in the creation of their human and environmental reality. Power is being aware of what one is choosing to do, feeling free to do it, and doing it intentionally.

The interrelationship of the concepts of awareness, choices, freedom to act intentionally, and involvement in creating change constitutes power. Such manifestations can be measured by the Barrett Power as Knowing Participation in Change Tool using semantic differential technique to rate each of the power concepts on a set of bipolar adjective scales (Barrett, 1983, 1986). See Figure 2 for an example of the scoring guide for one of the power concepts. The words in capital letters represent higher frequency or more powerful aspects of the bipolar adjective pairs; the words in lower case letters represent lower frequency or less powerful indicators.

The Barrett Power as Knowing Participation in Change Tool is used in both phases of the Rogerian practice methodology. While it is used to assist in pattern manifestation appraisal in the first phase, it is used to promote knowing participation in change in the second phase of delibera-

Figure 2
Scoring Guide

	my INVOLVEMENT IN CREATING CHANGE is												
constrained	1	:	2	:	3	:	4	:	5	:	6	:	7	FREE*
ORDERLY	7	:	6	:	5	:	4	:	3	:	2	:	1	chaotic
unpleasant	1	:	2	:	3	:	4	:	5	:	6	:	7	PLEASANT
worthless	1	:	2	:	3	:	4	:	5	:	6	:	7	VALUABLE
IMPORTANT	7	:	6	:	5	:	4	:	3	:	2	:	1	unimportant
INTENTIONAL	7	:	6	:	5	:	4	:	3	:	2	:	1	unintentional
superficial	1	:	2	:	3	:	4	:	5	:	6	:	7	PROFOUND
following	1	:	2	:	3	:	4	:	5	:	6	:	7	LEADING
shrinking	1	:	2	:	3	:	4	:	5	:	6	:	7	EXPANDING
INFORMED	7	:	6	:	5	:	4	:	3	:	2	:	1	uninformed
SEEKING	7	:	6	:	5	:	4	:	3	:	2	:	1	avoiding
ASSERTIVE	7	:	6	:	5	:	4	:	3	:	2	:	1	timid
VALUABLE	7	:	6	:	5	:	4	:	3	:	2	:	1	worthless

*Words in capital letters represent higher frequency end of scales. On a color chart, higher frequency is represented by blue and lower frequency by red.
From "A Nursing Theory of Power for Nursing Practice" by E.A.M. Barrett, 1989. In Riehl-Sisca (Ed.), *Conceptual Models for Nursing Practice*, 3rd ed. (p. 213). Norwalk, CT: Appleton & Lange. Used with permission of the publisher.

tive mutual patterning. In both of these phases it is important not to think of people as being "sick." Value labels are avoided. It is equally important to help clients set aside derogatory value labels that have been ascribed to them by others or self. Health, as well as illness, is value-related and ultimately defined by the individual as that individual perceives it to be.

PRACTICE VIGNETTES

Mary[1] was a client who had participated in creating a situation at work that was similar to her previous marital situation that had ended in divorce 8 years before. After several months of discussion in health patterning sessions, she decided she was in another so-called "bad marriage" and needed to divorce her job. Despair characterized her decelerated field rhythms. She

---

[1]Names and other identifying information have been changed to protect client anonymity and consent to discuss aspects of their lives has been obtained.

was suicidal but didn't want to die or to be hospitalized as she had been following her divorce. She did exercise her option to take antidepressant medication. I referred her to a psychiatrist for a medication consultation. He prescribed Elavil and recommended hospitalization for what he labeled from the DSM III taxonomy a "Major Depression, Recurrent." Mary adamantly refused hospitalization. Instead, she and I planned what in retrospect could be termed a "healthy withdrawal." In the traditional health care system Mary probably would have been labeled noncompliant. After a month she discontinued the Elavil due to the side effect of tachycardia.

Creatively and courageously Mary resigned from her job. However, with mutual consent the company president "laid her off" and she was able to collect money from unemployment insurance during her transition period. Mary proceeded to create a temporary healing cocoon. She yearned for a peaceful and nurturing environment. I was aware that her sense of hopelessness and suicidal ideas might escalate when she stopped working and had lost contact on a daily basis with her usual world. Withdrawal and creating a cocoon are not traditional nursing interventions for this type of rhythmic pattern. This, nevertheless, was her informed choice, and my role as advocate and counselor was to support her through the experience of transition.

The care plan designed by the two of us patterned her environment in a different way. It included a systematic program of exercise with deep breathing, relaxation, and three miles of walking each day in the winter weather. She allowed as much sunlight into her apartment as possible and spent 30 minutes a day rocking near a window with the sunlight directly on her. As she sat and rocked she sometimes concentrated on experiencing peacefulness or visualized success in a new business position. In addition to meditation, Mary listened to music of her preference that she found soothing or energizing each day. She also listened to an innovative power imagery audiotape that I developed and recorded specifically for her between office visits to reinforce her evolving conception of power as knowing participation in change.

Power imagery is an example of the innovative imagery modality that uses power theory to enhance the capacity to participate knowingly in change. The tape was designed to stimulate an increasing awareness of thoughts, feelings, and actions connected with Mary's current life experiences and included suggested affirmations to facilitate expression of her intentionality for well being. For example, the following affirmation was used, "Say to yourself aloud, I forgive myself and absolve myself of all guilt, here and now, and forever. Say it again slowly and let yourself feel it. I forgive myself and absolve myself, here and now, and forever." Open-ended exploration of higher frequency choices (free, valuable, informed, expanding, seeking, assertive, leading, intentional, important, pleasant, orderly, and profound) provoked creation of possibilities and encouraged her to design new ways of involving herself in creating change. The imagery also provided a structure for visualizing success in obtaining employment that would facilitate further actualization of developmental potentials for unitary change.

Mary's feelings of hopelessness and helplessness began to subside quickly after she resigned from her job. Her change in environment was also accompanied by a sense of unburdening relief. For several months she increased her office visits to twice weekly and also made at least one phone call daily to reach out for support to one of her friends or adult children. She began to experience nurturance in the temporary respite from her demanding business world.

The pattern manifestations that constituted Mary's power profile changed from lower to higher frequency power. Power profile, of course, refers to a person's unique interrelationship of the power indicators of awareness, choices, freedom to act intentionally, and involvement in creating changes. Over a period of 6 months Mary experienced a power profile transition that can be described as a major pattern transformation. Toward the end of the last month she looked for and found a new job and got on with the business of living her life. A year later, after receiving a major promotion in her new position, her rhythms continued to be harmonious with her environment.

The Power as Knowing Participation in Change Tool was used during both phases of the Rogerian practice methodology. Pattern manifestation appraisal involved asking Mary to complete the tool (see Figure 3). Then scores were computed for awareness, choices, freedom to act intentionally, and involvement in creating changes. Based on the ratings of the bipolar adjective pairs of the semantic differential power scores, current pattern manifestations were defined. These manifestations were described to the client as unpleasant but expanding *awareness, choices* that were viewed as superficial although important. In addition, her *freedom to act intentionally* was experienced as constrained as well as avoiding, and her *involvement in creating changes* was manifest as chaotic and worthless.

In the deliberative mutual patterning phase, power profile scores as well as adjective indicators for awareness, choices, freedom to act intentionally, and involvement in creating change were discussed to individualize Mary's learning of power theory. Patterning probabilities were established which potentially could be actualized by enhancing Mary's ability to knowingly participate in change in a variety of ways. As a result, Mary selected new actions based on more powerful choices; for example, resigning from her

Figure 3
Example of Scoring

my INVOLVEMENT IN CREATING CHANGE is

	1	2	3	4	5	6	7		
constrained	:	X :	:	:	:	:		FREE	2
ORDERLY	:	:	:	:	X :	:		chaotic	3
unpleasant	:	:	X :	:	:	:		PLEASANT	3
worthless	:	X :	:	:	:	:		VALUABLE	2
IMPORTANT	:	:	X :	:	:	:		unimportant	5
INTENTIONAL	:	:	:	X :	:	:		unintentional	4
superficial	:	:	X :	:	:	:		PROFOUND	3
following	:	:	:	:	X :	:		LEADING	5
shrinking	:	X :	:	:	:	:		EXPANDING	2
INFORMED	:	:	X :	:	:	:		uninformed	5
SEEKING	X :	:	:	:	:	:		avoiding	7
ASSERTIVE	:	:	X :	:	:	:		timid	5
+* VALUABLE	:	:	:	:	:	X :		worthless	46

*Retest item noted as positive (+) indicated same response to the scale as when the scale appeared earlier in the rating of this concept. A positive sign suggests reliability while a negative (−) sign suggests lack of consistency (reliability) of response. The retest item is not included in the score.
From "A Nursing Theory of Power for Nursing Practice," by E.A.M. Barrett, 1989. In Riehl-Sisca (Ed.), *Conceptual Models for Nursing Practice*, 3rd ed. (p. 213). Norwalk, CT: Appleton & Lange. Used with permission of the publisher.

---

job, activities designed to accelerate her field rhythms, and eventual seeking of more synchronous employment.

Evaluation by means of the client's reported experience was an ongoing means of validating effectiveness of the unitary human field modalities. In addition, the Ference Human Field Motion Tool (Ference, 1979, 1986) was used as an evaluation measurement instrument since it is an index of unitary human change. It has been demonstrated in research to be related to power (Barrett, 1983), the capacity whereby one knowingly participates in the nature of change by actualizing some potentials for human change rather than others.

This example illustrates that Mary intuitively knew that she could take care of her health and the nurse–client mutual process of deliberately patterning the client's environmental field assisted her to do so. Nursing care facilitated knowing participation and Mary emerged from the trauma of her despair.

It should be noted that the nurse as a four-dimensional presence experienced in the client's environment also has power which can be used to assist the client in knowing participation in change. In health patterning, the nurse enhances the client's power as an outcome of the nurse–client mutual process. Health patterning is fine tuning to enhance knowing participation and other means of actualizing potentials for human change.

The second case example concerns Susan. Her pattern manifestations were related to cultural relocation trauma. Susan was from Europe. When Susan came to see me the first time, she looked shocked and frightened as I introduced myself. Susan immediately began to cry. Within a few minutes she explained that she had seen me before. She said about a month before she had seen me in a dream in which she was on an ocean liner and I was her traveling companion. She remembered both of us standing on the deck, leaning against the railing and looking out into the dark waters with the bright moonlight glistening across the surface of the sea.

Susan went on to say that this was not the first time she had experienced a dream that had come true and she wanted to know if that sounded "crazy." I replied that it didn't. Susan remarked that she was relieved since *she* knew it was true and if I couldn't believe her then how would she ever trust me. She asked if I had ever seen her before or had known her in another life. I replied that I had not.

Rogers' (1983) theory of paranormal events accounts for Susan's dream as a precognitive experience. What was in her four-dimensional present hadn't happened yet in three-dimensional clock time. Her experience of the present simply extended beyond the "average" or "usual" present. It was an example of relative present or infinite now which is multidirectional and, therefore, could equally account for experiences of déjà vu as well as precognition.[2]

To continue, I would like to share two examples from my practice of what might be termed "four-dimensional" knowing. This special type of knowing participation in change or power also appears in Rogers' theory of paranormal events. As the health patterning process evolves, it seems that clients increasingly experience four-dimensional knowing.

First, there is Diedre, who experienced, as she called it, an "intercontinental communication." For two weeks she had been having dreams of a woman who was dying in Santo Domingo. Diedre had lived with this woman during her 4 years in high school. After the first dream, she called and learned that indeed the woman had suddenly become quite ill. Then one morning Diedre awoke after having dreamed that the woman had died

---

[2] The *relative present* or *infinite now* are terms used by Rogers (1970) to describe what is currently in a person's awareness. Such terms are not defined by clock or calendar time and their meaning can vary considerably among people. According to Rogers, some people are aware in their relative present of events usually considered as past or future by others.

and that her spirit was hovering over her bed telling Diedre farewell. At that moment the phone rang. It was Diedre's mother calling from her home in Africa to tell her that the woman in Santo Domingo had died two hours before.

As Diedre recounted this experience during our next meeting together, I asked her to bring the woman into the room and to have a dialogue with her. I asked her to "Let her be here. Let yourself see her. Talk to her. Tell her what you want her to know." Diedre was able to do this quite easily as we often use this type of non-temporal, non-spatial communication style. It is simply a way of making contact in a four-dimensional system. As Diedre talked to the woman and recounted times that she vividly remembered, the tears began to flow. She openly grieved and shared this experience with me.

Second, there is Barbara, who had discovered a lump in her breast. She came in for a session the day before she was scheduled to have a lumpectomy. This was on November 4. When the session was over and as Barbara was walking out the door, she turned to me and said, "I don't know why, but November 22 is going to be a good day." The next day the lumpectomy was performed. Barbara had previously decided that she wanted to have the lumpectomy and that regardless of what the frozen section might indicate she wanted no further immediate surgery. In case of a malignancy she wanted time to carefully consider the various options available to her. The day after the lumpectomy, her surgeon came to her room and told her that the pathology report had revealed cancer cells. And then he said, "I've tentatively scheduled you for further surgery on November 22." When she told me about this, I asked her if she recalled what she had said to me when she was leaving on November 4th. She didn't remember and so I reminded her that she had said, "I don't know why, but November 22 is going to be a good day." On November 22, Barbara had a modified radical mastectomy. The pathology report indicated that 38 lymph nodes were examined and no cancer cells were present. November 22 was indeed a good day and somehow she knew it would be at a time when she could not have known *why* it would be.

These examples illustrate that four-dimensional knowing transcends the three-dimensional parameters of time and space. As clients increasingly embrace and celebrate their unique human-environmental process, could it be that this type of awareness or knowing is more often manifest? Rogers' theory of the paranormal provides a framework to account for these experiences.

Further work in developing current Rogerian theories is needed. Of course, many new Rogerian theories need to be generated and tested through basic research as well. Likewise, use of the theories in practice requires further illustration and testing through applied research.

CONCLUSION

The goal of my work in nursing practice is to enhance clients' ability to share in the creation of their reality by way of their knowing participation. This process of assisting clients in developing and using power is termed "health patterning."

The health patterning approach to nursing practice is only limited by knowledge of the Rogerian system, creativity in using that knowledge, and to some extent by the state-of-the-art of development in this continually evolving science. This abstract system of thought constitutes substantive nursing knowledge and is a basis for nursing practice.

The dynamic interface of science and art presents scholars with the challenge of explicating imaginative possibilities for the well being and betterment of all people. Indeed, Rogers' Science of Unitary Human Beings is a nursing science vision for the emerging century.

REFERENCES

Barrett, E.A.M. (1983). An empirical investigation of Martha E. Rogers' principle of helicy: The relationship of human field motion and power. *Dissertation Abstracts International, 45* (University Microfilms No. 84-06, 278)

Barrett, E.A.M. (1986). Investigation of the principle of helicy: The relationship of human field motion and power. In V.M. Malinski (Ed.), *Explorations on Martha Rogers' science of unitary human beings* (pp. 173–184). Norwalk, CT: Appleton-Century-Crofts.

Barrett, E.A.M. (1988). Using Rogers' science of unitary human beings in nursing practice. *Nursing Science Quarterly, 1*(2), 50–51.

Barrett, E.A.M. (1989). A nursing theory of power for nursing practice: Derivation from Rogers' Paradigm. In J. Riehl (Ed.), *Conceptual models for nursing practice* 3rd ed. (pp. 207–217). Norwalk, CT: Appleton & Lange.

Ference, H.M. (1979). The relationship of time experience, creativity traits, differentiation, and human field motion. *Dissertation Abstracts International* (University Microfilms No. 80-10, 281)

Ference, H.M. (1986). The relationship of time experience, creativity traits, differentiation, and human field motion. In V.M. Malinski (Ed.), *Explorations on Martha Rogers' science of unitary human beings* (pp. 95–105). Norwalk, CT: Appleton-Century-Crofts.

Rogers, M.E. (1970). *An introduction to the theoretical basis of nursing.* Philadelphia: F.A. Davis.

Rogers, M.E. (1983). *Science of unitary human beings: A paradigm for nursing.* Unpublished manuscript.

Rogers, M.E. (1986). Science of unitary human beings. In V.M. Malinski (Ed.), *Explorations on Martha Rogers' science of unitary human beings* (pp. 3–8). Norwalk, CT: Appleton-Century-Crofts.

9

Intentionality in the Human-Environment Encounter in an Ambulatory Care Environment

Suzanne D. Thomas

Rogers' (1986) Science of Unitary Human Beings offers a *scientific* basis for the study of nursing and for the use of nursing knowledge with clients in the holistic promotion of health. This chapter discusses how Rogers' work is used in an ambulatory primary care setting as a basis for practice and for the development of a mid-range theory synthesized from logical extensions of nursing science. Cases are used as illustrations. Identifying data in the cases are changed to protect clients' anonymity.

A NURSING SCIENCE-BASED PRACTICE

A science-based practice expresses clear linkages between science and practice. The purpose of this section is to identify the philosophical and theoretical framework for a science-based nursing practice in a primary care environment.

Scholarly practitioners think about phenomena experienced in clinical situations as concepts. Concepts label phenomena; knowledge concerning the phenomena is applied by practitioners using the scientific system of thought.[1] Principles and theories of science provide a perspective for the

---

[1] A scientific system of thought, or a science, is an organized set of principles, concepts, and theories relating to a central focus. Rogerian science focuses on unitary human beings.

interpretation of experiences and guide analysis and interpretation of data and actions throughout an encounter. Interpretation of the meaning and significance of experiences is guided by the philosophical structure underlying the scientific system (Burns & Grove, 1987).

The philosophical position of Rogerian scientists is one of holism. Holism is expressed in the definition of human beings as unitary. A unitary human being is indivisible and different from the sum·of its parts. The unitary human being is both the distinguishing focus of nursing science and the basic unit of study (Rogers, 1980, p. 329).

The ultimate value of a science is judged by its usefulness to practitioners for identifying and classifying information, providing explanations, and enabling practitioners to forecast probable outcomes of actions under known conditions (Carter, 1985; Brinberg & McGrath, 1985). To be judged useful, theory must move from a way of thinking about phenomena of importance to a way of manipulating variables that enables testing of research hypotheses for the generation of knowledge (Hacking, 1983). The historical significance of the nurse's caregiving role in human society (Donahue, 1985) supports the necessity for nursing science to be clinically useful.

What distinguishes a professional practice from a routine application of a set of skills is the scientific knowledge base on which the professional practice is founded. Professional nursing practice provides a means of generating and testing hypotheses derived from the scientific system.

Three criteria for judging the usefulness or value of a scientific system are its scope, parsimony, and differentiation (Brinberg & McGrath, 1985). Rogers' nursing science is both global in scope and parsimonious in its definition of principles and concepts. Application of nursing science with clients requires the nurse to differentiate human and environmental field pattern manifestations. Thus, differentiation requires linking principles and concepts of the abstract system with empirical knowledge. Mid-range theories facilitate tests of broad abstract scientific principles.

Rogers' (1988) system supports development of multiple theories in nursing science. Thus, theory development involves inductive and deductive logic. Yin's (1984) multiple case study design is consistent with Rogers' position. Development of the Human Environment Encounter Model, reported elsewhere (Thomas, 1988), involved a synthetico-deductive process using Yin's multiple case study design that links it to Rogers' system as well.

An empirical understanding of nursing science involves both a pragmatic and a limiting perspective. Pragmatically, an empirical understanding of nursing science facilitates the testing of practice-related research hypotheses. However, there is some loss of both parsimony and scope through linking abstract concepts and principles to culturally grounded empirics. Thus, a report such as this, which purports to demonstrate how to use nursing science, is limited to the scholar's present visions and must not be considered a final solution to abstract puzzles.

APPLICATIONS OF NURSING SCIENCE IN PRIMARY NURSING CARE

Nursing science is applied in primary nursing care with logical extensions of the concepts and principles to specific conditions and situations arising in practice. For example, the nurse is a human energy field; the client is a human energy field. Each is to the other an energy form of the environmental energy field. The clinic setting, staff, and clients are energy forms of the nurse's environmental field. Each energy form serves as an empirical referent of the changing pattern manifestations of the environmental field. Each nurse and each client has a unique, recognizable field pattern (Thomas, 1987, 1988). The nurse and the environmental field are integral, "in continuous, mutual process" (Rogers, 1986, p. 6). Continuous, mutual process explains the nature of the human-environmental relationship (Thomas, 1988). Nurses and clients, that is, energy fields, are continuously changing. In the principle of helicy, Rogers (1986) defines the nature of change as "continuous, innovative, and probabilistic" (p. 6). Thus, the nurse–client continuous, mutual process is characterized by continuous, innovative, and probabilistic change (Thomas, 1988).

Barrett's (1983, 1986, 1988) theory of Power as Knowing Participation proposes that nurses and clients knowingly choose to participate in change. Deliberate choice to participate in change is an act of power. If the nurse deliberately chooses to participate in change with the intention of assisting clients to move toward a more desirable condition of health, that is a form of nursing therapy. A nurse knowingly takes deliberate actions to promote a client's health. By taking deliberate action a nurse increases the probability that certain, highly valued changes will occur. Information about the client's pattern and the dynamics of the changes taking place allows the nurse to forecast with varying degrees of confidence the likelihood that a desired outcome will occur. However, in a relative universe, the nurse does not predict outcomes with certainty. The nurse does not control care. Instead, the nurse and the client are knowing participants in change for the client's well being.

Nurses and clients share the human characteristic of intentionality. Intentionality is defined as a person's world view, by which experiences are valued and intuited as reality (Thomas, 1987, 1989). A nurse's intentionality as a helping, healing professional also includes a scientific knowledge base of practice, a commitment to serve the well being of the client, and willingness and ability to confront oneself (Krieger, 1979). When a nurse takes a deliberate action to help a client, the nurse's action is framed in intentionality. The Human Environment Encounter Model links with Barrett's theory through intentionality. Freedom to act intentionally is a dimension of power (Barrett, 1983, 1986). The nurse deliberately uses power to promote the client's health.

CASES ILLUSTRATING THE HUMAN ENVIRONMENT ENCOUNTER MODEL

Concepts and dynamics of the Human Environment Encounter Model are presented in two cases. Interpretive notes are shown in parentheses.

A female client with vaginal candidia moniliasis was told by another practitioner to use medicated vaginal tablets, to douche with vinegar and yogurt, and then to douche with soda. The client visited this nurse in clinic for follow-up. The client believed the overgrowth of yeast had increased. Intuitively, the nurse knew from the chart and history what the problem was. Intuition is a broad-based, deep grasp of the facts and of the situation (Benner & Tanner, 1987). Intuition is continuous, immediate comprehension of the nurse–client process. In some cases intuition is experienced as a sudden insight. However, intuition does enable the nurse to continuously know what is happening (Thomas, 1987).

Inspection revealed a bright red, swollen, tender, almost weeping vulva. The nurse chose a virginal size Graves speculum, which had been warmed on the heating pad. Tension was building. The nurse's energy was intensely focused on the client's need for comfort while noting her inflamed tissues. The client's muscles were tense. She had to concentrate to relax her legs and perineum.

As the nurse gently placed the speculum into the client's vagina, she asked, "Can you stand that?" The client replied in astonishment, "Stand up?" The nurse laughed and said, "No. I meant, 'Can you tolerate that?'" The client responded from her orientation. The nurse had deliberately refocused the communication toward positive potentials.

Then the client laughed and said, "Yes. It's okay." (Her response told the nurse a high degree of mutuality was established.) Then the nurse said humorously, "Now I want you to do a back flip!" At that both laughed until they had tears rolling down their faces and the tension was dispelled from their encounter. According to Parse (1987), this was an example of laughter at the ridiculous possibilities in the situation (Parse, 1987). The nurse had deliberately used humor to release tension.

Meanwhile, the nurse quickly took the specimen and removed the speculum before they finished laughing. Empathy was established in the tremendous rush of energy during their laughter. Raile (1983) defined empathy as a feeling manifestation of the human field. To the nurse, empathy felt like a connectedness to the client, with a marked increase in available energy and a greater intuitive understanding of the client's intentionality.

The nurse examined the tissue specimen microscopically, and found numerous white blood cells and epithelial cells, indicating a moderate to severe inflammatory reaction. Her anger returned when she considered that the inflammation was a response to the treatment.

When the nurse returned to the examining room, the client was dressed and seated beside the desk. The nurse explained that she was having an inflammatory reaction and instructed her to stop all douching. A more appropriate treatment was substituted.

The nurse did not want the client to sense her anger, and in an attempt to hold back her strong feelings, she began to hesitate and stutter. The nurse experienced turbulent energy field pattern manifestations as she attempted to divert her anger. There was no way to hold back experience. It flows and it becomes turbulent if you attempt to divert it.

The dynamics of the nurse–client process began with the nurse deliberately focusing her energies on the client's needs and positive potentials in the situation, while acknowledging the presence of negative potentials. It was critical not to elicit a painful reaction that might have reduced the probability of establishing empathy. But it was important for the nurse to acknowledge that the client could have a painful reaction if the examiner was not extremely careful with the speculum.

Intuition provided the scenario for deliberate humor. The growing tension, the client's snapped reply, and the natural awkwardness of the situation fueled a hearty mutual laugh that resulted in a high degree of empathy in the experience of womanhood.

From the empathic perspective, it was then difficult for the nurse to divert her anger. Stuttering speech validated how difficult it was to hold back experience in the empathic relationship, yet ethics required that the nurse not reveal her full perspective.

A second case offers another example of the model. Some clients are skeptical of the nurse's abilities to provide care. This client asked many questions to assess the nurse's knowledge and abilities. Her challenging orientation was clear in her curt tone of voice, her responses to questions with multiple questions, and the way she positioned her body to avoid being face to face with the nurse—she was angled away with her face partly turned back toward the nurse.

Knowing that it was imperative for the client to have faith in her provider's abilities, the nurse answered all the questions as best she could. The nurse's orientation was in motion toward establishment of faith and trust in the helping relationship, understanding all along that it would be difficult to overcome the client's skepticism.

As the nurse examined her breasts, the client asked how the nurse could tell "grainy" tissue from "fat globules." The nurse cited characteristics and emphasized differences between "grainy" and "fat tissue" which enabled her to clinically evaluate the tissues. The nurse explained that she knew by constant interaction with other clinicians during her early work as a clinician, and that this had gradually become kinesthetic knowledge which she translated with a set of terms to describe the phenomenon: glandular breast tissue. The nurse's energy was intensely focused upon presenting herself to the client as a scholarly and highly competent nursing professional in her effort to establish credibility.

All this took place in a matter of 1 to 2 minutes as the nurse examined the client's breasts and demonstrated self-breast examination. Intense experience may encompass more "time" than chronological time indicates. Thus, experiential time or time experience is relative to the intensity of the felt experience (Rawnsley, 1977). In this example, the intensity of the experience compressed the nurse's chronological time perspective and exemplified, in Ference's (1979, 1988) phrase, "accelerated human field motion."

After the final string of adjectives, the nurse laughed and said, "That's jargon for, 'you have normal breast tissue and it feels like this.'" With that, the nurse put the client's hand on the area over her gland at eleven o'clock on her right breast. Intuitively, the nurse had reached a turning point in the relationship. Her energy was rapidly being depleted. It was the client's choice now whether or not she wanted to establish an empathic, trusting relationship with the nurse. In effect, the nurse said silently "I have shown you I am knowledgeable. You do not have to quiz me any further. I am changing my response to you. It is time for you to decide if you want to work with me or not." Thus, the nurse deliberately participated in change (Barrett, 1983, 1986) for the well being of the client, while inviting the client to participate with her. This was an example of the nurse's intentionality guiding therapeutic actions.

The client laughed. They both relaxed and the nurse completed the examination with the client's help. The nurse felt a partnership had been melded and empathy established. The nurse also felt very comfortable with the client. The client continued to ask questions, but not with such a challenging tone. The change in tone, the relaxation, and the sense of going forward in a partnership validated the empathic relationship. If the client had chosen to continue her distant, challenging intentionality, however, the nurse would have shielded herself from a skepticism that was, moment by moment, depleting her energy.

In other cases clients were unable to recognize the choice or chose not to enter an empathic relationship with the nurse. With a destructive, chaotically turbulent client, the nurse deliberately distanced herself from the client. With a client who exhibited rapid, unstable changes in her field pattern, the client did not appear to recognize that the nurse was reaching out to her. And one client recognized the invitation to choose an empathic relationship with the nurse but was too afraid to change her dysfunctional patterns to engage in a therapeutic relationship. Most, however, chose to enter the empathic relationship with the nurse.

Here the nurse's orientation, intuition, and valuing are demonstrated in a difficult situation with a challenging, skeptical client. Tension builds from the nurse's intense focus on the client's pattern manifestations and the desire to develop a therapeutic relationship despite expressed skepticism. The nurse deliberately changes her responses. The client must now decide whether or not to choose an empathic partnership or a relationship of distance and distrust. If the client chooses empathy, a partnership is formed.

Cases illustrate the flow of experiential, behavioral, and sensory information necessary for nurse–client process. Nurses participate in the dynamics of experience with clients. Integrality is a theme of the nurse–client encounter. Intentionality is an experiential concept, as are human field motion, power as knowing participation, nurse–client empathy, and client empowerment for self-health care.

Experiential concepts are those that describe scientific knowledge through observation or participation in situations (Mish, 1984). Experiential concepts are similar to maps of situations shared in common with others that can be validated in recorded case notes. Rarely does experiential information appear on a client's chart. However, experiential information is essential for the nurse to provide expert care (Benner, 1984).

Behavioral information is the observation and interpretation of another's behavior. Behavioral knowledge is the knowledge of what another person does and the usual meaning associated with that action. Self-health care actions are behaviors, which can be observed and validated, and they are often recorded in nursing notes.

Sensory information is perceived by the physical senses—vision, hearing, taste, touch, and smell. Sensory, behavioral, and experiential concepts are empirical referents of the human and environmental energy field patterns. Nursing is a holistically focused science, and meaning is found in pattern manifestations of energy fields, not in particular empirical referents. As the understanding of holistic patterns grows, so will grow the sophistication of empirical pattern referents and their reconceptualization from a multi-dimensional view.

HUMAN-ENVIRONMENT ENCOUNTER MODEL

The encounter of the human and environmental energy fields is marked by continuous, innovative, probabilistic change (Thomas, 1988). Changes in patterns are increasingly complex and diverse. Rogers' principle of resonancy (1986, p. 6) is logically extended to the human environment encounter through examination of pattern manifestation changes that provide the empirical referents signifying degrees to which clients are achieving the desired conditions of health.

The goal of nursing is to promote health (Rogers, 1988). An important dimension of health promotion is the client's power to provide self-health care (Malinski, 1986). Empowering clients to better provide self-health care promotes health. Thus, the efficacy of a nurse's deliberate actions on behalf of the client can be evaluated by the degree to which the client is empowered for self-health care.

Rogers' idea that the universe is four-dimensional puzzles some practitioners, yet, in reality, space and time are one. For this scholar, evidence of four-dimensionality is seen in the continuous motion of the universe (Ference, 1988). For example, a three-dimensional representation of a human field would show width, depth, and length of the field over time. A four dimensional representation of the same human field would show a fluid energy form in continuous motion, undergoing continuous, innovative, probabilistic changes in the direction of increasing diversity (Thomas, 1988).

Ference's theory of motion (1988) is synthesized from nursing science. Ference (1979) states that human field motion is a "multidimensional, experiential position" (p. 4). The Human-Environment Encounter Model (Thomas, 1988) links with Ference's theory of motion in this conceptualization of four-dimensionality as a universe in continuous motion, thus adding a stronger foundation for nursing science.

A second logical extension of a multidimensional universe is the conceptualization of the human-environment encounter in the ever-present now. The sense of clock time speeding or dragging is experiential evidence of human and environmental field motion.

An intense experience with a client can seem like a long or short period of clock time, when in fact the experience is characterized by changes in field motion. Measurement of clock time provides information about the earth's position relative to the sun. Measurement of field motion (Ference, 1979) provides information about the relative rate and quality of the human-environment process. Each is useful information, although their meanings have very different implications for nursing practice.

The following case illustrates a client's empowerment for self-health care. A client visited his nurse for health promotion counseling. He wanted to lose weight, begin an exercise program, and carry out recommendations from a recent health risk appraisal.

Health risk appraisal is a method of assessing an individual's risk of dying from certain diseases or accidents within a 10-year period based on the individual's health-related behaviors, history of illnesses and inherited factors (Robins & Hall, 1970; Hall & Zwemer, 1979; Wiley & Camacho, 1980; Breslow & Enstrom, 1980). Reviewing one's chances of dying in the near future elicits often negative, fearful reactions and avoidance behaviors. As a result, there is a low success rate for changing health-related behaviors from a health risk appraisal report (Beery, Schoenbach, & Wagner, 1986).

Although prevention is disease focused, health promotion is focused on helping the client to optimize potentials for well being (Thomas, Hathaway, & Arheart, in press). To an uninformed observer, these two different processes can appear identical. However, the focus of the process and the intentionality of the practitioner and client vary significantly. Although the stated purpose of the encounter described was disease prevention, the nurse's focus and intentionality were health promoting.

The nurse deliberately centered (Krieger, 1979) and focused energies toward the encounter with the client. At the beginning of the session, the nurse reviewed the risks and prevention strategies detailed in the health risk appraisal, then asked, "Do you want to change any of these factors for yourself?"

The client began a discussion of how he wanted to make a number of changes in his life. However, he was having a great deal of difficulty making changes. His approach was to trap himself into performing the desired behaviors. His orientation was toward self-control and self-imposed forceful changes in his behaviors. And he couldn't quite force himself to begin an exercise program or to lose weight. The nurse's orientation was one of self-love and acceptance. Forceful changes were philosophically alien. The client wanted the nurse to help him trap himself into doing what was "good" for himself.

While the client was telling about trapping himself, the nurse envisioned a man chasing, catching, and beating a small child into fearful obedience. The nurse shared this vision with the client and asked if it fit what he was saying. The client agreed that it did. The nurse expressed great sadness and gently suggested that the client not approach himself that way. He visibly relaxed into his chair, gave a deep sigh, and seemed relieved to be free of the vision.

The nurse invited the client to envision the man and the child in the scene in a loving way, hugging and walking hand in hand together. As the nurse extended the vision to one in which the man considered the child's needs from a loving perspective, the client grasped the allegorical meaning. He was to love himself and consider his needs from a self-loving perspective.

Together they discussed the client's pattern identifying several changes he might try as first steps toward seeking improved well being while maintaining a deep sense of attunement to his inner self.

Eventually, the client lost weight and participated in regular, vigorous exercise. He frequently told the nurse how much her care had meant to him. He was empowered by learning to love himself. He described the session as a "life-changing" encounter. The nurse felt a deep sense of satisfaction that the client was so empowered by learning to love himself.

CONCLUSION

In conclusion, the nurse and the client are energy fields in continuous, mutual process. The nurse–client process is characterized by continuous, innovative, probabilistic change. The nurse acts deliberately to increase the probability that desired changes will occur while understanding that, in a relative universe, the nurse does not control outcomes of care. Instead, the nurse forecasts with varying degrees of confidence the likelihood that desired conditions of well being will occur to mark pattern changes in the nurse–client process. The nurse deliberately participates in changes focused on optimizing the client's potential well being. The client is invited to be a willing, knowledgeable participant for changes in his or her own well being. Efficacy of deliberate changes is measured in the degree of nurse–client empathy established and the client's degree of empowerment for self-health care.

REFERENCES

Barrett, E.A.M. (1983). *An empirical investigation of Martha E. Rogers' principle of helicy: The relationship of human field motion and power*. Unpublished doctoral dissertation. New York University, New York. (University Microfilms 84-06278)

Barrett, E.A.M. (1986). Investigation of the principle of helicy: The relationship of human field motion and power. In Malinski, V. (Ed.), *Explorations on Martha Rogers' science of unitary human beings* (pp. 173–184). Norwalk, CT: Appleton-Century-Crofts.

Barrett, E.A.M. (1988). Practice applications: Using Rogers' science of unitary human beings in nursing practice. *Nursing Science Quarterly, 1*, 50–57.

Beery, W., Schoenbach, V.J., & Wagner, E.H. (1986). *Health risk appraisal: Methods and programs, with annotated bibliography.* Washington, DC: DHHS Publication No. (PHS) 86-3396.

Benner, P. (1984). *From novice to expert.* Menlo Park, CA: Addison-Wesley.

Benner, P., & Tanner, C. (1987). Clinical judgment: How expert nurses use intuition. *American Journal of Nursing, 87*(1), 23–31.

Breslow, L., & Enstrom, J.E. (1980). Persistence of health habits and their relationship to mortality. *Preventive Medicine 9*, 469–483.

Brinberg, D., & McGrath, J.E. (1985). *Validity and the research process.* Beverly Hills: Sage Publications.

Burns, N., & Grove, S.K. (1987). *The practice of nursing research: Conduct, critique and utilization.* Philadelphia: W.B. Saunders.

Carter, M.A. (1985). The philosophical dimensions of qualitative nursing science research. In Leininger, M.M. (Ed.) *Qualitative research methods in nursing* (pp. 27–32). Orlando, FL: Harcourt Brace.

Donahue, M.P. (1985). *Nursing: The finest art.* St. Louis: C.V. Mosby.

Ference, H.M. (1979). *The relationship of time experience, creativity traits, differentiation and human field motion: An empirical investigation of Rogers' correlates of synergistic human development.* Unpublished doctoral dissertation. New York University, New York. (University Microfilms 80-10281)

Ference, H.M. (1988). A theory of motion. *Proceedings.* Nursing Science Institutes. Carmel, CA: Nightingale Society.

Hacking, I. (1983). *Representing and intervening: Introductory topics in the philosophy of natural science.* Cambridge: Cambridge University Press.

Hall, J.H., & Zwemer, J.D. (1979). *Prospective medicine: Health hazard appraisal.* Indianapolis: Methodist Hospital.

Krieger, D. (1979). *The therapeutic touch: How to use your hands to help or heal.* Englewood Cliffs, NJ: Prentice-Hall.

Malinski, V. (1986). Nursing practice within the science of unitary human beings. In Malinski, V. (Ed.), *Explorations on Martha Rogers' science of unitary human beings* (pp. 25–34). Norwalk, CT: Appleton-Century-Crofts.

Mish, F.C. (Ed. in chief) (1984). *Webster's ninth new collegiate dictionary.* Springfield, MA: Merriam-Webster.

Parse, R.R. (1987). The lived experience of laughing [Abstract]. *Proceedings.* American Nurses' Association, Council of Nurse Researchers. October, 1987.

Raile, M.M. (1983). *The relationships of creativity, actualization, and empathy in unitary human beings.* Unpublished doctoral dissertation. New York University, New York. (University Microfilms 83-13874)

Rawnsley, M. (1977). *Relationship between the perception of speed of time and the process of dying: An empirical investigation of the holistic theory of nursing proposed by Martha Rogers*. Doctoral dissertation, Boston University.

Robbins, L., & Hall, J.H. (1970). *How to practice prospective medicine*. Indianapolis: Methodist Hospital.

Rogers, M.E. (1980). Nursing: A science of unitary man. In J.P. Riehl & C. Roy (Eds.), *Conceptual models for nursing practice* (2nd ed.) (pp. 329–337). Norwalk, CT: Appleton-Century-Crofts.

Rogers, M.E. (1986). Science of unitary human beings. In Malinski, V. (Ed.), *Explorations on Martha Rogers' science of unitary human beings* (pp. 3–8). Norwalk, CT: Appleton-Century-Crofts.

Rogers, M.E. (1988, October). *Opening speech*. Paper presented at the Nursing Science Institutes, sponsored by the Nightingale Society, Scottsdale, AZ.

Thomas, S.D. (1987). Intentionality in the nurse/client encounter [Abstract]. In E.A.M. Barrett (Symposium Chair), Rogerian science-based practice: Patterning the health of humankind (p. A6). *Proceedings of Scientific Sessions*. 29th Biennial Convention, Sigma Theta Tau, International.

Thomas, S.D. (1988). Light wave frequency, intentionality and nursing care. *Nursing Science Institutes 1988 (Monograph)*. Carmel, CA: Nightingale Society.

Thomas, S.D. (submitted). Development of the human-environment encounter model.

Thomas, S.D., Hathaway, D.K., & Arheart, K. (in press). Development of the general health motivation scale. *Western Journal of Nursing Research*.

Wiley, J.A., & Camacho, T.C. (1980). Life-style and future health: Evidence from the Alameda County study. *Preventive Medicine 9*, 1–21.

Yin, R.K. (1984). *Case study research: Design and methods*. Beverly Hills: Sage Publications.

10

Nursing Care of the Elderly: Futuristic Projections

Martha Raile Alligood

This chapter presents projections for nursing interventions with the elderly developed from a research program spanning several years. It centers around hypotheses derived from Rogers' principles of helicy and integrality (Rogers, 1980, 1986). The studies have focused on the measurement of variables, developed as operationalizations of these principles, in samples of the adult lifespan, 18–92 years of age (Raile, 1983; Alligood, 1986, 1989). The goal of this work was to develop knowledge, through research, to be implemented in science-based nursing practice.

This chapter is organized under three major headings: an introduction and review of the theoretical and research base including a discussion of the movement from the Science of Unitary Human Beings to its practice applications; a presentation of implications of the research findings for the science and for nursing practice; and futuristic projections of two nursing interventions based on the research findings.

INTRODUCTION AND REVIEW OF THEORETICAL AND RESEARCH BASE

Rogers' Science of Unitary Human Beings (1986) provides a conceptual system from which to derive hypotheses of the nature and direction of unitary developmental change. Rogers' postulates helicy, integrality, and resonancy as principles descriptive of the nature and direction of their change. Research designed to test propositions derived from the principles in persons across the lifespan develops knowledge of unitary human development. These principles are stated by Rogers (1986) as follows:

> Principle of Helicy: The continuous, innovative, probabilistic increasing diversity of human and environmental field patterns characterized by nonrepeating rhythmicities.
>
> Principle of Integrality: The continuous mutual human field and environmental field process.
>
> Principle of Resonancy: The continuous change from lower to higher frequency wave patterns in human and environmental fields.

In previous research conducted by this author, relationships were proposed and tested among empirical indicants of helicy (i.e., creativity and actualization) and an empirical indicant of integrality (i.e., empathy). "Empirical linkages were developed to operationalize the human characteristics suggested by Rogers' homeodynamic principles in order to test for the presence of human field pattern manifestations and their proposed relationships. Creativity and actualization were used to operationalize innovativeness and diversity. A measure of empathy was used to assess the principle of integrality" (Alligood, 1989, p. 109) (see Figure 1). The theoretical definitions are stated as they were operationalized. According to Raile (1983), creativity is a manifestation of innovative human field pattern characterized by a tendency toward variety measured by the Similes Preference Inventory (Pearson & Maddi, 1966). Actualization is a manifestation of increasing diversity of human field pattern characterized by evolving human potentialities measured by the Personal Orientation Inventory (Shostrom, 1974). Empathy, again according to Raile, is a human field pattern manifestation emerging from the mutual human-environmental process as feeling attributes measured by the Hogan Scale (Hogan, 1969). The theoretically proposed relationships among the indicants were tested in 236 persons 18–60 years of age resulting in clear support for the three study hypotheses (Raile, 1983; Alligood, 1986, 1989).

Building on the findings of support, a second study was conducted repeating the methods of the original study with this exception: the age of the sample was over 60 years. Using a descriptive design, the study was conducted with a cross-sectional survey of 47 men and women who were 61–92 years of age and residing in four different states. Subjects volunteered at churches and church-affiliated retirement apartments to complete a demographic form and three paper and pencil measures: the Similes Preference Inventory (Pearson & Maddi, 1966), the Personal Orientation Inven-

Figure 1

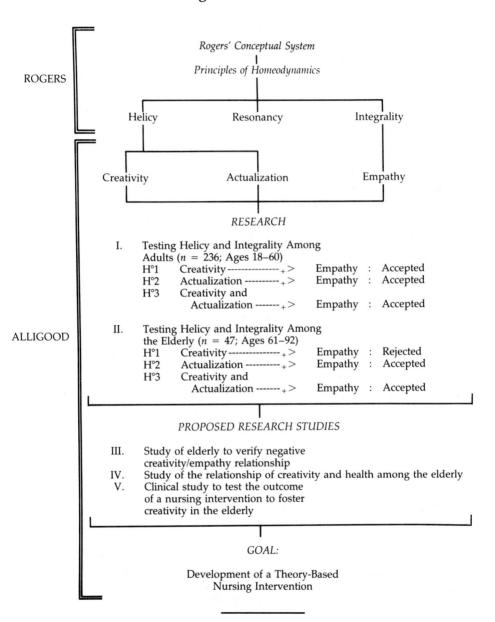

Table 1
Hypotheses, Correlation Coefficients, and Percentage of Covariance
First Study ($n = 236$)

Hypothesis	Correlation Coefficient	Percent of Covariance
1 = Creativity/Empathy	.27*	7
2 = Actualization/Empathy	.39*	15
3 = Creativity + Actualization/Empathy	.46*	21

*p = <.001

tory (Shostrom, 1974), and the Hogan Scale (Hogan, 1969). The three hypotheses predicting positive relationships among creativity, actualization, and empathy were tested to answer the research question: Will the findings of support for the predictive ability of hypotheses derived from helicy and integrality in persons 18–60 years of age hold true in a sample of persons beyond 60 years?

Data were analyzed computing the Pearson product-moment correlation coefficients and multiple correlations for the relationships among creativity, actualization, and empathy. Whereas in the original study the hypotheses were accepted and the findings supported the proposed relationships, in the study of the elderly group the findings differed as illustrated in Table 2.

Hypothesis 1 was rejected since the relationship between creativity and empathy was negative with a correlation coefficient of $r = -.32$ significant at $p = > .01$ level. Hypothesis 2 was accepted with a substantial positive correlation of .68 between actualization and empathy, significant at $P = > .001$ level. Subsequent analyses were conducted to verify the negative relationship between creativity and empathy including: Kendall's Tau, Spearman's Rho, and the substitution of the logarithm of the Similes Preference Inventory (Log SPI) for the Similes Preference Inventory (SPI). These nonparametric analyses verified the pattern of relationship found in the parametric analyses using Pearson's r.

In summary, characteristics were derived from the principles (helicy and integrality) and defined theoretically and operationally. These characteristics became the empirical indicants of the studies (creativity, actualization, and empathy) that tested the relationship among the characteristics as predicted by the theory. The goal of this work was to test a theory of human development and produce knowledge for nursing practice. Figure 1 illustrates the program of research derived from Rogers' conceptual system to test hypotheses postulated in accordance with Rogers' principles of helicy and integrality. Resonancy is assumed in these studies and not tested.

Table 2
Hypotheses, Correlation Coefficients, and Percentage of Covariance
Second Study ($n = 47$)

Hypothesis	Correlation Coefficient	Percent of Covariance
1 = Creativity/Empathy	− .32*	9
2 = Actualization/Empathy	.68**	46
3 = Creativity + Actualization/Empathy	.69**	48

*p = <.01
**p = <.001

The movement from theory to practice is not an easy one. Cross (1981) has noted, "The systematic accumulation of knowledge is essential to progress in any profession . . . however, theory and practice must be constantly interactive. Theory without practice is empty and practice without theory is blind" (p. 110) suggesting the interdependence between theory and practice.

Development of theory-based practice is discussed by several authors including Chinn and Jacobs (1987), Aggleton and Chalmers (1987), Duldt and Griffin (1985), and Barrett (1988). Chinn and Jacobs describe the process of identifying empirical indicators for abstract concepts. Their description of the process approximates my own experience when they suggest it is both an inductive and deductive process with the aim of testing existing conceptualizations and the pursuit of hunches about events and relationships.

The identification of empirical indicators for the conceptualizations set forth by Rogers (1986) in the principles of helicy and integrality was a vital step in this movement from abstract theory to testing of the proposed relationships. Chinn and Jacobs (1987) describe the validation of theory in practice as an important stage that involves validation of theoretical propositions. In this instance Rogers' (1986) homeodynamic principles are identified as the genesis of testable propositions. Whereas principles have been identified as the heart of a theory, they are in reality propositions that are tentative until demonstrated to be true (Duldt & Griffin, 1985).

Aggleton and Chalmers (1987) included Rogers as a developmental model in their general discussion of nursing models. They reasoned that a developmental model would prescribe the need for a nursing intervention in the case of ill health or disease that threatens the developmental process. Following their reasoning, the role of the nurse would be to maintain or restore patterns of normal development or maturation. Their logic is im-

portant to the thesis of this chapter, since findings from research designed
to test principles of human development among the elderly might also have
the capacity to identify a developmental need in the elderly for nursing
intervention (Raile, 1983; Alligood, 1986, 1989).

Barrett (1988) discusses science-based practice using Rogers' system.
She has proposed appraisal of the manifest behavior pattern and mutual
patterning of behavior as two major phases of a Rogerian nursing methodology developed through her practice. She clearly illustrates the use of
the conceptual system in her practice through case presentations. Barrett
describes science-based practice as the use of substantive knowledge developed through research and logical analysis.

Finally, there are those who incorporate nursing diagnosis in their discussion of the movement from theory to practice (Thompson, McFarland,
Hirsh, Tucker, & Bowers, 1986; Gordon, 1987; Guzzetta, Bunton,
Prinkey, Sherer, & Seifert, 1988). Thompson et al. suggest that practice
builds on observable manifestations, application of theory, nursing interventions, and evaluation of outcomes in relation to specific phenomenon.
Therefore, they specify the theory base and clinical application for specific
nursing diagnoses. Although they include a functional pattern of individual-environmental interaction and include two diagnoses: (1) "potential for
injury" (p. 198) and (2) "impaired home maintenance management" (p.
199), reference is not made to nursing science as a basis for that pattern but
to theoretical models from other disciplines. It is interesting to note, however, that although the theoretical basis for these diagnoses is not nursing
science, the two diagnoses included for the pattern of individual-environmental interaction have a higher incidence of application among the elderly. Likewise, when this author tested Rogers' (1986) theory, based on
person-environment process, it was among the elderly that findings of support for the principle of unitary human development were mixed, a finding
which could suggest a person-environment pattern disturbance.

Gordon (1987) discusses the development of theory-based practice, including nursing diagnosis, and describes Rogers (1970) as proposing a "life
process model." Gordon identifies unitary human beings as Rogers' client
focus and the pattern of client-environment interaction as her diagnostic
focus. The goal of nursing is to help clients pattern toward healthful behàv-
iors to realize their "creative-formative potentialities" (p. 73). Guzzetta et
al. (1988) also discuss the movement from theory to practice. They advocate the use of nursing models as a practice guide for structure and terminology, assessment parameters, data organization, nursing diagnoses,
patient outcomes, plans, interventions, and evaluation. The conceptual
model is presented as a precursor to theory that develops from extensive

testing and use in clinical practice. Their development of the "Unitary Person Assessment Tool," based on the NANDA Nursing Diagnosis Taxonomy 1, is noted here for its application to practice (p. 14).

Rogers' Science of Unitary Human Beings has been viewed as a developmental or life process model for nursing. The use of logical reasoning and research findings has facilitated the movement toward science-based practice (Barrett, 1988) aimed at assisting unitary human beings throughout the life process. The work of Thompson et al. (1986) and the linkage to the person-environment pattern facilitates movement into the decision-making process of nursing diagnosis. Gordon (1987) demonstrates forward thinking in the identification of a client focus, a diagnostic focus, and proposed outcomes when using Rogers' (1970, 1980, 1986) model for practice. Guzzetta et al. (1988) have worked toward unitary person assessment and nursing diagnoses based on the work of NANDA. It should be noted that they do not view person or environment in the same manner as the four-dimensional world view of the Science of Unitary Human Beings. However, the ideas of these researchers have contributed to the description of the movement from theory to its practice applications.

IMPLICATIONS FOR THEORY AND PRACTICE

With this background, I will consider the findings from the second research study I conducted from two perspectives: first, the perspective of implications for theory including methodology; second, the perspective of implications for nursing care of the elderly or application.

Theoretically, it is necessary to consider the possibility that the finding of a negative creativity/empathy relationship is a manifestation of unitary human development not reflected in the current characteristics, principles, or research measures. This perspective then raises several questions. First, are the homeodynamic principles operational across the lifespan of human development as presently stated? Since the manifestation of increased diversity (actualization) related substantially (Garrett, 1958) to empathy suggesting greater diversity in the elderly group, one would also expect the creativity/empathy relationship to reflect increased innovativeness rather than relating negatively.

Second, are field patterns increasingly diverse and innovative as Rogers has postulated? The findings of the first study supported that premise in the 18–60-year-old sample. However, among the elderly, in the second study, the findings were mixed. Increased diversity was present but increased innovativeness was not. This finding must be explored in future studies but two possible answers will be addressed here. The first concerns a consideration of methodology. Is it that the Personal Orientation Inventory (POI) had the capacity to capture manifestations of increased diversity but the Similes Preference Inventory (SPI) did not have the capacity to measure increased innovation of unitary human development? As I have mentioned elsewhere (Alligood, 1986), tools from other disciplines can be useful to us in these beginning studies. As I stated, "The uniqueness of the nursing perspective in our discipline is not only the way in which the variable is measured, but also the selection of the variables and their proposed relationships" (p. 159). Also, the use of psychometric instruments may provide a knowledge base for future tool development in the Science of Unitary Human Beings. Presumably these measures would not be as precise as measures developed in the Science of Unitary Human Beings but would capture the essence of the variable. In this phase it is not only considerations of how to measure that are important to the methodology but also what to measure. Given the limitations of this phase of development of the science, possible methodology problems are acknowledged. The answer to the dilemma of this perspective remains hidden in future studies and in the development of tools consistent with the science.

Perhaps a more plausible theoretical implication of this finding is that the human characteristics, as understood through the principles, are unitary manifestations emerging from the mutual human-environment process and can, therefore, be considered indices of health and the need for nursing intervention. If so, then the findings from this research suggest the need for a nursing intervention aimed at facilitating the expression of the innovative creativity of human development. This leads to the second perspective for consideration, the implications for nursing care of the elderly. If the principles are operational across the lifespan the positive actualization/empathy relationship suggests greater diversity in the elderly and the negative creativity/empathy relationship may suggest pattern change manifest as the need for creative expression among the elderly.

The fact that this phenomenon of unitary human development has been demonstrated in a segment of our society for whom present care practices involve major physical environmental changes should come as no surprise. Although physical changes are the most obvious, there are other unitary manifestations of those changes. The fact that contemporary society refers to retirement as "putting one out to pasture" is noteworthy here. The impact of major life changes such as retirement, moving from one's home to a retirement home, or moving from a larger to a much smaller place is significant. Equally important is the probable lack of meaning that daily activities, and the feelings associated with them, have for elderly human beings. Considering these factors, it is not surprising that the negative finding fell between creativity as innovativeness and empathy as the feeling attributes of the person-environment process. Furthermore, given the linkage to Rogers' Principles of Unitary Human Development, it seems logical that this negative creativity/empathy relationship would impact development or health (Reed, 1983).

Since the Rogerian conceptual system is a developmental or life process model, the knowledge derived from research of the system is knowledge about unitary human development. Furthermore, developmental models suggest the need for nursing intervention when phenomena threaten the developmental process. Here the nurse would attempt to restore normal patterns of development and maturation. Gordon (1987) views Rogers' system as a life process model and suggests nursing seeks to help the client maintain a pattern of living that coordinates with the emerging pattern. Patterns that do not permit movement toward well being or health require nursing attention. Gordon further suggests the goal of the nursing intervention to be promotion of the client's progress toward maximum health potential by: (1) strengthening mutual interaction, (2) recognizing potentialities of the client and the environment, and (3) helping the client use conscious personal choice. Similarly, Barrett (1988) has said that power is essential in the health patterning process and has linked power as knowing participation to making choices.

The goals for nursing identified by Gordon (1987) and the two diagnoses identified by Thompson et al. (1986) as well as the guidelines for Unitary Person Assessment set forth by Guzzetta et al. (1988) are useful in projecting possible interventions and outcome measures for clinical studies. For example, it may be possible in the future to identify persons at risk in the area of potential for injury or impaired home maintenance management. Or, interventions may be designed to empower the elderly by encouraging conscious personal choice.

Other studies indicated from a review of the implications of this research include repeating the study of the elderly to see if the relationship is replicated, and, if so, to identify other demographic characteristics of persons manifesting a negative creativity/empathy relationship. Unitary nursing interventions could be identified to enhance creativity while also measuring the impact of the intervention on health and development. How might creativity be enhanced in persons in accordance with the Rogerian Science of Unitary Human Beings?

PROJECTED FUTURISTIC NURSING INTERVENTIONS

I will discuss, however, two proposed interventions as future nursing modalities: guided reminiscence and humor. Commonly noted as universal phenomena, this author is proposing them as unitary manifestations of the field pattern of the mutual process of persons and environment. Guided reminiscence has the capacity to facilitate remembrance of meaningful times. Earlier periods of higher creativity can become the relative present pattern for the elderly by calling to remembrance meaningful life experiences, if creativity needs are met through being productive and feeling needed. Guided reminiscence, therefore, is suggested as an independent nursing intervention to enhance creativity.

Bulechek and McClosky (1985) include the reminiscence therapy. developed by Hamilton (1985) as an independent nursing intervention with three components: memory, experiencing, and social interaction. Hamilton suggests that memory, with its function of organizing past experiences, provides a sense of continuity from past to present and, thus, contributes to a higher level of wellness. Other disciplines have studied reminiscence but focused on the nature of reminiscence (Butler, 1963). In contrast, nurses have explored reminiscence as a nursing intervention with a beneficial outcome for the client derived from the activity itself. For example, Chennelly (1979) studied aged persons who recently moved to a senior apartment complex. She found clients who received reminiscence therapy exhibiting a significantly higher rate of satisfaction with their new environment than the clients who did not reminisce. Likewise, Ryden (1981) wrote in support of reminiscence as a nursing intervention. Based on Rogers' concept of four-dimensionality, I am proposing the use of reminiscence to facilitate memory of past accomplishments and times of productivity as a way to enhance creativity in a person's relative present. In the Science of Unitary Human Beings, the time of the creative accomplishment is irrelevant. The nurse facilitates the memory of experiences and the sharing of those memories.

Humor is another unitary behavioral manifestation of the person-environment process. As an individual experience in which persons can relate what is being heard to their own past, humor also emerges from the mutual, interactive process between person and environment. In addition, the linkage between humor and creativity is well established (The Positive Power of Humor & Creativity, 1987). In fact, Rogers has suggested laughter as a nursing intervention (Fawcett, 1989) and Snyder (1985) discusses humor as an independent nursing intervention. Snyder (1985) identifies 10 theories of humor from other disciplines, most of which focus on explaining humor.

Humor began to be linked to health when Normal Cousins (1979) wrote of the positive health benefits of humor that he learned from his own illness. However, despite this link, no nursing studies of humor were located. Therefore, humor is proposed as a nursing intervention to be tested in the elderly with an outcome measure of increased creativity. With the numbers of elderly and the life expectancy in the United States increasing, there is a critical need for better understanding human development of the elderly (Reed, 1983). The Rogerian framework is useful to study the relationship of environmental changes to health and well being. Since present care of the elderly often means subjecting them to major environmental changes, the elderly are an appropriate focus for these studies.

Rogers (1986) has postulated aging to be a developmental process. I am suggesting that the finding of a negative relationship between empathy and creativity in this age group has developmental implications for nursing care. In studies conducted by this author, this manifestation was seen among this age group although not among others (see Table 2). In the elderly, the need for a nursing intervention that will foster creativity is probably more related to their role in society than to their age, however.

CONCLUSION

In conclusion, I have reviewed a research study designed to test propositions derived from the principles of helicy and integrality in persons 18–60 years of age. A second study designed to test the same propositions in persons over 60 was presented with a finding of a negative relationship between creativity and empathy. The implications of applying theory to practice have been discussed. The findings have been explored from the perspective of the theory and from the perspective of nursing care of the elderly. Two independent nursing interventions have been proposed for clinical testing with the elderly and an outcome of increasing creativity. This program of research would suggest the elderly need increased creative expression to facilitate the mutual person-environment process of unitary human development (Reed, 1983). Based on the finding of a negative creativity/empathy relationship among the elderly, nursing interventions to facilitate creative expression have been identified. Guided reminiscence recalls past creativity to the relative present based on Rogers' concept of four-dimensionality. Humor also fosters creativity through memory and experience of thought and feeling. Guided reminiscence and humor, therefore, are proposed as independent nursing interventions aimed at unitary human development in the elderly. I have suggested that Rogers' principles of unitary human development are explanatory indices of human developmental change and health.

REFERENCES

Aggleton, P., & Chalmers, H. (1987). Models of nursing, nursing practice and nursing education. *Journal of Advanced Nursing, 12,* 573–581.

Alligood, M.R. (1986). The relationship of creativity, actualization, and empathy in unitary human development. In V. Malinski (Ed.), *Explorations in the science of unitary human beings* (pp. 145–160). Norwalk, CT: Appleton-Century-Crofts.

Alligood, M.R. (1989). Rogers' theory and nursing administration: A perspective on health and environment. In B. Henry, M. DiVincenti, C. Arndt, & A. Marriner (Eds.), *Dimensions of nursing administration: Theory, research, education, and practice.* Boston: Blackwell Scientific Publications.

Barrett, E.M. (1988). Using Rogers' science of unitary human beings in nursing practice. *Nursing Science Quarterly, 1,* 50–51.

Bronkema Hamilton, D. (1985). Reminiscence therapy. In G.M. Bulechek & J.C. McClosky (Eds.), *Nursing interventions: Treatments for nursing diagnoses* (pp. 139–151). Philadelphia: W.B. Saunders.

Bulechek, G.M., & McClosky, J.C. (1985). *Nursing interventions: Treatments for nursing diagnoses.* Philadelphia: W.B. Saunders.

Butler, R.N. (1963). The life review: An interpretation of reminiscence in the aged. *Psychiatry, 26,* 65–76.

Chennelly, S. (1979). *Reminiscing: A coping skill for the elderly.* Unpublished master's thesis, University of Rochester, Rochester, NY.

Chinn, P., & Jacobs, M. (1987). *Theory and nursing* (2nd ed.). St. Louis: C.V. Mosby.

Cousins, N. (1979). *Anatomy of an illness as perceived by the patient: Reflections on healing and regeneration.* New York: Norton.

Cross, K.P. (1981). *Adults as learners.* Washington, DC: Jossey-Bass.

Duldt, B.W., & Giffin, K. (1985). *Theoretical perspectives for nursing.* Boston: Little, Brown and Company.

Fawcett, J. (1989). *Analysis and evaluation of conceptual models of nursing* (2nd ed.). Philadelphia: F.A. Davis.

Garrett, H. (1958). *Statistics in psychology and education.* New York: David McKay Company, Inc.

Gordon, M. (1987). *Nursing diagnosis: Process and application* (2nd ed.). New York: McGraw-Hill.

Guzzetta, C., Bunton, S., Prinkey, L., Sherer, & Seifert, P. (1988). Unitary person assessment tool: Easing problems with nursing diagnoses. *Focus on Critical Care, 15*(2), 12–24.

Hogan, R. (1969). Development of an empathy scale. *Journal of Consulting and Clinical Psychology, 33,* 307–316.

Pearson, P.H., & Maddi, S.R. (1966). The similes preference inventory: Development of a structured measure of the tendency toward variety. *Journal of Consulting Psychology, 30,* 301–308.

Raile, M. (1983). The relationship of creativity, actualization, and empathy in unitary human development: A descriptive study of M. Rogers principle of helicy (Doctoral dissertation, New York University). *Dissertation Abstracts International, 44,* 449B. (University Microfilms No. 83-13, 874)

Reed, P. (1983). Implications of the life-span developmental framework for well-being in adulthood and aging. *Advances in Nursing Science, 6,* 18–25.

Rogers, M.E. (1980). Nursing: A science of unitary man. In J. Riehl, & C. Roy (Eds.), *Conceptual models for nursing practice* (pp. 329–337). New York: Appleton-Century-Crofts.

Rogers, M.E. (1970). *An introduction to the theoretical basis of nursing.* Philadelphia: F.A. Davis.

Rogers, M.E. (1986). Science of unitary human beings. In V. Malinski (Ed.), *Explorations in the Science of Unitary Human Beings* (pp. 3–8). New York: Appleton-Century-Crofts.

Ryden, M.B. (1981). Nursing intervention in support of reminiscence. *Journal of Gerontological Nursing, 7,* 461–463.

Shostrom, E.L. (1974). An inventory for the measurement of self-actualization. *Educational and Psychological Measurement, 24,* 207.

Snyder, M. (1985). *Independent nursing interventions.* New York: John Wiley & Sons.

The positive power of humor and creativity (1987). *Second Annual National Conference For: Human Resource Managers, Managers, Nurses, Therapists, Counselors, Social Workers, Teachers, Parents, Physicians, Dentists & Clergy.* Albany, NY: Russell/Sage.

Thompson, J.M., McFarland, G.K., Hirsch, J.E., Tucker, S.M., & Bowers, A.C. (1986). *Clinical nursing.* St. Louis: C.V. Mosby.

11

Chronological Age as an Anomalie of Evolution

W. Richard Cowling, III

The dependence on chronological age as a referent for determining the developmental progress of human beings is widespread among the clinical disciplines. This dependence and emphasis on age as a developmental referent influences theoretical as well as practice perspectives. Of specific concern is the use of the age referent as a major theme in the development of nursing science and practice. However, it is important that the reader understand the distinction between nursing science and practice as knowledge because nursing practice encompasses the creative use of nursing science but extends beyond it. Consequently, age as a developmental referent influences the generation of the science used in practice and influences the actions associated with practice that go beyond the science. In this regard, Rogers (1970, 1980) has proposed a conceptual perspective of human evolution that emphasizes alternative indices of development to chronological age. Pattern is postulated as the primary indicator of human evolution as manifest in a variety of experiential, perceptual, and behavioral cues.

CHRONOLOGICAL AGE

Because most gerontological research is primarily based on testing the relationship of chronological age to a number of variables associated with human behavior and perception, a false view of human development has arisen. The context of this research is clearly chronological age-relatedness. Furthermore, the research is based on what Allport (1960) has characterized as actuarial prediction (i.e., prediction based on group norms), rather than clinical prediction, (i.e., which is prediction based on individual experience). This is a particularly important distinction for nursing knowledge; for nursing knowledge requires judgments to act in behalf of human patterning in individual situations or contexts.

A preponderance of research has linked age to variables of human perception and behavioral change (Levison, 1981; Ludwig, 1982; Moore, Richards, & Hood, 1984; Nebes, Madden, & Berg, 1983; Pearce & Denney, 1984; Raskin, Maital, & Bornstein, 1983). These include temporal perception, visual perception, spatial perception, learning styles, cognitive styles and processes, and perceptual-motor capabilities. It is difficult to summarize this research in any meaningful way due to the criticisms launched against it because of its failure to take into consideration such factors as the role of experience, ecological validity of tasks, and cohort effects (Akiyama, Akiyama, & Goodrich, 1985). But, in general terms, the literature suggests a steady decline or stabilization in these areas associated with advancing age. However, many suggest that the trends for groups do not hold for individuals. As a result, in order to make meaningful assumptions about its relevance to nursing practice, one must examine the context of this research.

PATTERN PERSPECTIVE

The Science of Unitary Human Beings provides an alternative theoretical vantage point from which to view human evolution: as emerging field patterning that is a manifestation of human-environmental field process. Emerging patterning proceeds four-dimensionally rather than linearly. Thus, chronological age as a marker of human development is inconsistent with the tenets of unitary nursing science. Furthermore, it becomes relatively clear that when using the conceptual and theoretical perspectives of this science that practice stems more readily from pattern-related rather than age-related development. In overly simplistic terms, practice decisions are less age-appropriate and more pattern-appropriate. However, a caveat here is that the elderly as a group may have pattern age-specific trends. As in any science, then, it is important to distinguish generalizing from knowledge of a group to other groups and inferring that such knowledge is relevant to an individual.

What is the nature of a nursing science of human evolution that is pattern-based rather than chronological age-based? What is the knowledge now emerging that is generated from testing theories from this science? What are the practice implications of scientific knowledge and practice knowledge consistent with the Science of Unitary Human Beings?

The aim of nursing science from a unitary perspective would be to capture the features of emerging patterning and to seek to understand the ways in which knowledge of these features can facilitate a pattern emergence conducive to the individual's well being. Conceptually, Rogers (1986, 1987, 1988) has argued that the best indicators of human development are time perception, spatial perception, imagination, and human field motion. Change is postulated in the direction of timelessness, spacelessness, imaginativeness, transcendence, and motionlessness (Malinski, 1986). Several studies have been developed to test the relationships among these indices of human patterning (Alligood, 1986; Cowling, 1986; Ference, 1986; Rawnsley, 1986). The results, generally speaking, suggest diversity in co-varying trends among individuals. The major question that pervades this research is what are the best ways (i.e., measurement techniques) to capture indices of unitary patterning. No doubt, the development of the science is dependent on addressing this question more completely and thoroughly. It is evident that indices of patterning are experiential in nature. In other words, unitary patterning is experienced by the individual and the individual can have awareness of his or her patterning. The observation of another individual's patterning may also be possible, but more difficult to attain with particular clarity. As a result, the self-reported perception and other expressions of experience to a clinician in practice, or similarly to an investigator in a research situation, provides a critical link to an individual's unitary pattern.

However, it seems that the phenomena of concern to all people who care for the elderly are similar. For instance, several disciplines share a concern about phenomena associated with successful aging, in particular the maintenance of health as well as increasing wellness potentials. There is also shared concern about environmental phenomena that may influence conditions such as depression, activity and energy decline, incontinence, and confusion. However, difference can exist in the conceptualizations provided by varying theoretical perspectives that guide these disciplines. In other words, those disciplines interested in the well being of the elderly may have interest in the same territory but utilize different maps.

From the perspective of unitary nursing science and practice, the phenomena of concern includes experience, perception, and expressions. Pattern-based practice deals with such phenomena as the focal point of assessment and intervention rather than chronological age as the major referent for clinical decision making.

PRACTICE EXAMPLES

Several examples of pattern-based practice will make this concept clearer. Confusion, depression, incontinence, and sleeplessness are all common clinical problems associated with gerontological nursing practice.

A 75-year-old client diagnosed as having Alzheimer's disease wanders around the unit of a nursing home often interacting with staff and clients as if she were still managing a dress shop she owned 20 years ago. She has difficulty focusing on three-dimensional referents in her environment (i.e., what time it is, her spatial location, and animate and inanimate objects in her physical environment). Consequently, it is often difficult to get her focused on such activities as eating, bathing, and dressing which are essential to her physical comfort. Also, she expresses some painful emotions related to sadness and anxiousness.

The important distinctions between practice based on chronological age and pattern follow. From a chronological age perspective, three-dimensionality is an important construct. For instance, time is linear, the client is 75 years old and she is out of touch with reality as she focuses on a period in her life when she was 55 years old. Her major problem is in relating to three-dimensional referents in her physical environment that influence her general comfort and well being. Her sadness and anxiousness are problematic and require treatment aimed at alleviation, such as medication, distraction, or social participation. One way to help her be more comfortable would be to use reality orientation to help her adapt to her physical environment.

From a pattern perspective, however, the client's experience goes beyond the three-dimensional. She is experiencing a chronologically earlier time period—her relative present. Her perception varies but appears to incorporate feelings of discomfort now and then. For instance, she grows disturbed when people enter and exit the room. She speaks to them about purchasing hats or dresses. Her body movements and verbalizations are examples of pattern expressions. The aim of the nursing assessment would be to capture the features of the pattern through focusing on the parameters of experience, perception, and expression. Considering the pattern manifestations (experience, perception, expressions) as a whole, a dominant feature of this person's emergent pattern is fearfulness.

Focus would center on this pattern characteristic and the individual's perceptions. Fearfulness is evident from the expressions of voice, movement away from individuals, cowering posture, hostility at attempts to distract from the perception, a wandering search for safety, and general withdrawal to more isolated areas of the room. The experiential, perceptual, and expressive features are not dependent on three-dimensional referents. These features transcend this particular time and space. By attending to her fearfulness, rather than to orientation, a different patterning may be possible. For instance, if fear is acknowledged, its expression allowed, and attention is given to transforming such fearfulness, patterning more conducive to the well being of the client may be facilitated.

Depression is another common example of a clinical problem associated with age. From a chronological perspective, age-related losses subject the individual to depression. Intervention would then focus on adaptation to age-related changes. From a pattern perspective, focus would center on the experience of growing older, the perception of growing old, and the expressions of growing old for that individual. These features of the person's pattern would provide a picture of the major themes and characteristics that exist. Working with these through creative imagery may facilitate patterning that is more conducive to well being.

Incontinence is another of a clinical phenomenon that consumes much time in nursing practice. From an age-related perspective, incontinence is viewed in the context of physiological changes associated with aging. From a pattern perspective, incontinence has meaning that goes beyond the physical event. Both perspectives have relevance for caring for the client suffering from incontinence, however. Certainly the physical dimensions of incontinence are problematic and warrant attention. The pattern perspective would view the experience, perception, and expression surrounding the incontinence as relevant as well.

Sleep alterations such as insomnia that result in restlessness and discomfort comprise another commonly reported problem with the elderly. From a three-dimensional perspective, sleep is viewed as a physiological process with psychological consequences. For instance, one gerontological text (Matteson & McConnell, 1988) describes internal factors (degenerative central nervous system changes, sensory impairments, illness, and ineffective individual coping) and external factors (the physical environment and drugs). From a pattern perspective, nursing care might focus on assisting the client to identify what he or she experiences at the time of sleeplessness, what are his or her perceptions of the experience, and in what forms are these expressed. The nurse might even request an elaboration of the experience in the form of a journal or drawings that reflect the experiential elements of this individual's sleeplessness. Attention in nursing care could be given to an expanded awareness of the experience of sleeplessness and suggesting activities that would be more consistent with comfort and well being. Appropriate nursing interventions might include helping the person accept diverse sleep behaviors, using the sleeplessness time to practice guided imagery that accomplishes greater relaxation and well being, and creating new activities that promote sleep. Much of this can be accomplished through helping the client become more aware of his or her unique pattern.

CONCLUSION

Chronological aging has been a major referent of gerontological nursing assessment and practice. The use of varying theoretical perspectives derived from other disciplines have guided the development of gerontological nursing practice. These continue to have value in organizing and elaborating gerontological nursing practice. However, a pattern perspective based on the Science of Unitary Human Beings offers an alternative approach. Further research and clinical trials using the pattern-based practice approach are warranted. Some examples of clinical practice situations have been reviewed with the aim of comparing the pattern perspective with three-dimensional perspectives. Additional specification of clinical phenomena and practice situations described theoretically from varying perspectives can have value in identifying research questions and indicating potential practice strategies.

REFERENCES

Akiyama, M.M., Akiyama, H., & Goodrich, C.G. (1985). Spatial development across the life span. *International Journal of Aging and Human Development, 21*(3), 175–185.

Alligood, M.R. (1986). The relationship of creativity, actualization, and empathy in unitary human development. In V. Malinski (Ed.), *Explorations on Martha Rogers' science of unitary human beings* (pp. 145–154). Norwalk, CT: Appleton-Century-Crofts.

Allport, G. (1960). The general and unique in psychological science. *Journal of Personality, 30*, 405–422.

Cowling, W.R., III. (1986). The relationship of mystical experience, differentiation, and creativity in college students. In V. Malinski (Ed.), *Explorations on Martha Rogers' science of unitary human beings* (pp. 131–141). Norwalk, CT: Appleton-Century-Crofts.

Ference, H.M. (1986). The relationship of time experience, creativity traits, differentiation, and human field motion. In V. Malinski (Ed.), *Explorations on Martha Rogers' science of unitary human beings* (pp. 95–105). Norwalk, CT: Appleton-Century-Crofts.

Levison, W.H. (1981). A methodology for quantifying the effects of aging on perceptual-motor capability. *Human Factors, 23*(1), 87–96.

Ludwig, T.E. (1982). Age differences in mental synthesis. *Journal of Gerontology, 37*(2), 182–189.

Malinski, V. (1986). Further ideas from Martha Rogers. In V. Malinski (Ed.), *Explorations on Martha Rogers' science of unitary human beings* (pp. 9–14). Norwalk, CT: Appleton-Century-Crofts.

Matteson, M.A., & McConnell, E.S. (1988). *Gerontological nursing: Concepts and practice.* Philadelphia: W.B. Saunders.

Moore, T.E., Richards, B., & Hood, J. (1984). Aging and the coding of spatial information. *Journal of Gerontology, 39*(2), 210–212.

Nebes, R.D., Madden, D.J., & Berg, W.D. (1983). The effect of age on hemispheric asymmetry in visual and auditory identification. *Experimental Aging Research, 9*(2), 87–91

Pearce, K.A., & Denney, N.W. (1984). A lifespan study of classification preference. *Journal of Gerontology, 39*(4), 458–464.

Raskin, L.A., Maital, S., & Bornstein, M.H. (1983). Perceptual categorization of color: A life-span study. *Psychological Research, 45*, 135–145.

Rawnsley, M.M. (1986). The relationship between the perception of the speed of time and the process of dying. In V. Malinski (Ed.), *Explorations on Martha Rogers' science of unitary human beings* (pp. 79–89). Norwalk, CT: Appleton-Century-Crofts.

Rogers, M.E. (1986). Science of unitary human beings. In V. Malinski (Ed.), *Explorations on Martha Rogers' science of unitary human beings* (pp. 4–23). Norwalk, CT: Appleton-Century-Crofts.

Rogers, M.E. (1987). Rogers' science of unitary human beings. In R.R. Parse (Ed.), *Nursing science: Major paradigms, theories, and critiques* (pp. 139–146). Philadelphia: W.B. Saunders.

Rogers, M.E. (1988). Nursing science and art: A prospective. *Nursing Science Quarterly, 1*, 99–102.

12

Visionary Opportunities for Knowledge Development in Nursing Administration

Cynthia Caroselli-Dervan

At one time, people who were in need of health care epitomized the concept of submission with virtually no choices. As a matter of course, they accepted the negation of their identities as they were issued depersonalized wristbands. They accepted diagnostic labels, relinquished the power of decision making, and soon found that all information relative to their situations was "classified." No questions were elicited, no guarantees were offered, and no challenges to authority were recognized.

Fortunately, times have changed. At no other point in the history of civilization has the average individual been confronted with so many options related to lifestyle, as well as to health care. The same may be said of the individual nurse—roles have expanded and multiplied. Alternative work hours and patterns have evolved, and varied approaches to education are available. The health care environment has become highly technical, giving rise to new client populations. Yet this growing diversity is not without its risk or its price. Ethical dilemmas regularly confront the nurse and beckon new issues to be addressed.

The environment has experienced a technological, punctuational evolution. The inflationary cost of health care and diagnosis-related reimbursement constitute a familiar reality. Increased consumer expectations have compelled caregivers to justify fees, to certify quality, and to share the locus of decision making.

Simultaneously, as Sheridan (1983) has stated, "increased types and numbers of providers create a new competitive environment" (p. 36). This allows the client the opportunity to choose not only on the basis of the provider's personal style, but also with concern for discipline, preparation, and fee. Investor-owned health care facilities, with a philosophy and intent similar to that found in other service industries, are commonplace. The image of the hospital and hospital industry as "big business" has gained acceptance.

Consequently, as more health care exists today, there is more health care to manage. Nursing administrators represent the largest constituency providing health care and are in a unique position to change the face of health care delivery. However, old approaches to planning and problem solving offer little assistance in creating new approaches for dealing with this new enterprise.

Innovative visionary opportunities describe the mission of the nurse manager in light of Rogers' conceptual system, the Science of Unitary Human Beings (Rogers, 1986). While in this paper I offer few strategies, I do suggest that the reader consider the options that become possible when nursing management is examined from the Rogerian perspective. Undoubtedly, more questions will be raised than answered.

PARADIGM SHIFTS

Perhaps the one constant of the time in which we live is its evolutionary nature. Philosophies and beliefs once perceived as infallible are now viewed in a critical light, laying the basis for substantial paradigm shifts. These paradigm shifts have taken various forms and, in many instances, have wide-ranging implications.

For example, there is the move from a world view formed by Cartesian philosophy to world view framed by quantum physics. The Cartesian view is reductionistic, mechanistic, and analytic. "It consists in breaking up thoughts and problems into pieces and in arranging these in their logical order" (Capra, 1982, p. 59). According to Cartesian philosophy, the person is viewed as the summation of parts, and, in an absolute sense, there is differentiation between mind and body. Nothing in the universe is left to chance or innovation. Events are perceived to plod along with unending sameness. In this system, the whole may be discerned by study of the parts.

This Cartesian view of reality persisted with far-reaching effects until the first three decades of this century when quantum theory was formulated (Capra, 1982). With the sweep of revolutionary change, reductionism was replaced by a sense of unified wholeness in which "nature does not show us any isolated basic building blocks, but rather appears as a complicated web of relations between the parts of a unified whole" (p. 81). In this paradigm, the individual cannot be understood by analyzing component parts. The distinction between mind and body fall by the wayside and a sense of all-pervasive interconnectedness emerges.

Similiar shifts are seen in other paradigms. Health care delivery has moved from a prevailing view characterized by benevolent spending, charitable distribution of resources, and a nonprofit perspective to a view determined by the exigencies of quality assurance, cost containment, legalism, and a motivation for profit. Another relevant example is found in nursing, which has moved from a procedural, pre-scientific, and subservient occupation to a unique, scholarly, research-based profession.

Conceptualizations of management and administration have undergone similiar changes. The traditional, classical view of the nature of management was derived from the social philosophy of Max Weber (1954). He saw the work life of the employee as separate and irrelevant to the domestic life and vice versa. In fact, the employee was seen as a functional tool for task completion, and not as an individual. The most desirable stance that a manager could take was to approach each worker in an identical and uniform fashion. Reminiscent of the Cartesian view of human beings as machines, Weber's work also may have been the progenitor of the assembly-line mind set.

Recently, however, and as a result of the paradigm shift previously mentioned, the prevailing mode of managerial thinking is more concerned with individual wholeness. As more attention is focused on the personhood of the worker, managers are more concerned with the worker's life *in toto*. The popularity of other models such as Theory Z evolved, and center around the notion of work as an integral component of the worker's life (Ouchi, 1981).

Nursing and nursing administration, indivisible from these paradigm shifts, have attempted to address similar concerns. Much attention has been focused on the unique nature of nursing. In order to manage situations of increasing complexity, nursing administrators need intellectually based, scientifically developed knowledge. Whereas the administrative role has passed from attendance taking to operational accountability, so too have the conceptual underpinnings of administrative nursing practice moved from behavioral proverbs to theoretically derived concepts.

USING ROGERS' SYSTEM

When viewed within Rogers' (1986) Science of Unitary Human Beings, such theory development can continue in an exciting and uniquely integral way. This can then be used to describe and define nursing in the bureaucratic organization of the hospital.

Rogers (1986) views human beings as energy fields. In fact, the field is what underwrites the unity of human beings. As such, a field is more than a summation of parts. In keeping with this conceptual system, an institution's nursing service is viewed as an energy field in mutual process with its environment.

As the largest constituency in virtually all health care institutions, nursing service must be seen as more than employees and staffing schedules, more than a body count of functionaries required to staff a shift. All shifts and all nurses should be viewed as interdependent. In keeping with Rogers' (1986) notion of irreducibility, the behavior and characteristics of the nursing service cannot be predicted from knowledge of the behavior and characteristics of one nurse, one unit, or one shift. Thus, since Rogers (1986) sees energy fields as infinite, the idea of a universe of open systems invalidates causality. The "quick fix" management intervention, therefore, so appealing to Western ways of knowing, is viewed as mechanistic and naive. Conversely, participatory management is viewed as an indicant of open systems and congruent with Rogers' (1986) conceptual system.

Pattern identifies energy fields and is the distinguishing characteristic of a field that changes continuously and innovatively (Rogers, 1986). In managerial parlance, pattern has been referred to as the corporate climate and, most recently, this continuous innovation has been equated with excellence (Peters & Waterman, 1982). It is this distinguishing characteristic, or pattern, that unfailingly presents itself to the observer and that often acts as a powerful incentive or deterrent to the recruitment and retention of staff. Leader expectations are related in some way to actual worker performance, and are readily apparent to the observer. New roles and new structures are coordinate with an innovative pattern of evolving managerial thought.

Four-dimensionality, a concept within Rogers' (1986) system, describes a nonlinear domain without spatial or temporal attributes and may be considered an inherent characteristic of the visionary administrator. In this light, the nursing executive who is bound to linear thinking, to space and time, is all the more mired in tradition rather than enriched by it. This kind of manager is too busy "putting out fires" to plan for the future. Change itself can be viewed as harmful and undesirable here. By contrast, the visionary leader embraces change with its innovation and creativity.

Rogers (1970) makes a strong case for a universe of open systems in which "people are inseparable from the natural world" and in which people and environment are in continuous mutual process with one another (p. 46). In attempting to operationalize this, one quickly sees the usefulness of the principle of integrality in formulating a theory of nursing management. This principle speaks of the continuous mutual human field and environmental field process (Rogers, 1986). Clearly, nursing is integral with the health care delivery system, both continuously evolving as a unified process. It is hard to conceptualize one without the other, just as it is difficult to conceive of a hospital without nurses.

Integrality eschews the particular approach to problem solving in favor of a perspective of innovation that implies continuous evolution of both the nursing and organizational energy fields. As an indicant of mainstream managerial thought, Peters and Waterman (1982) appear to subscribe to the principle of integrality when they note that "there is no such thing as a good structural answer apart from people considerations, and vice versa" (p. 9). Furthermore, they advocate the consideration of organizational variables as interdependent.

Integrality can be useful in assisting the nurse executive to implement primary nursing. The casual observer may see this model of care delivery as relevant only to the nursing service. However, in a universe of open systems, all energy fields are in continuous mutual process. Thus, every other constituency (or energy field) in the organization is involved with this evolving emergent. For example, a cursory look at the day-to-day realities of client care demonstrates that the attending physician must communicate directly with the primary nurse, rather than with the head nurse (Marram, Schegel, & Bevis, 1974). This is a change in medical practice, and can serve as an indicant of change in the practice of other disciplines. These changes could also include modifications in staffing patterns, materials management, accounting, discharge planning, and even in the structure of the physical plant. Particular thinking must be avoided in order to remain holistic in viewing an organization as more than the sum of its parts. Other examples of practice changes related to the implementation of primary nursing may be enumerated. However, even a "common sense" approach bears out the notion that a change in daily operations by the largest constituency in the organization will hold some implications for all other constituencies.

A CASE IN POINT

Staff turnover and retention have become preeminent issues as the nursing personnel shortage grows ever more severe. Consider the following scenario in regard to a theoretical application of concepts to practice.

Baxter 3 is a 30-bed neurosurgical unit in Big Deal Medical Center. Unlike other institutions, this hospital has experienced no recent layoffs, anticipates no plans for expansion, and, in general, has experienced no major changes for some time. Baxter 3 has a professional staff of caregivers, 23 to 40 years of age, who are assisted by several unit aides for the performance of tasks that do not involve direct client care. The staffing patterns are considered lean but adequate, and have been stable for over a year and a half. Yet over the course of the last 8 months, this stable tenure of staff has changed. Five nurses left the unit for the following reasons: one nurse transferred to pediatrics to fulfill a career goal; another left the unit to assume a supervisory position; one has returned to school to obtain a master's degree and joined the hospital's per diem pool; one nurse stated that, since she had worked on Baxter 3 for over 4 years, she felt the need of a new challenge; and, finally, one nurse had major travel plans that extended well beyond the hospital's leave-of-absence policy.

An individual's view of and subsequent approach to this situation is contingent upon that individual's conceptual system, which provides the choice of management intervention. Two divergent approaches appear that represent two mutually exclusive paradigms.

The traditional perspective examines this situation in particular form and attempts analysis of these so-called "acceptable" reasons for termination. Five discrete events are discerned. A reductionistic stance looks at cause and effect and assumes that the nurses who remain on the unit are secure, since they choose to continue in the setting.

A Rogerian approach considers the situation holistically and looks for synthesis, rather than analysis. The terminations, as manifestations of pattern, are seen as evolutionary emergents. The continuous mutual process is looked at from the stance of nonlinear acausality. It is assumed, by virtue of integrality and irreducibility, that the remaining nurses are also involved in this process.

Intervention in the traditional mode would seek to regain equilibrium and effect adaptation through a strategy of recruitment and replacement. The assumption is "business as usual."

Intervention in a Rogerian mode would require learning more about these evolutionary emergents. Linear causation is not possible since equilibrium and adaption are irrelevant in light of Rogers' (1986) principle of helicy. Rather, continuous, innovative change is reflected by creative, increasingly complex nonrepeating rhythmicities. As stated earlier, the behavior and characteristics of the unit's staff cannot be predicted from knowledge of the behavior and characteristics of one nurse, and vice versa. Since all energy fields, or staff members, are in continuous mutual process, all experience the phenomenon of staff turnover. In this way, the nurse executive must see not five terminations, but an emerging pattern of field manifestation. The situation is more than the sum of its parts. In contrast to the traditional approach of recruitment and replacement, the Rogerian approach attempts both replacement and retention. The assumption here centers around the emergence of a more diverse environmental field.

It is important to note that the managerial perspective of causality is the predominant *modus operandus* in health care organizations. Pseudoscientific approaches espouse *the* management intervention that resolves all conflicts. Highly centralized, bureaucratic structures utilize linear problem solving, and stifle the direction of managerial thinking from pragmatic to being imaginative and visionary.

VISIONS OF THE FUTURE

The operative word must be "vision." To avoid the mistakes of the past, the nurse administrator must acknowledge the needs of personnel who require the opportunity to influence their own practice (Scott, 1984). In effect, the nurse manager must operationalize participatory management by facilitating power sharing. This is a courageous move. It requires the abandonment of androcentric definitions of power that speak of domination and submission in favor of those characterized by mutuality.

Barrett (1983) has developed such a theory of power. Derived from Rogers' (1986) principle of helicy, Barrett views power as "the capacity to participate knowingly in the nature of change characterizing the continuous patterning of the human and environmental fields. . . . Power is being aware of what one is choosing to do, feeling free to do it, and doing it intentionally" (Barrett, 1983, p. 138). This is a far cry from Lewin's (1951) mathematical definitions of power, and from others that conjure up notions of Machiavellian machinations (Etzioni, 1961; Galbraith, 1983).

The time is long past when such causal approaches are useful or productive. Nursing and environmental field patterns change continuously and with such acceleration that the nurse administrator must be free enough and creative enough to envision a glimpse of the future. The Science of Unitary Human Beings is a conceptual system that provides a workable means of revolutionizing nursing management as well as a useful framework for considering the mission of the nurse executive: of confronting uncertainty, guiding change, and nurturing the mutual process that enhances the creativity of a rich and diverse energy field.

Rogers' work has provided an opportunity for vision that can furnish answers to some of those unimagined, unanticipated questions. It is important not to squander this opportunity. The stakes are high, the risks are great, but the prospects are revolutionary.

REFERENCES

Barrett, E.A.M. (1983). *An empirical investigation of Martha E. Rogers' principle of helicy: The relationship of human field motion and power.* Unpublished doctoral dissertation, New York University. (University Microfilms Publication No. 84-06-278)

Capra, F. (1982). *The turning point: Science, society, and the rising culture.* New York: Simon and Schuster.

Etzioni, A. (1961). *A comparative analysis of complex organizations: On power, involvement, and their correlates.* New York: The Free Press.

Galbraith, J.K. (1983). *The anatomy of power.* Boston: Houghton Mifflin.

Lewin, K. (1951). *Field theory in social science.* New York: Harper Press.

Marram, G.D., Schegel, M.W., & Bevis, E.O. (1974). *Primary nursing: A model for individualized care.* St. Louis: C.V. Mosby.

Ouchi, W. (1981). *Theory Z: How American business can meet the Japanese challenge.* Reading, MA: Addison-Wesley.

Peters, T.J., & Waterman, R.H. (1982). *In search of excellence: Lessons from America's best run companies.* New York: Harper & Row.

Rogers, M.E. (1970). *An introduction to the theoretical basis of nursing.* Philadelphia: F.A. Davis.

Rogers, M.E. (1986). Science of unitary human beings: A paradigm for nursing. In V.M. Malinski (Ed.), *Explorations on Martha Rogers' science of unitary human beings.* Norwalk, CT: Appleton-Century-Crofts.

Scott, P.P. (1984). Executive career planning. *Nursing Economics, 2,* 60.

Sheridan, D.R. (1983). The health care industry in the marketplace: Implications for nursing. *Journal of Nursing Administration, 13,* 36–38.

Weber, M. (1954). *On law in economy and society.* Cambridge: Harvard University Press.

Nursing Service as an Energy Field: A Response to "Visionary Opportunities for Knowledge Development in Nursing Administration"

Judith A. Rizzo

As a nurse administrator I am pleased not only to discuss Caroselli-Dervan's chapter but also that she has related Rogers' framework to nursing administration in a relevant manner.

Certain important points have been made; I will note several separately and then address ideas as they flow.

1. The health care environment has become increasingly complex and diverse.

2. Nurse administrators are in a position to change the face of health care delivery.

3. The Cartesian view, which is reductionist and mechanistic, has been replaced in the scientific world by a sense of irreducible wholeness. The era of benevolent spending in health care has moved to a period of economic constraint forcing cost containment. The health care environment is heavily regulated, litigation abounds, and the supply of health care workers has diminished.

4. Nursing and nursing management are indivisible from the paradigm shifts noted.

5. Administrative nursing practice has moved from behavioral proverbs to theoretically derived concepts.

6. An institution's nursing service can be viewed as an energy field the behavior and characteristics of which cannot be predicted from a knowledge of the parts, that is, one nurse, one unit or one shift.

7. Pattern identifies the energy field and often acts as a powerful incentive or deterrent to the recruitment of staff. New roles and new structures speak to an innovative pattern of evolving managerial thought.

8. The nurse executive bound to linear thinking, relative to space and time, is too busy "putting out fires" to plan futuristically.

9. The visionary leader embraces change seeing its inherent potential for innovation and creativity.

10. The nurse manager must operationalize participatory management by facilitating power sharing. The definition is not one of domination and submission but rather Barrett's (1983) definition of power as knowing participation in change.

While Caroselli-Dervan's statement that the health care environment has become increasingly complex seems somewhat obvious, it is important to note that the more recent nursing administration literature supports her view. Beyers (1988), in the publication *Current Strategies for Nurse Administrators*, states that the diversity found in nursing administration is simply and clearly a reflection of the diversity in health care itself. Gilmore and Peter (1987), speaking specifically of hospitals, note them to be "growing more complex and changing at a faster rate than ever before" (p. 11). It seems apparent there is agreement with Rogers that change occurs in the direction of complexity or diversity.

Caroselli-Dervan makes the point that nurse administrators are in a position to change the face of health care. She further notes that science has shifted its paradigm from reductionism to wholeness and views nursing as indivisible from this shift. In acute care settings, the medical model still permeates the environment with cause and effect reasoning. It is also probably not unfair to state that physicians generally continue to view the patient as a summation of parts, even though it is not possible to arrive at a picture of a whole human being by adding together arterial blood flow, gall bladder, and state of mind.

Nurses work closely with their physician colleagues and in this mutual process, more often than not, participate in this particulate view of patients. There are, however, some hopeful signs that indicate nurses do indeed look at the totality of the person and that such a view will begin to pervade the health care environment with the potential to change prevailing views in the medical community.

Caroselli-Dervan states that an institution's nursing service can be viewed as an energy field and indicates that the pattern that identifies the field—in this case the nursing service—acts as a powerful incentive or deterrent to recruitment. This is an interesting analogy that I will operationalize by a brief example. The pattern of the nursing service could be one of management by participation in which the primary nurse is able to make autonomous decisions and involve his or her primary patients and their significant others. Patterns evolve continuously and change is inherent in that evolution. Since change is integral to the patterning process, it loses its threatening aspects and becomes a normal part of the life process.

Caroselli-Dervan's point related to the nurse executive, bound to linear thinking, relative to space and time, as being too busy "putting out fires" to plan futuristically may be a trifle strong. While I would agree that visionaries embrace change as having the inherent potential for innovation and creativity, I am unclear that a linear view obviates the ability to have vision or plan. In this sense, then, while I enthusiastically endorse views such as Rogers' (1970) conceptual system, I need to be mindful that it is just that—a view. Rogers' nonlinear, acausal system provides a way of viewing humans and the world which can be of some use toward valuable outcomes. There is, however, a need to continue to acknowledge that those who view the world differently, specifically in a causal way, are still capable of achieving significant outcomes.

Caroselli-Dervan provided an example of dealing with staff retention and recruitment from a Rogerian wholistic perspective. Current nursing administration literature speaks to the issue of recruitment and retention and those speaking are likely to be cause and effect thinkers. Yet there is in their writings some of what Caroselli-Dervan refers to as wholism. Wall (1988) states that "A nurse recruited must become a nurse retained for the nursing shortage to decrease" (p. 25). She goes on to note that there are no simple or quick solutions to the nursing shortage. She states that a program which combines recruitment and retention can provide a base for problem identification which then is able to direct the thinking of hospital administration to the need to make changes in the work environment. Wall takes a wholistic view by considering nurses in relation to their environment, and viewing retention as a positive outcome of that nurse-environment mutual process.

Vanevenhoven, Stull, and Pinkerton (1988) note "We have only begun to understand, measure, and enhance job satisfaction of professional nurses" (p. 78). They go on to say that nurse administrators must realize that their

approach to job satisfaction needs to be dealt with creatively and in a mul-
tifaceted way in order to achieve optimal outcomes for nurses and patients
alike. The above helps to illustrate that causal thinkers have the ability to
view the whole. There is room here for a blending of thinking which is
where, I believe, we in nursing stand today.

Finally, the true significance of Caroselli-Dervan's chapter is her belief
that nursing administration has moved from behavioral proverbs to theoretically derived concepts. Henry, O'Donnell, Pendergast, Moody, and
Hutchinson (1988) stated recently that despite the fact that there is not yet
a wealth of nursing administration research, scientific productivity is increasing. They cite the number of doctoral programs and an ethos among
nurse executives which is supportive of research as a sign that an increasing
number of projects of high quality can be expected in the future.

They also express their anticipation of new experiments which they believe will challenge organizational norms and policies as they relate to environmental change. DeGroot, Ferketich, and Larson (1987) note that our
survival as a profession hinges "on our ability to develop and test theory,
and our related success in fulfilling the major purpose of theory, namely,
the description, explanation, and prediction of the phenomena central to
nursing practice" (p. 38). Henry (1988) cites diligent inquiry and the understanding of complexity as the corner stones of theory-based nursing administration. She notes that the task of nursing administration is to assess
theoretical perspectives in both nursing and organizational science and then
devise questions and develop methodologies that blend and test theory from
each of those fields. She continues by saying that "perspectives of power
may generate much needed information" (p. 167), noting that there is little
research in nursing that tests theories of power in organizational or political
contexts. She believes that information is needed about the kind of volun-
tary cooperation and negotiations that occur between consumers and
professionals in a variety of environments.

Barrett (1983) has provided a theory of power based on Rogers' framework and an instrument to measure it. Trangenstein (1988) and Dzurec
(1986) have used the tool to date. Barrett (1983) defines power as "the
capacity to participate knowingly in the continuous changing patterning of
the human and environmental fields" (p. 5). From Barrett's perspective,
individuals have the capacity to rearrange their environment intentionally
as well as to fulfill their potential by exercising choice. Nurse administrators would do well to consider Barrett's theory of power relative to their
individual organizations.

The literature indicates a growing concern for theory-based knowledge. I
would emphasize that it is important for nursing administration to derive
its theories from *nursing* and not from just any conceptual frameworks.

Over the last 30 years, there has been much discussion in the nursing literature as to whether nursing is a science, whether nursing theory is essential to the development of nursing knowledge, whether nursing should borrow its knowledge from other disciplines, and whether any of it matters at all.

Rogers (1970) spoke of nursing's need for a conceptual framework from which to derive and develop nursing theory. "The emergence of a science of nursing demands a clear, unequivocal conceptual frame of reference" (p. 84). Newman (1980) saw the purpose of a conceptual framework as providing a focus which is able to direct one's questions as well as the theories one tests.

Fawcett (1978) believed that when published nursing research is not linked to theory, the message may be that a theoretical base is not necessary. She noted that only since the late 1960s have the behavioral sciences integrated theory and research, and believed that it should not be surprising that the fledgling science of nursing has not yet accomplished such an integration.

Nurse scholars have a responsibility to move nursing science beyond its fledgling phase. Nursing, as a science, will not mature if nurse scholars do not tend to its development and derive nursing theory from nursing conceptual frameworks. This theory can then be tested in research and applied in practice. This book is evidence of evolution, or is it revolution, toward that goal.

REFERENCES

Barrett, E. (1983). An empirical investigation of Martha E. Rogers' principle of helicy: The relationship of human field motion and power. *Dissertation Abstracts International, 45*, 615A. (University Microfilms No. 8406278)

Beyers, M. (1988). Corporate level nursing administration. In M. Stull & S. Pinkerton (Eds.), *Current strategies for nurse administrators* (pp. 3–15). Rockville, MD: Aspen.

DeGroot, H., Ferketich, S., & Larsen, P. (1987). Theory development in a non-university service setting. *Journal of Nursing Administration, 17*(4), 38–44.

Dzurec, L. (1986). The nature of power experienced by individuals manifesting patterning labeled schizophrenic: An investigation of the principle of helicy. *Dissertation Abstracts International 47*, 4467B. (University Microfilms No. 8701004)

Fawcett, J. (1978). The relationship between theory and research: A double helix. *Advances in Nursing Science, 1*(1), 49–62.

Gilmore, T., & Peter, M. (1987). Managing complexity in health care settings. *Journal of Nursing Administration, 17*(1), 11–17.

Henry, B. (1988). Research issues for nurse administrators. In M. Johnson (Ed.),

Series on nursing administration Vol. 1 (pp. 155–176). Menlo Park, NJ: Addison-Wesley.

Henry, B., O'Donnell, J., Pendergast, J., Moody, L., & Hutchinson, S. (1988). Nursing administration research in hospitals and schools of nursing. *Journal of Nursing Administration, 18*(2), 28–31.

Newman, M. (1980). *Theory development in nursing.* Philadelphia: F.A. Davis.

Rogers, M.E. (1970). *An introduction to the theoretical basis of nursing.* Philadelphia: F.A. Davis.

Trangenstein, P. (1988). Relationships of power and job diversity of job satisfaction and job involvement: An empirical investigation of Rogers' principle of integrality. *Dissertation Abstracts International, 49*, 3110B. (University Microfilms No. 8625655)

Vanevenhoven, R., Stull, M., & Pinkerton, S. (1988). The nursing shortage and staff nurse retention. In M. Stull & S. Pinkerton (Eds.), *Current strategies for nurse administrators* (pp. 65–80). Rockville, MD: Aspen.

Wall, L. (1988). Plan development for a nurse recruitment-retention program. *Journal of Nursing Administration, 18*(2), 20–26.

Unit III
Visions of Rogers' Science-Based Research

Nursing's contribution to the future of humankind will be no greater than the scholarly research through which the theoretical basis of nursing practice becomes explicit.

Martha E. Rogers

13

Rogerian Patterns of Scientific Inquiry

Elizabeth Ann Manhart Barrett

> We have to remember that what we observe is not nature itself but nature exposed to our method of questioning.
>
> *Werner Heisenberg*

At the beginning of the 1980s, scholars were addressing the issue of whether or not conceptual models of nursing could serve as the basis for research (Barrett, 1980). For example, while researchers in the 1960s and the early 1970s at New York University investigated constructs considered relevant to understanding the unitary person, it was not until 1977 when Rawnsley framed her study solely within the Science of Unitary Human Beings that hypotheses were derived from this framework (Ference, 1986). Since that time much progress has been made by Rogerian researchers (Malinski, 1986).

In the 1980s, the literature has witnessed the generation of numerous research studies based in a variety of nursing conceptual models. In fact, Phillips (1988b) recently asked nurse researchers to "consider seriously the question of whether we can afford to continue using non-nursing models and theories to do research. The time has come to take the stance that nursing theory development and research must be within the framework of nursing models to advance nursing practice" (p. 49).

Today, we have moved beyond the question of whether or not the Science of Unitary Human Beings can be further developed and tested through research to ask what methods will serve us best in these efforts. Questions concerning the appropriateness or adequacy of the traditional scientific method as a mode of inquiry for nursing emerged as common themes in the nursing research literature during the 1980s (Moccia, 1988).

A major thrust of the 1990s is likely to be the development of new research methodologies specific to the discipline of nursing and, perhaps, to the Science of Unitary Human Beings. In 1976, Paterson and Zderdad proposed phenomenological nursology as a unique research method for their conceptual model of Humanistic Nursing. Leininger's (1985, 1988) unique ethnonursing methodology has been developed over a number of years to study her conceptual model of Cultural Care Diversity and Universality. In 1987, Parse proposed a unique research methodology for her conceptual model of Man-Living-Health. Parse noted that nursing scholars are developing the tradition of nursing science and, thus, need to "create, critique, and test research and practice methodologies congruent with the belief systems of the nursing theories and framework" (Parse, 1988, p. 45).

While researchers are at an early stage of inquiry into Rogerian ways of knowing, it is clear that the development and testing of knowledge concerning the Science of Unitary Human Beings is the pursuit of Rogerian researchers. Frequently, two questions are posed: (1) Is a quantitative study feasible using Rogers' Science of Unitary Human Beings? (2) Is a qualitative study feasible using Rogers' Science of Unitary Human Beings? Allow me to suggest that the answer to both questions is neither "yes" *nor* "no"; rather, it is "yes" *and* "no." In other words, the answer is "it all depends." The position taken in this chapter is that different methods can be used at different times for different purposes to answer different questions. This is consistent with the predominant position of the discipline itself (Munhall & Oiler, 1986a; Phillips, 1988b). According to Moccia (1986), "Nursing's quest for the perfect method is being abandoned as researchers recognize that there are a variety of ways to investigate questions, and that the nature of the question is a significant factor in choosing from among the alternatives" (p. 147).

PHILOSOPHICAL ASSUMPTIONS OF ROGERS' SCIENCE OF UNITARY HUMAN BEINGS

Rogerian epistemology and ontology guide the aforementioned research. While some qualitative and quantitative methods are appropriate for use in this system, others are not. The question will determine the approach to be taken in answering it. Qualitative approaches are broadly defined to include historical research and various types of philosophical inquiry such as the dialectic, hermeneutics, metaphysical analysis, and foundational inquiry as well as phenomenology, grounded theory, ethnography, case study method, and other qualitative methods.

Moccia (1985) identifies the dialectic as a method of philosophical inquiry that has potential for contributing to the understanding of Rogers' Science of Unitary Human Beings. The dialectic shares a unitary world view, provides coherence between the world view and the method of inquiry, and includes assumptions of the nature of existence that are similar to nursing's (Moccia, 1986). Both Hegel and Marx identified a dialectic that is different from other methods in several ways, however. One significant difference is their argument that the whole *as a totality* can never be known because of the difference between reality and appearances. Both Hegel and Marx maintained that there is always a difference between the way things "really" are and the way they "seem" to be (cited by Moccia, 1986, p. 149). This rings true for Rogerian researchers who study manifestations of field patterning as indicants of irreducible, four-dimensional energy fields. Such difficulties do not negate the value of research but rather caution researchers to understand the limitations of research endeavors.

Whereas science deals with specific phenomena of concern, philosophy, especially metaphysics, encompasses the entire universe (Sarter, 1988a). Nursing defines its domain with a number of implicit or explicit metaphysical assumptions. However, nursing has yet to agree on a unique disciplinary perspective for viewing phenomena although the Science of Unitary Human Beings provides such a perspective (Sarter, 1988a).

Holism as a Research Dilemma

One metaphysical issue related to nursing science is reductionism versus holism. Parse, Coyne, and Smith (1985) propose that nursing conceptual models constitute two paradigms: the totality paradigm, where the whole is defined as the sum of the parts, and the simultaneity paradigm, where the whole is defined as more than and different from the sum of the parts. They further maintain that quantitative methods are appropriate for the totality paradigm models and qualitative methods are appropriate for simultaneity paradigm models such as Rogers' Science of Unitary Human Beings. Other researchers simply propose that qualitative methods are holistic and quantitative methods are reductionistic (Munhall & Oiler, 1986a). Both Parse, Coyne, and Smith (1985) and Munhall and Oiler (1986a) argue that the philosophical underpinnings of qualitative methods are congruent with holism and, thus, qualitative methods are more appropriate for developing nursing science.

The position taken here is that neither type of method truly captures the whole. Limitations are inherent in both types of methods. Yet there are ways to quantitatively measure manifestations of irreducible wholes (Rogers, 1989). In Rogerian science, for example, field pattern identifies the whole. Questions that relate to parts are not valid in this regard. Measurement instruments developed by Ference (1979), Barrett (1983), and Paletta (1988) were designed to measure manifestations of irreducible human energy fields in mutual process with irreducible environmental energy fields.

Sarter (1988a) identifies these metaphysical assumptions as based on but not limited to scientific knowledge; she defines the need for scholars to study such issues through metaphysical analysis. She notes that the task of developing appropriate metaphysical underpinnings for nursing science is in its infancy. In metaphysical analysis the question studied will dictate the approach taken in answering it (Sarter, 1988a). "It is," Sarter explains, "important to present all major positions taken on a question, to interpret and critically analyze these varying points of view, and then to justify the position taken by the researcher according to a specific set of criteria" (p. 189).

Moccia's (1985) and Sarter's (1988c) work using philosophical inquiry illustrates the usefulness of such methods to enhance understanding in the Science of Unitary Human Beings. Similarly, by using a variety of qualitative and quantitative methods we remain open to greater possibilities for generation and validation of the knowledge base of Rogerian science.

Sarter (1988b) argues that nursing's intellectual endeavors are twofold: (1) to develop scientific theories and (2) to develop a philosophical foundation as a larger context in which to situate its theories. Furthermore, she notes that Rogers' Science of Unitary Human Beings is nursing's first attempt at grand scale philosophizing. "Rogerian science attempts to describe the entire universe, while focusing in depth on unitary man within that universe" (p. 52). Hence, for Rogerian researchers the crucial consistency lies between the research question or problem statement and the philosophical base of the Science of Unitary Human Beings.

While nurse theorists who embrace the totality paradigm define the whole as the sum of the parts (biopsychosociocultural person), Rogers (1989; Sarter 1988a) insists that examining such parts will not encompass an understanding of the whole (unitary person). Rogerian science thus posits the universe as evolving in a process of continuous change in the direction of increasing diversity in a four-dimensional reality (Rogers, 1970, 1980, 1986; Sarter, 1988a).

Rogers' Epistemological Holism and the Research Tradition

Rogers' epistemological holism provides direction for the development of the Rogerian research tradition. As Sarter (1988b) proposed, for Rogers, "all forms of experience, from sensory to mystical, objective and subjective, are accepted as legitimate sources of knowledge" (p. 53). Since this science "emphasizes the synthesis of objective and subjective data" (p. 54), it may provide a direction for the development of a unique Rogerian research methodology. Certainly, it guides current use of various methodologies to answer research questions. Munhall and Oiler (1986b) quote Lauden who noted that "there are times when two or more research traditions, far from mutually undermining one another, can be amalgamated, producing a synthesis which is progressive with respect to both the former research traditions" (p. 20).

Meleis (1989) pointed out that while existing world views of different approaches to developing knowledge may be incompatible, "what nursing ought to be doing is developing our own world view rather than looking at theories that have been developed by other disciplines." This, of course, is exactly what Rogers has done.

Rogers, of course, bases her developments on the previous work of philosophers von Bertalanffy, de Chardin, B. Russell, and Polanyi (Sarter, 1988b). Her system, however, is a new and unique product. Within it, only research questions consistent with Rogers' concepts and principles are appropriate for study. In general, if the purpose of the research is to determine relationships or differences among phenomena, then quantitative methods provide precise ways of measuring patterns via numerical data. However, if the purpose is to study the meaning of lived experiences, then the rich critical description (Bolster, 1983) of qualitative methods provides a way to do that through narrative data. In neither instance is a focus on particular parts of people valid. In fact, for Rogers (1970), parts do not exist in a whole. As a result, research questions require congruence with this Rogerian world view.

Beginning nearly 30 years ago, Rogers has consistently proposed that nursing's phenomenon of concern is people and their world (Rogers, 1961, 1964, 1970, 1980, 1983, 1986, 1989). Recently, Munhall (1989) put it this way: "Nursing is concerned with some fundamental questions about the nature of human beings, the nature of the environment and the interaction between the two" (p. 21). This domain is not only the unique focus of nursing as a discipline but also constitutes the substantive knowledge base of the Science of Unitary Human Beings whereby irreducible unitary humans and their environments are defined in the context of energy fields, openness, pattern, and four-dimensionality.

What nurse researchers believe about health, illness, and nursing derives from what they believe about the nature of reality (Sarter, 1988c). The philosophical underpinnings of research pertaining to Rogerian science reflect the assumptions about unitary human beings in mutual process with their environments.

METHODS AS TOOLS OF SCIENCE

Methods are the tools of science just as a thermometer, stethoscope, and other instruments are tools of practice. These methodological tools are not to be confused with the phenomena of interest. Nor are they to be confused with tools that are research instruments used to quantitatively measure theoretical constructs. Just as one cannot take a temperature with a stethoscope, one cannot solve a research dilemma with an incorrect puzzle-solving method. Methods are the nuts and bolts of procedural operations for the systematic processes used to answer research questions. Greater diversity of methods allow for solving more diverse types of puzzles.

For our purposes here, whether or not qualitative or quantitative methods are selected depends on the particular phenomenon being studied, the particular question being asked, and the congruence of available methods with Rogerian science. For example, a quantitative causal modeling design using path analysis is not appropriate if the purpose is to establish causal relations since Rogerian science is acausal. However, a quasiexperimental design is a useful means of testing the effectiveness of a unitary human field practice modality, such as Meehan's (1988) work on the effects of therapeutic touch on the pain of postoperative clients. One would not, on the other hand, use quasiexperimental or any other type of design to study the effectiveness of a behavior modification program since, theoretically, behavior modification posits causality. It would be incongruent with Rogerian science and inappropriate for study.

It is interesting to note that quasiexperiments have also been used in the social sciences to study "open systems by searching for acausal configurations of multiple interdependencies rather than direct linear relations" (Morgan, 1983d, p. 23). In addition, canonical correlation which, according to Dzurac and Abraham (1986), "has been widely used in research on holistic phenomena" (p. 60) is a multivariate quantitative strategy that explores the relationship between two sets of interdependent variables.

Advantages and Disadvantages of Types of Methods

Each family of methods has advantages. For example, quantitative methods allow for the possibility of generalization of findings beyond the sample studied. Qualitative methods often reject the notion of generalization and treat every human situation as "novel, emergent and filled with multiple and often contradictory meanings that cannot be understood through observation at a distance" (Morgan, 1983d, p. 26).

Each type of method also presents its own difficulties to the Rogerian researcher. While qualitative methods are often considered more consistent with holism (Munhall & Oiler, 1986b; Parse, Coyne, & Smith, 1985), one major difficulty is that they are often "to the extent possible atheoretical" (Munhall, 1988, p. 3). However, whether from a qualitative inductive beginning or a quantitative deductive beginning, the study must eventually link in some meaningful way with the Science of Unitary Human Beings. For example, in Parse's (1987) research methodology, phenomenological data are analyzed by translating the data from the language of the subjects to the language of the researcher. In this manner findings are interpreted in relation to Parse's Man-Living-Health conceptual model. In instances of other qualitative approaches such as the development of grounded theory, unless at some point the emerging theory links with the Science of Unitary Human Beings, it is not a valid strategy for Rogerian scientists.

While the lack of congruence of quantitative methods with Rogerian philosophical holism must be acknowledged, it does not require rejection of this approach. Rather, it requires that the research question be congruent with the science by focusing on manifestations of irreducible wholes and not parts and that interpretation of findings reflect limitations in the method.

To abandon the quantitative method until we have more extensively examined its usefulness does not seem wise. Jacobs (1986) noted that "although traditional scientific theory sought to explain reality and relied on underlying notions of causality that are seriously questioned, if not rejected today, there is no reason to embrace the notion that events in empirically observed reality cannot be meaningfully related" (p. 45).

An accepted research dictum cautions that "correlation is not causation" (Munro, 1986, p. 64). As a result, correlational approaches are compatible with the acausal nature of Rogerian science. Researchers know the difficulty in constructing testable theorems that accurately reflect relationships among manifestations of unitary persons in mutual process with their environments. Yet, by using various descriptive and in some instances quasiexperimental designs, efforts to deductively develop and test theory consistent with the Science of Unitary Human Beings are proceeding (Malinski, 1986).

Using Multiple Modes of Inquiry

Both qualitative and quantitative inquiry are appropriate for use by the Rogerian scientist. This position is consistent with Phillips' (1988b) comments that "a specific model and the research question guide the choice of method. Various research methods are appropriate for all nursing models. Nursing models provide a multiplicity of ways to perceive phenomena that require different research strategies. This broadens the possibility of providing greater scope to the knowledge base of nursing" (pp. 48–49).

Reeder (1988) gave additional credence to this position when asked the following question. "Given a particular position on holism, specifically Rogers' Science of Unitary Human Beings, is there an irreconcilable philosophical incongruence in use of quantitative methods?" She replied, "No, quantitative methods can be used." Reeder went on to say that the Rogerian researcher begins by asking a different question that first frames the focus in four-dimensional holism rather than in a three-dimensional context. She continued by noting that after the researcher describes the phenomena in terms of the Rogerian conceptual model, he or she then employs quantitative methods for measurement purposes. Reeder (1984) also advocates use of qualitative methods by Rogerians and has conducted philosophical inquiry in relation to this science.

Support for the position that both types of methods are appropriate is further gained from Munhall's (1989) reminder that "the exclusive use of any approach to science would, as stated by Kuhn, systematically eliminate those kinds of questions that cannot be stated within the concepts and tools of one paradigm" (p. 24).

Munhall & Oiler (1986a) proposed a nonlinear qualitative–quantitative schema in which qualitative methods of discovery and theory generation constitute a first level of activity and quantitative methods of validation constitute a second level of activity. They state that they have taken this position not because they could "substantiate the compatibility of the two world views but because the two world views both can be substantiated, not in truth per se but in problem solving according to the task at hand" (p. 38).

Both perspectives, qualitative and quantitative, allow for different types of knowledge to increase our understanding of the phenomena (Munhall & Oiler, 1986a). The qualitative–quantitative nonlinear linkage can be complementary rather than competing or antagonistic. It becomes a case of "and" rather than "either/or."

Tripp-Reimer (1985) also proposed that qualitative and quantitative research approaches may not be opposing methodologies. Rather, they can provide complementary data sets that together provide a more complex picture than can be obtained by either method singly. Each has limitations and advantages.

Qualitative studies are often exploratory and tend to be hypothesis generating. They are used appropriately when an investigator knows little about the phenomenon or when a fresh perspective on an area well investigated is desired. On the other hand, the researcher needs quantitative methods when the goal is to know how much, how often, or to what extent the phenomenon is occurring (Tripp-Reimer, 1985).

Qualitative studies may be precursors to quantitative investigations in certain instances (Munhall & Oiler, 1986a; Tripp-Reimer, 1985). Qualitative data also provide a generalized background for interpreting statistical results in later studies. Results can be compared to see if there is a "fit" between the two types of data.

After critiquing various nursing perspectives, Cowling (1986) also concluded that multiple modes of inquiry are necessary for the advancement of nursing science. His cogent critique of G. Morgan's work identified insights that shed light on the current state of nursing as a science. Cowling agreed with Morgan's position that any one insight provides only a partial view of a phenomenon and that any particular research approach may also be limited in its ability to illuminate the phenomena. An expanded perspective and flexibility of approach with greater attention to the links between theory and method as well as broadening the range of methodologies were suggested.

Morgan's (1983e) position is useful not only for science, in general, but also for the Science of Unitary Human Beings. He proposed that we "replace the view that science involves a quest for certain knowledge that can be evaluated in an unambiguous way with the view that it involves modes of human engagement on which we can and should reflect, and about which we can converse to improve our understanding and practice" (p. 18).

Rogerian scientists investigate their phenomena of interest within a particular frame of reference. However, they can investigate these phenomena in different ways using different methodologies as puzzle-solving strategies. The same phenomenon is capable of yielding knowledge of many different kinds. Science is concerned with actualizing potentialities of possible knowledge (Morgan, 1983). Rogerian science allows for research diversity. There are numerous appropriate paths of action.

In this light, I will discuss an example from my research concerning the development and testing of a theory of Power as Knowing Participation in Change that was derived from Rogers' Science of Unitary Human Beings. Quantitative methods were used to construct an instrument that measured the theoretical power construct, to establish the instrument's reliability and validity, and subsequent hypothesis testing (Barrett, 1983). In another study (Barrett, in progress), a qualitative descriptive exploratory design is being used to flesh out the theory through analysis of data obtained during semistructured interviews.

Similarly, Schultz (1987) called for holistic approaches to the systematic study of nursing phenomena. Specifically, she proposes a synthesis of patterns of knowing and methods of inquiry. According to Schultz, "this synthesis of inquiry can occur through using both the qualitative and quantitative paradigms to generate or obtain evidence, which can then be combined in a single text" (p. 135).

Morgan (1983d) cautions against the temptation to seek simple answers to the question of methods. Rather, he suggests analyzing research strategies in ways that move us "beyond method" (p. 41) by analyzing themes and issues that separate and unite the various research approaches.

Researchers are knowledge makers (Moccia, 1988; Morgan, 1983g). These knowledge generators deal with the actualization of possible knowledge since what is learned is connected with the particular research method used. One research approach may be more effective for a specific purpose than for another, yet ultimately the different strategies accomplish different goals.

According to Morgan (1983g), the different "voices" of the various research strategies converse about the nature of knowledge. Knowledge claims, of course, are tentative. In dealing with the issues that diversity of methods presents, Morgan (1983b) asks if we should "attempt to evaluate assumptions, search for common ground, adopt a criterion of usefulness, engage in dialectics, or decide that anything goes?" (p. 380). He (1983g) questions whether or not we should follow Feyerabend's (1975) notion that "anything goes" (p. 370). Feyerabend's advocacy of methodological anarchism rejects the idea that one form of knowledge can be judged as superior to another. Researchers who know what they are doing, why they are doing it, and how they might do it differently if they so choose are also likely to recognize the limitations of various methods (Morgan, 1983c).

The Science of Unitary Human Beings, like other sciences, is a changing endeavor dealing with a changing universe. What we know is an incomplete representation of an increasingly diverse four-dimensional reality. The phenomena of interest, unitary human beings in mutual process with their environments, are rich in potentialities. Multiple patterns of scientific inquiry facilitate understanding of the complex diversity of people and their world.

Quantum physics ushered in an entirely new holistic direction in science. "Modern physics can show the other sciences that scientific thinking does not necessarily have to be reductionistic and mechanistic, that holistic and ecological views are also scientifically sound" (Capra, 1982, pp. 29–30). It seems important to note that the major paradigm shift to holism was not accompanied by abandonment of traditional quantitative research methods, including experimental designs. Rather, different questions were asked about the phenomena that were conceptualized from an entirely different theoretical perspective reflecting a new world view.

The idea of a conscious pluralism regarding research activities was summarized by Morgan (1983b) when he asked, "What is to be gained by limiting our perspective?" (p. 390). Such a pluralism ultimately involves choice and the "existential dilemma as to what we should do or not do in our research" (p. 390). The range of choices open to Rogerian researchers requires critique of the nature as well as knowledge claims and consequences of various research methodologies (Morgan, 1983a). A "goodness of fit" between the phenomenon being studied, the research question, the particular method selected and the Science of Unitary Human Beings is essential.

The Link Between Philosophy of Science and Method

Contrary to Parse's (1987, 1989) and Munhall and Oiler's (1986c) position, Goodwin and Goodwin (1984) argue that research methodology is not necessarily linked with a particular philosophy of science. Perhaps the artificial dichotomy between philosophy and science is a particular perspective that "arises from failure to acknowledge multiple potential philosophies of science underlying research" (Dzurec & Abraham, 1986, p. 57).

It is unfortunate that quantitative and qualitative methods have been inexactly and artificially dichotomized. A polarization between the two perspectives has created a false separatist versus combinationist debate (Duffy, 1987b; Porter, 1989) that usually obscures more than it reveals.

Perhaps Sarter's (1988a) categorization of methods that were based on Carper's (1978) patterns of knowing are more appropriate for structuring the domain of nursing knowledge. Sarter (1988a) defines the paths to nursing research knowledge as empirical, personal, esthetic, ethical, and intellectual/interpretive. These paths cross philosophy of science boundaries by including both qualitative and quantitative approaches in the same category. For example, Sarter (1988a) includes both grounded theory and meta-analysis as empirical routes to knowledge. Could it be that inquiry should simply be regarded as inquiry regardless of method or philosophical commitments (Goodwin & Goodwin, 1984)?

In a similar fashion, Holter (1988) discusses Habermas' three distinctive clusters of sciences: empirical-analytic, historical-hermeneutic, and critically oriented. Knowledge created from critically-oriented sciences combines the other two forms of knowledge by recognizing their limitations and need for greater synthesis.

Porter (1989) discussed the similarities of quantitative and qualitative methods as opposed to the more frequent discussion of differences. She explored issues of the philosophical paradigm, the purpose of the inquiry, the research question, and the nature of the phenomenon under consideration. She too cited Habermas' perspective of critical theory as a human science alternative to the quantitative–qualitative dichotomy or the merging of methods. Porter proposed that it is critical to differentiate the philosophical from the methodological. Arguing that there is not a necessary linkage between paradigm and method, a researcher is free to use concurrently any appropriate philosophical underpinnings and any method. More importantly, Porter maintains that the separation of philosophical issues from methodological issues enables researchers to recognize more clearly the influence of the operative paradigm on the entire research process (Porter, 1989).

A number of methodologists also convincingly indicated that a link between philosophy of science and method is not an inherent requirement. Goodwin and Goodwin (1984) maintain that the notion that qualitative and quantitative research strategies represent distinctly different and mutually exclusive philosophical perspectives is a myth. Rather, they argue that the qualitative–quantitative distinction primarily concerns differences in methods of data collection, analysis, and interpretation. Moreover, it is possible to approach the study of a phenomenon with a certain philosophical orientation regardless of which method is being used. This is important since Rogerian researchers who may employ quantitative methods are not logical positivists. Their choice of research procedures flow from the research question as well as Rogers' epistemology and ontology. Methods are puzzle-solving tools.

Reichardt and Cook (1979) also maintain that the central issue in the methods debate is not research strategies per se but a contrast between conflicting paradigms. Since one must choose between these mutually exclusive world views, does it follow that one must also choose between the research methods that are linked to each paradigm? Reichardt and Cook propose that the philosophy of science perspective that specifies an incompatibility between qualitative and quantitative methods is in error. They argue that the assumptions that link the philosophy of science and a particular method as well as forced choice between qualitative and quantitative paradigms are incorrect; thus, the conclusion that researchers must choose between methods does not hold.

Reichardt and Cook (1979) also propose that just as the methods are not linked logically to the attributes of the philosophy of science at hand, the attributes are not linked logically to each other. For example, qualitative procedures are not necessarily subjective and quantitative procedures are not necessarily objective. Neither are qualitative procedures necessarily exploratory, grounded, and inductive nor are quantitative methods always confirmatory, ungrounded, and deductive. Reichardt and Cook quote Glaser and Strauss (1967, pp. 17–18), experts on grounded theory, who state, "There is no fundamental clash between the purposes and capacities of qualitative and quantitative methods of data . . . . We believe that each form of data is useful for both verification and generation of theory, whatever the primacy of emphasis." Nor are qualitative studies necessarily acausal; findings from some qualitative studies have reportedly been characterized by causal links (Kidder, 1981). These examples demonstrate that the logic of the task cuts across method (Reichardt & Cook, 1979).

It has been argued that both types of research methods can be associated with the attributes of either quantitative or qualitative methods. This does not mean that world view is unimportant in selecting a method; nor does it deny that certain research strategies are usually associated with specific philosophies of science. The major point, however, is that philosophies of science are not the sole determinant of choice of methods (Reichardt & Cook, 1979). That method and paradigm have been linked in the past does not mean that it is necessarily wise to do so in the future. Of course, researchers can still debate over which methods are preferred given a particular philosophical view and research situation. It is also important that the debate regarding methods not be confused with the debate regarding world view.

The congruence with holism is a frequently given reason by nurse researchers who select qualitative methods. Currently, the pendulum may be swinging from preference for quantitative methods toward qualitative approaches. This is true for other disciplines as well as nursing. However, when qualitative procedures have been put to the test as thoroughly as quantitative methods have been scrutinized, it is likely that the former will be found to be just as fallible (Overholt & Stallings, 1979). There is no single best approach. Although all methods are inadequate means of describing the whole, certain methods are useful for certain purposes. Methodologies specific to the Science of Unitary Human Beings are needed.

Methodological Triangulation

This discussion of methods would be incomplete without posing the question, "Do we or do we not triangulate?" Methodological triangulation is the use of multiple research methods in the study of the same phenomenon within a single research project (Duffy, 1987a). Triangulation, a blending of methods, is an entirely different issue than using different types of methods to answer different questions about a phenomenon.

Researchers who accept a paradigmatic distinction between methods usually reject the idea that the two types of methods can be used together. Yet, not all of the other researchers who reject the paradigm distinction acknowledge the usefulness of triangulation. There are also a growing number of researchers who find the paradigm issue of matching philosophy and method irrelevant and advocate combined use of the two methodologies (Goodwin & Goodwin, 1984). In other words, differing viewpoints abound.

Rogerian researchers will do well to head Phillips' (1988c) warning that "comprehensiveness of the research design can only be achieved when multiple measures are used within each method separately" (p. 5). The position taken here is that use of the two types of methods separately can be appropriate in different phases of the same study or in different studies. However, it is probably not logically sound to blend the two types of methods together (Phillips, 1988a). The rules and procedures for each are different. "Numerical and textual data cannot be combined in a meaningful analysis" (Phillips, 1988c, p. 4). In other words, qualitative data cannot be analyzed adequately using quantitative methods; nor can quantitative data be analyzed meaningfully using qualitative methods. In this type of triangulation "connections to a frame of reference cannot be made appropriately" (p. 4). It is not the use of different methods that is in error, but rather the simultaneous merging of methods.

An analogy from quantum physics illustrates the rationale for advocating use of both types of methods separately yet opposing mixing the methods together. Light can behave as a wave or as a particle depending on the way it is studied; however, it cannot behave as both a wave and a particle at any given time. "Both the 'particle picture' and the 'wave picture' are two complementary portrayals of the same reality, even if they cannot be charted at the same time. In other words, despite one's methods being limited to either/or, one's conception can embrace both and glimpse the whole"

(Morgan, 1984, pp. 288–289). In addition, "Just because you can see the picture only as a wave or particle at any given time doesn't mean it isn't both at all times" (p. 297). Reality is four-dimensional. This analogy also suggests the complementary nature of qualitative and quantitative methods as efforts to glimpse the whole. It raises the question, "Do multiple methods enhance understanding the complexity of the whole?"

DIRECTIONS FOR THE FUTURE

This discussion has been neither an exhaustive nor final view of the methods dilemma. Rather, it is a beginning attempt to respond to such issues from a Rogerian perspective. Nevertheless, we must move beyond the issue of qualitative versus quantitative methods and select ways to describe, understand, explain, interpret and in some instances probabilistically predict the science's unqiue phenomenon of concern, unitary human beings in mutual process with their environments. Regardless of the methods used, reductionism, mind–body dualism, and causal determinism are incompatible with the Rogerian world view that posits a four-dimensional universe of open systems (Rogers 1970, 1986).

Rather than proposing an inherent superiority of one method over another on the basis of intrinsic qualities it assuredly possesses or because of proposed incongruence between the conceptual model's ontology and methodology, let us continue pursuing research questions with the widest array of conceptual and methodological tools possible. This generation of nurse researchers will be educated in both the quantitative and qualitative traditions. They will be able to use the broadest range of methods to answer increasingly meaningful questions. They will recognize that all methods are limited and that discovery of a weakness is a challenge to improve the method rather than a reason to reject it (Reichardt & Cook, 1979). The challenge is to ask questions relevant to the phenomena of concern to the Science of Unitary Human Beings and to nursing, for indeed they are the same, and to persist in our endeavors despite the realization that our methods are flawed.

Rogers (1989) has provided research direction for the immediate future, proposing that both basic and applied research are needed. However, since applied research cannot go beyond the available, basic knowledge, there is urgent need for extensive basic research. Rogers outlines three priorities in the area of basic research. First, new questions reflecting holistic trends in science and society must be asked. Second, research instruments that measure or evaluate manifestations of unitary irreducible wholes need to be developed. Currently, there are at least three such instruments: Ference's

(1979) Human Field Motion Test, Barrett's (1983) Power as Knowing Participation in Change Tool, and Paletta's (1988) Temporal Experience Scales. Third, basic research on the nature of patterning (human field patterning and environmental field patterning) and the significance of wave frequencies in terms of continuous change is needed. In the area of applied research, studies of the effectiveness of noninvasive human field practice modalities in relation to human health are required (Rogers, 1989).

Simultaneously, we need to begin to explore possibilities of a unique Rogerian research methodology. Phillips (1988a, 1988c) called for new research methods that are relativistic rather than mechanistic and will uncover human-environment patterns of wholeness (Phillips, 1988a). If we alter the way we see, we will alter what we see, which will alter our understanding of people and their world. This commentary is prologue to the continuing search for and evolution of Rogerian patterns of scientific inquiry. Research is paramount in the version of Rogers' science-based nursing. According to Rogers (1964), "Nursing's contribution to the future of humankind will be no greater than the scholarly research through which the theoretical basis of nursing practice becomes explicit" (p. 94).

REFERENCES

Barrett, E.A.M. (1980, November). *Nursing conceptual frameworks as bases for research.* Paper presented at the Fall Research Day of Sigma Theta Tau, Upsilon Chapter, New York University, New York, NY.

Barrett, E.A.M. (1983). An empirical investigation of Martha E. Rogers' Principle of Helicy: The relationship of human field motion and power. *Dissertation Abstracts International, 45,* 615A. (University Microfilms No. 84-06, 278)

Barrett, E.A.M. (in progress). An exploratory descriptive study of power as knowing participation in change.

Bolster, A. (1983). Toward a more effective model of research on teaching. *Harvard Educational Review, 53,* 294–308.

Capra, F. (1982). *The turning point: Science, society and the rising culture.* New York: Simon and Schuster.

Carper, B. (1978). Fundamental patterns of knowing in nursing. *Advances in Nursing Science/Practice Oriented Theory, 1*(1), 13–23.

Cowling III, W.R. (1986). Methods: A reflective model. In P.L. Chinn (Ed.), *Nursing research methodology: Issues and implementation* (pp. 67–78). Rockville, MD: Aspen.

Duffy, M.E. (1987a). Methodological triangulation: A vehicle for merging quantitative and qualitative research methods. *Image: Journal of Nursing Scholarship, 19,* 130–133.

Duffy, M.E. (1987b). Quantitative and qualitative research: Antagonistic or complementary? *Nursing & Health Care, 6,* 356–357.

Dzurec, L.C. & Abraham, I.L. (1986). Analogy between phenomenology and multivariate statistical analysis. In P.L. Chinn (Ed.), *Nursing research methodology: Issues and implementation* (pp. 55–66), Rockville, MD: Aspen.

Ference, H.M. (1979). The relationship of time experience, creativity traits, differentiation, and human field motion: An empirical investigation of Rogers' correlates of synergistic human development. *Dissertation Abstracts International, 40,* 5206B. (University Microfilms No. 8010281)

Ference, H.M. (1986). Foundations of a nursing science and its evolution: A perspective. In V.M. Malinski (Ed.), *Explorations on Martha Rogers' science of unitary human beings* (pp. 35–44). Norwalk, CT: Appleton-Century-Crofts.

Feyerabend, P. (1975). *Against method.* London: New Left Books.

Glaser, B., & Strauss, A.L. (1967). *The discovery of grounded theory.* Chicago: Aldine.

Goodwin, L.D., & Goodwin, W.L. (1984). Quantitative versus qualitative research or qualitative and quantitative research? *Nursing Research, 33,* 378–380.

Holter, J.M. (1988). Critical theory: A foundation for the development of nursing theories. *Scholarly Inquiry for Nursing Practice, 2,* 223–232.

Jacobs, M.K. (1986). Can nursing theory be tested? In P.L. Chinn (Ed.), *Nursing research methodology: Issues and implementation* (pp. 39–53). Rockville, MD: Aspen.

Kidder, L.H. (1981). Qualitative research and quasi-experimental frameworks. In B. Brewer & B.E. Collins (Eds.), *Scientific inquiry and the social sciences* (pp. 226–256). San Francisco: Jossey-Bass.

Leininger, M. (1985). *Qualitative research methods in nursing.* Orlando, FL: Grune and Stratton.

Leininger, M. (1988). Leininger's theory of nursing: Cultural care diversity and universality. *Nursing Science Quarterly, 1,* 152–160.

Malinksi, V.M. (Ed.). (1986). *Explorations on Martha Rogers' science of unitary human beings.* Norwalk, CT: Appleton-Century-Crofts.

Meehan, T.C. (1988, October). Theory development. *Rogerian Nursing Science News: Newsletter of the Society of Rogerian Scholars,* pp. 4–7. (Available from Society of Rogerian Scholars, P.O. Box 362, Prince Street Station, New York, NY.)

Meleis, A. (Speaker). (1989, May 12). *Nursing science in the context of health: Panel discussion.* (Cassette Recording No. D11-507). Louisville, KY: Meetings International. Recorded at Nurse Theorist Conference, Discovery International, Pittsburgh.

Moccia, P. (1985). A further investigation of "dialectical thinking as a means of understanding systems in development: Relevance to Rogers' principles." *Advances in Nursing Science, 7*(4), 33–38.

Moccia, P. (1986). The dialectic as method. In P.L. Chinn (Ed.), *Nursing research methodology: Issues and implementation* (pp. 147–156). Rockville, MD: Aspen.

Moccia, P. (1988). A critique of compromise: Beyond the methods debate. *Advances in Nursing Science, 10*(14), 1–9.

Morgan, G. (1983a). Exploring choice: Reframing the process of evaluation. In G. Morgan (Ed.), *Beyond method* (pp. 392–404). Beverly Hills: Sage Publications.

Morgan, G. (1983b). Knowledge, uncertainty, and choice. In G. Morgan (Ed.), *Beyond method* (pp. 383–391). Beverly Hills: Sage Publications.

Morgan, G. (1983c). In research, as in conversation, we meet ourselves. In G. Morgan (Ed.), *Beyond method* (pp. 405–407). Beverly Hills: Sage Publications.

Morgan, G. (1983d). Research strategies: Modes of engagement. In G. Morgan (Ed.), *Beyond method* (pp. 19–42). Beverly Hills: Sage Publications.

Morgan, G. (1983e). Research as engagement: A personal view. In G. Morgan (Ed.), *Beyond method* (pp. 11–18). Beverly Hills: Sage Publications.

Morgan, G. (1983f). Toward a more reflective social science. In G. Morgan (Ed.), *Beyond method* (pp. 368–376). Beverly Hills: Sage Publications.

Morgan, G. (1983g). The significance of assumptions. In G. Morgan (Ed.), *Beyond method* (pp. 377–382). Beverly Hills: Sage Publications.

Morgan, R. (1984). *The anatomy of freedom: Feminism, physics, and global politics.* Garden City, NY: Anchor Books.

Munhall, P.L., & Oiler, C.J. (1986a). Epistemology in Nursing. In P.L. Munhall & C.J. Oiler (Eds.), *Nursing research: A qualitative perspective* (pp. 27–45). Norwalk, CT: Appleton-Century-Crofts.

Munhall, P.L., & C.J. Oiler (1986b). Language and nursing research. In P.L. Munhall & C.J. Oiler (Eds.), *Nursing research: A qualitative perspective* (pp. 3–25). Norwalk, CT: Appleton-Century-Crofts.

Munhall, P.L., & C.J. Oiler. (1986c). Philosophical foundation of qualitative research. In P.L. Munhall & C.J. Oiler (Eds.), *Nursing research: A qualitative perspective* (pp. 47–63). Norwalk, CT: Appleton-Century-Crofts.

Munhall, P.L. (1988). *Qualitative research proposals: Form in the service of substance.* Unpublished manuscript.

Munhall, P.L. (1989). Philosophical ponderings on qualitative research methods in nursing. *Nursing Science Quarterly, 2,* 20–28.

Munro, B. (1986). Correlation. In B. Munro, M. Visintainer, & E. Page (Eds.), *Statistical methods for health care research* (pp. 63-85). Philadelphia: Lippincott.

Overholt, G.E. & Stallings, W.M. (1979). *Ethnography in evaluation: Dangers of methodological transplant.* Paper presented at the Annual Meeting of the American Educational Research Association, San Francisco, CA.

Paletta, J.L. (1988). The relationship of temporal experience to human time. *Dissertation Abstracts International, 49,* 1621B. (University Microfilms No. 8812521)

Paterson, J.G., & Zderdad, L.T. (1988, Original publication, 1976). *Humanistic nursing.* New York: National League for Nursing.

Parse, R.R. (1987). Paradigms and theories. In R.R. Parse (Ed.), *Nursing science: Major paradigms, theories, and critiques* (pp. 1–12). Philadelphia: W.B. Saunders.

Parse, R.R. (1988). Creating traditions: The art of putting it together. *Nursing Science Quarterly, 1,* 45.

Parse, R.R. (Speaker). (1989, May 12). *Nursing science in the context of health: Panel discussion* (Cassette Recording No. D11-507). Louisville, KY: Meetings International. Recorded at Nurse Theorist Conference, Discovery International, Pittsburgh.

Parse, R.R., Coyne, A.B. & Smith, M.J. (1985). *Nursing research: Qualitative methods.* Bowie, MD: Brady.

Phillips, J. (1988a). The looking glass of nursing research. *Nursing Science Quarterly*, *1*, 96.

Phillips, J. (1988b). The reality of nursing research. *Nursing Science Quarterly*, *1*, 48–49.

Phillips, J. (1988c). Research blenders. *Nursing Science Quarterly*, *1*, 4–5.

Porter, E.J. (1989). The qualitative–quantitative dualism. *Image: Journal of Nursing Scholarship*, *21*, 98–102.

Reeder, F. (1984). *Nursing research, holism, and philosophies of science: Points of congruence between M.E. Rogers and E. Husserl.* Doctoral dissertation, New York University. (University Microfilms No. 84-21, 466)

Reeder, F. (Speaker). (1988, June 22). *Questions regarding phenomenology and other modes of inquiry* (Teleconference). New York: Modes of Inquiry for Nursing, (New York University, Division of Nursing Doctoral Seminar).

Reichardt, C.S., & Cook, T.D. (1979). Beyond qualitative versus quantitative methods. In C.S. Reichardt & T.D. Cook (Eds.), *Qualitative and quantitative methods in evaluation research.* (7–32). Beverly Hills: Sage Publications.

Rogers, M.E. (1961). *Educational revolution in nursing.* New York: Macmillan.

Rogers, M.E. (1964). *Reveille in nursing.* Philadelphia: F.A. Davis.

Rogers, M.E. (1970). *An introduction to the theoretical basis of nursing.* Philadelphia: F.A. Davis.

Rogers, M.E. (1980). Nursing: A science of unitary man. In J.P. Riehl & C. Roy (Eds.), *Conceptual models of nursing practice,* (2nd ed.) (pp. 329–337). New York: Appleton-Century-Crofts.

Rogers, M.E. (1983). *Nursing science: A science of unitary human beings. Glossary.* Unpublished manuscript, New York University, Division of Nursing.

Rogers, M.E. (1986). Science of unitary human beings. In V.M. Malinski (Ed.), *Explorations on Martha Rogers' science of unitary human beings* (pp. 3–8). Norwalk, CT: Appleton-Century-Crofts.

Rogers, M.E. (Speaker). (1989, May 12). *Nursing science in the context of health: Panel discussion* (Cassette Recording No. D11-507). Louisville, KY: Meetings International. Recorded at Nurse Theorist Conference, Discovery International, Pittsburgh.

Sarter, B. (Ed.), (1988a). *Paths to knowledge: Innovative research methods for nursing.* New York: National League for Nursing.

Sarter, B. (1988b). Philosophical sources of nursing theory. *Nursing Science Quarterly*, *1*, 32–59.

Sarter, B. (1988c). *The stream of becoming: A study of Martha Rogers' theory.* New York: National League for Nursing.

Schultz, P.R. (1987). Toward holistic inquiry in nursing: a proposal for synthesis of patterns and methods. *Scholarly Inquiry for Nursing Practice*, *1*, 135–146.

Tripp-Reimer, T. (1985). Combining qualitative and quantitative methodologies. In M. Leininger (Ed.), *Qualitative research methods in nursing* (pp. 179–194). New York: Grune & Stratton.

14

Structuring the Gap from Conceptual System to Research Design within a Rogerian World View

Marilyn M. Rawnsley

It is the desire to produce order out of chaos that impels us to search
for regularities and connections, to docket things and label them.
Emmett (1967, p. 128)

Now that science is looking, chaos seems to be everywhere.
Gleick (1987, p. 5)

Science strives to provide explanations of our world useful for identifying
and solving problems (Kaplan, 1964; Kuhn, 1970; Laudan, 1977; Phillips
1987). To achieve its ends, the activities of science are constructed according to an abstracted set of methods and processes that transcend the political, cultural, and historical identities of its participants. For those who
master its syntax, the language of science offers a universal mode of communication.

Within the shared universe of science, there are many disciplines that lay
claim to a specific territory of knowledge development. The territory or
domain of a discipline is established through the questions asked, the research traditions used to investigate these questions, and the theories developed from these processes to explain phenomena of interest. However, in
order to qualify as scientific, knowledge resulting from these activities

must meet two fundamental criteria: first, it must be useful in suggesting and solving domain problems; second, it must be intelligible to other speakers of scientific language. The first standard is met through explication of the relevance of the produced knowledge to contemporary or recurrent issues of concern to members of the discipline. The second is achieved through demonstration that the knowledge has been generated through processes that can be articulated to and recognized by the scientific community within and beyond the discipline. While emphasis on the first criterion is essential for the maturation of a given discipline, it is attention to the second that allows for continued membership of that discipline in the larger society of science.

Within the discipline of nursing, the Rogerian world view has claimed recognition as the Science of Unitary Human Beings. In order to establish the legitimacy of its claim, knowledge development within this framework must satisfy fundamental scientific criteria. Since it is a new science, demonstration of the domain significance of its knowledge is an appropriate concern of scholarly debate. But if it is to be accepted as valid science, then the methods and techniques through which that knowledge is developed, tested, and refined must be examined in reference to articulated processes. In this discussion, the process of moving from conceptual framework to research design is explained and discussed from the perspective of theory building. Emphasis is given to identifying problems for the researcher committed to the Rogerian world view and guidelines to facilitate progress in paradigm development are proposed.

BACKGROUND

The Rogerian Science of Unitary Human Beings (Rogers 1986, 1988) postulates a four-dimensional universe of human and environmental energy fields characterized by patterning that is continually innovative and diverse as individual fields resonate together in continuous mutual process unobstructed by boundaries of time, space or humanly derived constraint. This essentially optimistic world view seems, on the surface, to share similarities with other contemporary scientific views particularly those consonant with post-Newtonian physics (Malinski, 1986, pp. 15–23).

Within the discipline of nursing, however, the Science of Unitary Human Beings stands alone. In the branch of knowledge called nursing, in which manifest patterning is more readily recognized as motivated by action—outcome than generated from intellectual abstraction, the world view of the Rogerian conceptual system is unique. In fact, defining attributes of the Science of Unitary Human Beings approximate Kuhn's (1970) description of a paradigm, the model abstraction which revolutionizes a field of study.

Rogers (1970) introduced a radical world view into the discipline of nursing when she proposed a holistic mutuality of persons and environment that transcended commonly accepted notions of time and space. Serious contemplation of the implications of Rogers' writings demands a different conceptualization of the academic and service dimensions of nursing. If Rogers had formulated the discussion as a philosophical investigation of the nature of the relationship between individuals and their environment, then interpretation and incorporation into the foundational premises of professional education and practice would have been appropriate. But, in 1970, Rogers proposed her ideas as a theoretical basis for nursing thereby placing further evaluation of its validity and utility within the purview of science and its methods for developing, testing, and refining theory.

Evidence of the intentionality of this scholarly connection is apparent in the evolution of the conceptual system, that is, from a theoretical basis for nursing (Rogers, 1970) to a Science of Unitary Human Beings (Rogers, 1986, 1988). The chronology of scientific progress in the Rogerian framework is well documented in Malinski (1986). The problems associated with conducting scientific inquiry to examine hypotheses said to be derived from an abstract conceptual system are less adequately articulated.

According to Kuhn (1970), the radical view of phenomena apparent in a true paradigm generates new questions for study and new methods of investigation. Because this new conceptualization is visionary, methodologies appropriate from the perspective of an older world view are incapable of capturing the meaning of relationships postulated in this nonconforming view. New research strategies must be invented for this purpose.

However, while nursing's position in the domain of science is still being legitimized, it is unreasonable to expect its scholars to invent new research strategies that will be recognized by the larger scientific community. At this phase of its development as a scientific discipline, nursing is still earning the respect of its colleagues in science by demonstrating that it can speak the common language. The maturation of nursing as a science is being established within the larger scientific community through demonstration of competency in the methods of the dominant research tradition while within the discipline. At the same time, the Science of Unitary Human Beings is postulating a four-dimensional, unbounded universe of energy fields that cannot be captured by linear measures.

Where does such contradiction between abstract conceptual system and concrete method of inquiry leave the researcher who is committed to clarifying implications of the Rogerian conceptual system through empirical investigations? Perhaps wandering in a parallel universe (Briggs & Peat, 1984) exploring four-dimensional territory with three-dimensional maps.

An obstacle rarely addressed is the scientific sophistication of these conceptual cartographers. Although there is a cadre of nurse scientists who are, theoretically speaking, schooled in Rogerian thought, research framed within the conceptual system is largely representative of work accomplished in doctoral theses. Speculation about the reasons for this practice is beyond the scope of this discussion. But what is germane is an appreciation of the dilemma of doctoral candidates who are learning to speak acceptable science at the same time that they are attempting to advance knowledge according to a world view that transcends current methodologies. Given the double jeopardy of novice researchers operating under incongruous conditions, the progress made in developing the Science of Unitary Human Beings is remarkable.

Now, with two decades of studies as solid foundation, issues of design are being recognized as essential to continued progress. Although many studies purport to examine relationships postulated according to a Rogerian world view, the findings, including those that reach statistical significance, are not likely to constitute "necessary and sufficient conditions" (Emmett, 1967, pp. 70–79) for claiming validation of theoretical predictions. Speculation about the sources of difficulty have been explained as a function of the incongruity between world view and research tradition in studies designed by sincere but inexperienced researchers. While awaiting what may come to be a serendipitous breakthrough on investigative strategies, guidelines for strengthening the connections between a Rogerian description of phenomena and empirical research designs are worth reiterating.

PROCESS

The following discussion reflects a synthesis of ideas from the substantive work in theory construction of Dubin (1978) and Reynolds (1971). Modifying their explanations for purposes of structuring the gap between the Rogerian conceptual system and available research procedures seems reasonable at this stage in the development of nursing science.

Hypotheses are statements of predicted relationships among phenomena. When hypotheses are said to be theoretically derived—as opposed to arising inductively out of empirical observation—reasoning proceeds deductively from the abstract statements of a theoretical model to testing in the concrete world of experience. Evidence is found to be consistent or inconsistent with these theoretical predictions. The concepts and principles of the Science of Unitary Human Beings provides a descriptive rather than explanatory model of human energy fields. In light of its high level of abstraction and its concern with acausality, wholeness, and indivisibility of fields, the conceptual system is not formally structured to provide for direct derivation of empirically testable hypotheses. Therefore, it is the responsibility of the individual investigator to make apparent the logical links between the system and the hypotheses. This task is accomplished through articulation of the rules of correspondence as interpreted within a given study design.

A comparison of its structural components to Dubin's (1978) features of a theoretical model illuminates the problem in Figure 1.

Before proceeding with this explanation, it must be restated that, as the Rogerian conceptual system has evolved, it is characterized as "a conceptual system that underwrites the Science of Unitary Human Beings" (Rogers, 1986, p. 4) not as a theoretical model. Therefore, comparison with Dubin's scheme would be inappropriate for purposes of evaluation of adequacy. But since the goal is to clarify why empirically testable hypotheses cannot be derived directly from an abstact conceptual system, the illustration proves useful in identifying a possible source of confusion.

According to Dubin (1978), the nature of a model and the goals of science indicate whether reasoning should move in an inductive or deductive direction. That is, is the aim to understand about the process of interaction of the units in a system or is it to predict knowledge of the outcomes, either as values of a unit or the state of a system as a whole? In its present stage, the Science of Unitary Human Beings aims at understanding while empirical methods of research are structured toward prediction of values. Therefore, in order to operate within a quantitative research paradigm, the intrepid scholar must risk setting forth an individual interpretation of the implications of the conceptual system in propositional terms.

Reynolds (1971) cites three characteristics considered desirable for scientific knowledge: abstractness, intersubjectivity, and empirical relevance (pp. 13–18). While the abstractness of the Rogerian conceptual system is not in question, intersubjectivity and empirical relevance have been shown—in the comparison with Dubin's (1978) scheme—to be as yet undetermined. According to Reynolds (1971), intersubjectivity is reached through explicitness of detail that allows for agreement or disagreement with meaning, and logical rigor, which is gained by the use of systems of reasoning shared by other scientists. Empirical relevance refers to evaluation of the correspondence between the statements and the empirical data gathered to examine them.

This discussion centers on the use of agreed upon meaning in shared systems of reasoning; that is, explicitness and logical rigor in research designs that examine implications of the concepts and principles in the Sci-

Figure 1

Dubin (1978, pp. 7, 8)	*Rogers (1986, pp. 1–3; 1988, pp. 99–102)*
Theoretical structures:	
1. Units or variables in interaction	1. Energy fields, openness, patterning, four-dimensionality
2. Laws of interaction to specify relation of units	2. Principles of helicy, integrality, resonancy
3. Boundaries or conditions within which theory holds	3. Not specified
4. System states—in which units interact with each other differently	4. Not specified
5. Propositions—logical, true statements deduced from the model	5. Expository statements derived by researcher for a given study
Research operations:	
6. Empirical indicators or operational definitions of units in propositions	6. Operational definitions of units or variables in expository statements
7. Testable hypotheses derived from theoretical propositions	7. Testable hypotheses derived from expository statements

ence of Unitary Human Beings through empirical methods. But demonstration of intersubjectivity and empirical relevance of the statements and methods in any given study relies on the imagination and ability of the individual investigator. Making the connections between the abstract concepts and principles of the system and the research design explicit through propositional statements is the missing link in many studies framed in Rogerian thought. What seems clear from examining the theory-to-research process explained by Dubin (1978), however, is that investigators are moving directly to the research operations without the expository statements that are translated into testable hypotheses.

Deriving statements from such an abstract system in which system states and theoretical boundaries are not specified requires the investigator to take intellectual risks. By definition, propositions are said to be theoretically true and logically derived. But in view of the abstractness of the Rogerian conceptual system, the investigator is putting forth a personal interpretation of the logical implications of the concepts and principles for appraisal by the scientific community within and outside of nursing. The posture of the true scientist, involving creativity, courage, perseverance, and humility, is necessary for this task.

CONCLUSION

In conclusion, this discussion purported to offer direction for clarifying problems and processes inherent in designing scientifically credible research when moving deductively within the Rogerian framework. The question of inductive designs, including qualitative methods, which seem congruent with the goal of understanding the nature and direction of patterning diversity characteristic of unbounded, integral four-dimensional, resonating human and environment energy fields has not been addressed. This omission does not imply lack of concern for the integrity and relevance of these processes in the Rogerian framework; it simply means that depth discussion of these issues will be the focus of a future paper.

Meanwhile, those persons conducting research to advance knowledge in the Science of Unitary Human Beings need encouragement and support. It is through their efforts that new problems will become evident, designs will be refined or surpassed, and the discipline of nursing will continue to gain respect as a contributor to the self-correcting method of knowledge development known as science.

REFERENCES

Briggs, J.P., & Peat, F.D. (1984). *Looking glass universe.* New York: Simon & Schuster.

Dubin, R. (1978). *Theory building.* New York: The Free Press.

Emmett, E.R. (1967). *Handbook of logic.* Totowa, NJ: Littlefield, Adams & Co.

Gleick, J. (1987). *Chaos.* New York: Penguin Books.

Kaplan, A. (1964). *The conduct of inquiry.* Scranton, PA: Chandler.

Kuhn, T.S. (1970). *The structure of scientific revolutions.* Chicago: University of Chicago Press.

Laudan, L. (1977). *Progress and its problems.* Berkeley: University of California Press.

Malinski, V.M. (Ed.) (1986). *Explorations on Martha Rogers' science of unitary human beings.* Norwalk, CT: Appleton-Century-Crofts.

Phillips, D.C. (1987). *Philosophy, science and social inquiry.* New York: Pergamon Press.

Reynolds, P.D. (1971). *A primer in theory construction.* New York: Macmillan.

Rogers, M.E. (1970) *An introduction to the theoretical basis of nursing.* Philadelphia: F.A. Davis.

Rogers, M.E. (1986). Science of unitary human beings. In V.M. Malinski (Ed.), *Explorations on Martha Rogers' science of unitary human beings* (pp. 3–8). Norwalk, CT: Appleton-Century-Crofts.

Rogers, M.E. (1988). Nursing science and art: A prospective. *Nursing Science Quarterly, 1*(3), 99–102.

15

Theory Development[1]

Thérèse C. Meehan

The National Center for Nursing Research in NIH has funded a research project in which the theory being tested was generated by the Science of Unitary Human Beings (Meehan, 1987b). A brief description of the study and definitions of the independent and dependent variables are given, and the way in which the Science of Unitary Human Beings was presented as the theoretical rationale for the study is outlined. This will illustrate how the Science of Unitary Human Beings has been used to generate an applied research study.

Since the proposal was written, the choice of words to convey the model has changed and been updated; many of the most recent changes have not appeared yet in writing. A rewriting of the theoretical aspects of the proposal will serve to illustrate how the choice of words to convey the model has been changed and updated, and to put them into writing. This will allow readers to compare an outdated and updated presentation of the model. It will also provide them with the most current version of the Science of Unitary Human Beings to use as a basis for working in the system and evaluating work presented within the system.

[1]Reprinted with permission of *Rogerian Nursing Science News: Newsletter of the Society of Rogerian Scholars 1* (2), 4–8, 1988.

BRIEF DESCRIPTION OF THE STUDY

The purpose of the research project is to test the efficacy of therapeutic touch in decreasing selected stress-related reactions in patients who undergo major elective surgery, and thereby, in facilitating patients' recovery from surgery. Specifically, the project is designed to test the hypotheses that therapeutic touch will decrease preoperative anxiety; decrease postoperative tension-anxiety, fatigue, pain, and need for analgesic medication; and increase postoperative vigor, and feeling of readiness for discharge on the day of discharge. The design is for a comparative clinical trial employing equivalent experimental and control groups with repeated treatments and measures over the perioperative period.

A sample of 156 male and female patients scheduled to undergo major elective abdominal or pelvic surgery will be recruited as subjects. A randomized blocking procedure will be used to assign subjects to one of three treatment groups: an experimental group receiving therapeutic touch, a single-blind control group receiving mimic therapeutic touch, or a standard control group receiving standard nursing care and no study treatment.

Subjects will receive the assigned study treatment the evening before surgery and seven times during the postoperative period. Anxiety will be measured before and after treatment on the evening before surgery by the STAI-Y1 State Anxiety Questionnaire. Pain will be measured before and at four intervals following one treatment administered in conjunction with a p.r.n. analgesic on the first postoperative day using a Visual Analogue Scale. The time-lapse until receiving the next analgesic will be calculated. The amount and number of doses of analgesic medication received over the postoperative period will be calculated. Tension-anxiety, fatigue, and vigor will be measured on the evening before surgery and during the morning and evening of the first three postoperative days by the shortened form of the Profile of Mood States. Feeling of readiness for discharge will be measured on the day of discharge using a Visual Analogue Scale. The hypotheses will be tested using factorial analysis of variance, analysis of covariance, and repeated measures analysis of covariance.

The study variables were defined as follows:

Therapeutic touch: an intervention in which the nurse assumes a meditative state of consciousness and places her hands close to the body of the patient she intends to help. She then scans the body of the patient and gently attunes to his or her condition by becoming aware of differences in sensory cues in her hands. She then places her hands over areas of accumulated tension in the patient's body and redirects these energies.

In treating the patient with therapeutic touch the nurse: (1) assumes a meditative state of consciousness by shifting her awareness from a direct focus on her environment to an inner focus on what she subjectively perceives as the center of her life's energy and through which she attends to herself and the patient in a relaxed and gentle manner; (2) makes the specific intent to therapeutically assist the patient; (3) moves her hands, at a distance of 2 to 4 inches, over the body of the patient from head to feet attuning to the condition of the patient by becoming aware of differences in sensory cues in her hands; (4) focuses her intent on the specific direction of these energies, using her hands as focal points, for a period of 2 minutes; and (5) places her hands over the area of the solar plexus (just above the waist) and directs energy to the subject for approximately 2 minutes. The treatment time is 5 minutes. This definition is slightly modified from a definition developed by Quinn (1984), based on Heidt (1981), and followed by Keller and Bzdek (1986) and Meehan (1985).

Mimic therapeutic touch: a treatment in which the nurse imitates the physical movements of a nurse doing therapeutic touch, but during which she does not assume a meditative state of consciousness; there is no intention to therapeutically assist the patient, no attuning to the condition of the patient, and no conscious direction of energy. In treating the patient by mimic therapeutic touch the nurse: (1) makes the intention to repeat the movements which have been demonstrated to her (the movements of a nurse doing therapeutic touch); (2) focuses her intention on mentally subtracting from 100 by 7s; (3) moves her hands, at a distance of two to four inches, over the body of the patient from head to feet, while continuing to mentally subtract from 100 by 7s; (4) returns to the patient's head and repeats step 3, for a period of 2 minutes; and (5) places her hands over the area of the solar plexus (just above the waist) and begins counting backwards from 240, thus keeping her hands in the area of the solar plexus for about 2 minutes. The treatment time is 5 minutes. This definition is slightly modified from a definition developed by Quinn (1984) and followed by Keller and Bzdek (1986) and Meehan (1985).

Study treatment: the standard perioperative nursing care, which all patients would receive, without the addition of a specific study treatment.

Anxiety: a transient emotional state or condition of the human organism characterized by subjective, consciously perceived feelings of tension and apprehension, and heightened autonomic nervous system activity as measured by the STAI-Y1 Self-Evaluation Questionnaire (Spielberger, Gorusch, Lushene, Vagg, & Jacobs, 1983).

Acute pain: the patient's subjective report of intensity of hurting he or she is experiencing as measured by a Pain Visual Analogue Scale (Husskisson, 1974).

Time before receiving another analgesic: the amount of time in minutes between the time of administration of the p.r.n. narcotic given in conjunction with the study treatment and the time of administration of the next analgesic requested and received by the patient.

Amount of p.r.n. analgesic received: the number of milligrams of analgesic, prescribed by the patient's surgeon for p.r.n. postoperative pain relief, received by the patient between the time the patient entered the recovery room following surgery and the time of discharge, as estimated according to the table of Relative Potencies of Analgesics (Houde, 1979).

Tension-anxiety: a transient, fluctuating affective state of feeling associated with individual experience and reflecting a heightened skeletal muscular tension of both an observable and unobservable nature as measured by the shortened version of the Profile of Mood States (POMS), T subscale, developed by McNair, Lorr, and Doppleman (1971) and shortened by Shacham (1983).

Fatigue: a transient affective state of feeling associated with individual experience and representing a mood of weariness, inertia, and low energy as measured by the POMS F subscale.

Vigor: a transient affective state of feeling associated with individual experience and indicating a mood of vigorousness, exuberance, and high energy as measured by the POMS V subscale.

Readiness for discharge: the patient's subjective report of how ready he or she feels for discharge from the hospital on the day of discharge as quantitatively measured by Readiness for Discharge Visual Analogue Scale.

The theoretical rationale for the study was presented as follows: The Rogerian nursing conceptual model (Rogers, 1980) provides the nursing framework within which therapeutic touch has been researched and practiced to date. Rogers' model is based upon the assumptions that the human being is a unitary phenomenon, that energy fields are the fundamental units of the individual and environment, and that both are in a process of continuous, simultaneous interaction and change. Thus, it is posited that human beings are open systems of energy, and exchange of energy is the underlying dynamic of all human and environmental interaction. When a nurse treats a patient, each is viewed as an energy field within the other's environment. Experiences such as anxiety, pain, fatigue, and vigor are viewed as a function of the patient's unified nature in interaction with the environment. Changes in these experiences are viewed as a function of mutual energy exchange and repatterning of energy between patient and environment. It is posited that therapeutic touch derives its potential for therapeutic effect through the practitioner's actions of assuming a meditative state of consciousness, making the intent to help the patient or facilitate the patient's own natural healing process, and using her hands as a focus for perceiving and directing the transfer of energy. It is posited that the energy transfer, which is proposed to take place between nurse and patient, stimulates the patient toward greater wellness. This theoretical framework is held as a set of assumptions supported by the relativistic quantum field theories of contemporary physics (Bohm, 1973; Polanyi, 1965; Prigogine, 1976) and is in the early stages of testing in nursing science (Malinski, 1986). Mimic therapeutic touch is also viewed as an interaction in which an exchange of energy takes place between nurse and patient. However, the pattern of the energy exchange is posited to be different because the nurse does not assume a meditative state of awareness, does not attend to a perceived energy flow, and her intent is focused on repeating rote movements and counting numbers. It is posited that the energy transfer that is proposed to take place between nurse and patient does not stimulate the patient toward greater wellness. Any potential for therapeutic effect would arise from that assumed in the awareness of the patient. The rationale also focused upon mimic therapeutic touch as a single-blind control for placebo effect arising from the fact that a treatment is being given and the patient's expectation of therapeutic effect.

The rationale for the study treatment did not include any reference to the Rogerian model. Rather, the rationale focused only upon the fact that because human interaction is central to the nature of therapeutic touch, any experimental investigation of its effects cannot meet the double-blind criteria. Thus, the study treatment control group was intended to serve in lieu of a double-blind control group, and set a baseline for comparison against which the effectiveness of the therapeutic touch and mimic therapeutic touch could be judged.

REWRITING OF THE THEORETICAL ASPECTS OF THE PROPOSAL SO THAT IT IS CONSISTENT WITH THE MOST RECENT CHANGES AND UPDATING OF THE SCIENCE OF UNITARY HUMAN BEINGS

In the above outline of the way in which the Science of Unitary Human Beings was presented in the proposal, the definitions of the interventions and the explanation of the theoretical rationale for them are not always congruent with the Science of Unitary Human Beings as it is most currently stated. For example, the statement "individual and environment are in a process of continuous simultaneous interaction and change" should be changed to "individual and environment are in continuous, mutual process and innovative change." The statement that "exchange of energy is the underlying dynamic of all human and environmental interaction" should be changed to "mutual human-environmental process is the underlying dynamic of all human and environmental fields." The statement that experiences such as pain are a "function of the patient's unified nature in interaction with the environment" should be changed to "manifestations of the patient's unified field process with the environmental field." "Energy transfer" should be changed to "mutual process," and "energy exchange" should be changed to "energy process."

It should be made clear that the problem referred to in the literature as stress-related reactions in patients who undergo surgery was being reconceptualized within the Science of Unitary Human Beings model. In other words, the review of the stress literature was cited in support of phenomena which, from the point of view of the Science of Unitary Human Beings, were understood as manifestations of patient-environmental energy field patterning process, rather than reactions to stress or the relaxation response. The investigator then linked the theory of therapeutic touch, developed by Kunz and Krieger (1965–1972), to the Science of Unitary Human Beings. This theory proposes that therapeutic touch, as a nursing intervention, is a nurse–patient energy field interaction which promotes the patient's healing process and well being. The "nurse–patient energy field interaction" phrase in the theory was restated in the Science of Unitary Human Beings system as nurse-environmental/patient-environmental mutual process. The eight hypotheses being tested were generated deductively from the Science of Unitary Human Beings and inductively through nurses' experiences of perceiving themselves and their environments in terms of that same science.

The Science of Unitary Human Beings should have been presented as the theoretical rationale for all three of the interventions. The theoretical rationale would have been congruent with the model as it is currently stated if it had been presented as follows. From the perspective of the Science of Unitary Human Beings energy fields are the fundamental units of the human being and the human being's environment. Thus, the human being and the human being's environment are unitary phenomena and integral with one another in a continuous mutual process of energy field patterning and innovative change. Both are open systems of energy, and mutual human-environmental process is the underlying dynamic of all human and environmental field relationships. When a nurse treats a patient, she is viewed as an energy field pattern integral with the patient's environmental field patterning, and the patient is viewed as an energy field pattern integral with the nurse's environmental field patterning. In Rogers' words, "professional practice in nursing seeks to strengthen the coherence and integrity of the human and environmental fields, and to knowingly participate in patterning of the human and environmental fields for realization of optimum well being" (personal communication, June, 1988).

All three interventions would be viewed in the way that all professional nursing practice would be viewed: as knowledgeable, purposive patterning of patient-environmental energy field process. The operational definitions of therapeutic touch and mimic therapeutic touch indicate that, although the nurses use their hands in a manner that is specific and similar in appearance, as the mediating focus for the patterning of the mutual patient-environmental energy field process, the knowledge underlying the interventions and the purposive patterning of the interventions are quite different.

Therapeutic touch would have been better defined as a knowledgeable and purposive patterning of patient-environmental energy field process in which the nurse assumes a meditative form of awareness and uses her hands as a focus for the patterning of the mutual patient-environmental energy field process. The term "awareness" should have been used instead of "consciousness." In assuming a meditative form of awareness, the nurse would be more accurately described as shifting her awareness from parts of herself and her environment to (1) an awareness of herself as a unitary human being with the patient as an energy field pattern integral with her environmental field and (2) the patient as a unitary human being with herself as an energy field pattern integral with the patient's environmental field. Rather than "attuning to the condition of the patient," the nurse would be attuning to the patterning of the patient as a unitary human being. She would place her hands close to the patient's body, but rather than "scan the patient's body," she would scan the patient as an energy field or unitary human being. The nurse's perception of "accumulated tension in the patient's body" would be better described as her awareness of the patterning of the patient as an energy field or unitary human being. Phrases such as "directs energy," "redirects these energies," and "therapeutically assist the patient" would be changed to reflect the nurse's knowing participation in the purposive patterning and innovative change of the patient-environmental energy field process and her intent to facilitate the patient's comfort and well-being.

Mimic therapeutic touch would have been better defined as a knowledgeable and purposive patterning of patient-environmental energy field process in which the nurse focuses her attention on the parts of herself and her environment, on the parts of the patient, and on repeating rote movements and counting numbers. Study treatment would have been better defined as a knowledgeable and purposive patterning of patient-environmental energy field process in which the nurses carry out the perioperative care of the patients without the addition of either of the study interventions.

It should be made clear that the dependent variables, the experiences of anxiety, pain, fatigue, vigor, and feeling of readiness for discharge, are being viewed as unitary experiences, and as such, manifestations of patient-environmental energy field patterning process and innovative change. For patients who receive therapeutic touch, changes in their experiences of the dependent variables would be most accurately described as manifestations of innovative change which occur in the human-environmental energy field patterning process as the nurses administer the intervention. It would be posited that this particular purposive patterning of energy field process called therapeutic touch would manifest itself in the patient as less anxiety, pain, and fatigue, and greater vigor and readiness for discharge. For patients who receive mimic therapeutic touch, changes in their experiences of the dependent variables would also be described as manifestations of innovative change which occur in the human-environmental energy field patterning process as the nurses administer the intervention. However, it would be posited that this particular purposive patterning of energy field process called mimic therapeutic touch would be neutral in relationship to the patient and that any potential for manifestations of change toward greater well being in the patient would be a manifestation of purposive patterning on the part of the patient whose knowing participation in the patterning process is based upon the assumption that he or she is receiving therapeutic touch. This position is supported by the preliminary study findings. In the preliminary study, Meehan (1987a) found that approximately 30 percent of patients who received mimic therapeutic touch had a significant reduction in pain experience, an effect consistent with what is known to be expected from the placebo effect. For patients who receive study treatment, changes in their experiences of the dependent variables would be described as manifestations of innovative change which occur in the human-environmental energy field patterning process as nurses provide their usual nursing care without the addition of any study intervention. The manifestations of the particular purposive patterning of energy field process called study treatment would be viewed as baseline manifestations of patients' experiences of the dependent variables and serve as a standard against which the magnifestations of therapeutic touch and mimic therapeutic touch can be judged.

From the theoretical point of view, measurement of the dependent variables presents the most serious problem. There are no measurement instruments available which have been developed specifically to measure the dependent variables as manifestations of unitary human experience. Thus, the investigator takes the position that any human experience, feeling, or mood arises not from any part or parts of a human being, but (in the words of Whitehead [1978]) from their origin where they are inseparable: that is, in the investigator's view, from the unitary, energy field level. Thus, the experience of pain is considered to be a unitary phenomenon, and the Visual Analogue Scale measures the subjective experience of pain. The same argument would be made for feeling of readiness for discharge and the readiness for discharge Visual Analogue Scale. As can be seen from the definitions of anxiety, tension-anxiety, fatigue, and vigor, all include the idea that it is an experience, feeling, or mood that is being measured. However, theoretically speaking, this is the weakest link in the study. The issue of valid and reliable measurement of dependent variables in research generated from the Science of Unitary Human Beings is a large and serious one and will be addressed in future issues of this newsletter.

Finally, the updated version of the presentation of the study can be considered in relation to the model for theory development developed by Fawcett and Downs (1986) (see Figure 1). The conceptual-theoretical-empirical structure is illustrated in the diagram below.

[The author thanks Dr. Martha Rogers, Mrs. Dora Kunz, Dr. John Phillips, and Dr. Dolores Krieger for critique, editing, and suggestions for revisions.]

Figure 1
A Map of the Conceptual-Theoretical-Empirical Structure of the Study (After Fawcett and Downs, 1986, p. 88)

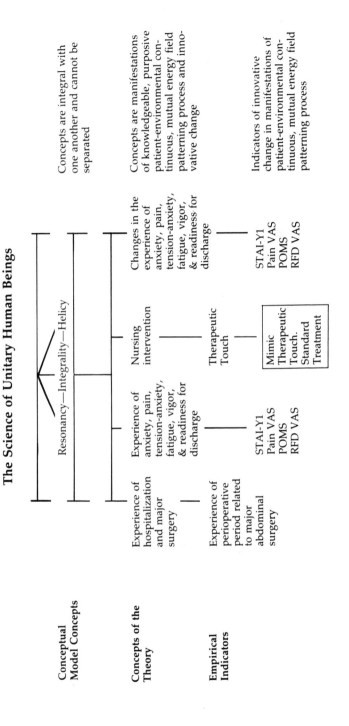

The Science of Unitary Human Beings

REFERENCES

Bohm, D. (1973). Quantum theory as indication of a new order in physical law. *Foundations of Physics*, *3*, 144–156.

Fawcett, J., & Downs, F.S. (1986). *The relationship of theory and research*. Norwalk, CT: Appleton-Century-Crofts.

Heidt, P. (1981). Effect of therapeutic touch on anxiety of hospitalized patients. *Nursing Research*, *30*, 32–37.

Houde, R. (1979). *Systemic analgesics and related drugs: narcotic analgesics*. In J.J. Bonica & V. Ventafridda (Eds.), *Advances in pain research and therapy*, Vol. 2. New York: Raven Press.

Husskison, E.C. (1974). The measurement of pain. *Lancet*, *9*, 1127–1131.

Keller, H., & Bzdek, V.M. (1986). Effects of therapeutic touch on tension headache pain. *Nursing Research*, *35*, 101–106.

Kunz, D., & Krieger, D. (1965–1972). The Pumpkin Hollow Foundation, Craryville, N.Y.

McNair, D.M., Lorr, M., & Doppleman, L.F. (1971). *Manual: Profile of mood states*. San Diego: Educational and Industrial Testing Service.

Malinski, V. (Ed.). (1986). *Explorations on Martha Rogers' science of unitary human beings*. Norwalk, CT: Appleton-Century-Crofts.

Meehan, M.T.C. (1985). *The effect of therapeutic touch on the experience of acute pain in postoperative patients*. Doctoral dissertation, New York University.

Meehan, T.C. (1987a). Secondary analysis. Unpublished data.

Meehan, T.C. (1987b). Therapeutic touch and surgical patients' stress reactions. (NRO 1676-01A1) Funded by the National Center for Nursing Research, NIH, July, 1988.

Polanyi, M. (1965). Life's irreducible structure. *Science*, *160*, 1308–1312.

Prigogine, I. (1976) Order through fluctuation: Self-organization and social systems. In E. Jantsch & C. Waddington (Eds.), *Evolution and consciousness: Human systems in transition*. Reading, MA: Addison-Wesley.

Quinn, J.F. (1984). Therapeutic touch as energy exchange: Testing the theory. *Advances in Nursing Science*, *6*, 42–49.

Rogers, M.E. (1980). Nursing: A science of unitary man. In J.P. Riehl & C. Roy (Eds.), *Conceptual models for nursing practice*. New York: Appleton-Century-Crofts, 329–338.

Sacham, S. (1983). A shortened version of the profile of mood states. *Journal of Personality Assessment*, *47*, 305–306.

Spielberger, C.D., Gorusch, R.L., Lushene, R., Vagg, P.R., & Jacobs, G.A. (1983). *STAI manual for the state-trait inventory*. Palo Alto: Consulting Psychologist Press, Inc.

Whitehead, A.N. (1978). *Process and reality*. D. Griffin & D. Sherburne (Eds.). New York: The Free Press.

16

The Relationships among the Experience of Dying, the Experience of Paranormal Events, and Creativity in Adults

Mary Dee McEvoy

Birth and death are considered universally significant events in an individual's life. Although events surrounding the birth experience, including pregnancy, delivery, and childhood development, have received attention, such is not as true of the death experience. Rather than strive to understand dying, our society has chosen largely to ignore it. Hence, relatively little research has been conducted to delineate pertinent aspects of dying. It is likely that the experience so vividly portrayed in Tolstoy's (1960) classic work *The Death of Ivan Illych* is implicitly more meaningful than the stage theories outlined by Kubler-Ross (1969) and Pattison (1977), and the psychological changes described by Lieberman (1965).

   The study described here was undertaken in an effort to understand dying from a new perspective. Its purpose was to examine the experience of dying within the conceptual model of unitary human beings described by Martha Rogers (1970, 1980, 1986, 1987). Rogers' conceptual model offers

---

This study was partially funded by the Women's Research and Development Fund of the City University of New York.

a unique way of viewing human experiences and, as such, was considered useful as a theoretical foundation.

THEORETICAL FRAMEWORK

Rogers' conceptual model is comprised of basic concepts, principles, and correlates of behavior. The basic concepts elucidate Rogers' views regarding the nature of the world, describing human beings and the environment as four-dimensional energy fields, patterned in a particular way and engaged in continuous, mutual process.

The principles Rogers' outlines flow from the basic concepts and postulate the nature of development such that development emerges from the mutual environmental field process as specified in the principle of integrality. Additionally, the principles postulate that the fields change in a particular fashion during development. Specifically, as specified in the principle of helicy, the field pattern increases in diversity and, as specified in the principle of resonancy, the energy waves increase in frequency.

A major thrust of this conceptual model is the nature of the human field pattern. However, human field pattern is an abstraction that manifests itself in correlates of behavior. The correlates of behavior postulate the human experience reflective of a particular field pattern. At this stage of model development, several correlates have been postulated, including timelessness, motion, and imagination. Table 1 outlines the concepts, principles, and correlates of behavior specified in the conceptual model of unitary human beings.

The components of the model—the concepts, principles, and correlates—are combined to develop the theoretical framework that guides the hypotheses to be tested. Using the method of theoretical analysis outlined by Newman (1979), the combination of principles and concepts used to frame this study of the experience of dying will be outlined.

In developing theoretical frameworks, Newman (1979) suggests that one examine the main theory and develop a corresponding auxiliary theory that is then operationalized for testing. Rogers' principles of integrality and helicy provide the theoretical underpinnings of this study.

The first proposition is that humans are continuously engaged in a developmental process, which includes dying (Rogers, 1970, 1980). Rawnsley (1986) also conceptualized dying as a developmental process when applying Rogers' principles in her study of the perception of time passing in those dying. Therefore, the description of the manner in which the human field changes during development is expected to be clearly evidenced during dying.

Table 1
Conceptual Model of Unitary Human Beings

Basic Concepts	Principles	Correlates of Behavior
Postulate the nature of the world	Postulate the nature of development	Postulate human experience related to the nature of development
Four-dimensionality	Development emerges from mutual human/ environmental field process (Integrality)	Timelessness
Energy fields		Increased motion
Human/environment process	Energy waves increase in frequency (Resonancy)	Imagination
Field patterning		
	Pattern increases in diversity (Helicy)	

The second proposition is based on the principle of integrality coupled with a view of the world as four-dimensional. Given this principle, persons as energy fields are open to a four-dimensional environment. Since we already have evidence that the world is four-dimensional (Freedman & van Nieuwenhuizen, 1985), energy fields integral or continuous with such an environment have the capacity for experiencing four-dimensionality. A correlate of behavior that exemplifies an experience of four-dimensionality includes paranormal events.

As previously defined, dying is a developmental process during which the integral four-dimensional human-environmental energy fields are in mutual process. Since the experience of paranormal events is a manifestation of a four-dimensional field, it may be anticipated that those engaged in four-dimensionality will experience paranormal events. Margenau (1970) supports this proposition by describing paranormal experiences as the ability to perceive within a four-dimensional universe, and states, "It is our human lot to look at the four-dimensional world through a slit-like opening. . . . Whenever the slit opens, and for some people the slit only opens at the time of death, you see more than a segmented three-dimensional slice of the four-dimensional universe" (p. 83). Wheatley (1976) further supports this proposition by viewing paranormal events as expressions of the relationship between humans and the environment.

The third proposition, derived from the correlates of patterning and the principle of helicy, is related to the experience of creativity. Creativity is of special interest relative to concepts advanced in the Science of Unitary Human Beings. Creativity is a manifestation of an innovative human field pattern integral with the environmental field. Field patterning undergoes change during development with change in the direction of diversity of field pattern manifesting increased innovation and creativity. As Rogers (1986) states, "Each environmental field is specific to it's given human field. Both change continuously, mutually and creatively" (p. 6).

Several studies have supported creativity as an important correlate of an innovative field pattern. Employing a canonical correlational design with 213 subjects, Ference (1986) found creativity and differentiation contributory to a canonical variate labeled "complexity–diversity." Cowling (1986), in examining the relationships between mystical experience, differentiation, and creativity, found that mystical experience and differentiation accounted for more of the variance of creativity than either variable alone (p < .001). Finally, Alligood (1986) found that creativity and actualization accounted for more of the variance of empathy than either variable alone (p < .001).

The potential relationship of complexity as an aspect of creativity has been supported by several authors (Cashdan & Welsh, 1966; Chambers, 1969; Crosson & Robertson-Tchabo, 1983; Eisenman & Robinson, 1967; Golann, 1963; Grove & Eisenman, 1970). Indeed, Barron (1952, 1953, 1955) has related the perceptual preference for complexity to creativity. The third proposition, then, is that during development creativity will be manifested as a reflection of a field pattern that is changing in the direction of increased diversity and complexity.

In summary, Rogers (1970, 1980, 1986, 1987) specifies that the human field pattern changes in a particular manner during development. Since dying is conceived as a developmental process, it is expected that manifestations of patterning will be highlighted during dying. Manifestations specifically examined in this study include those of the human-environmental field process within a four-dimensional universe reflected by the experience of paranormal events and manifestations of a diverse and innovative field pattern through creativity. Figure 1 outlines the main theory arising from Rogers' conceptual system and the corresponding auxiliary theory that forms the rationale for this study.

Figure 1
Theoretical Analysis

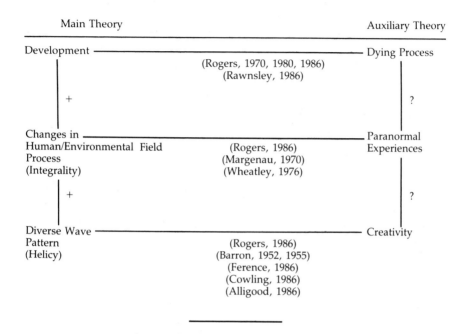

Main Theory   Auxiliary Theory

Development ——————————————————————— Dying Process
                        (Rogers, 1970, 1980, 1986)
                        (Rawnsley, 1986)

        +   ?

Changes in ——————————————————————— Paranormal
Human/Environmental Field   (Rogers, 1986)   Experiences
Process   (Margenau, 1970)
(Integrality)   (Wheatley, 1976)

        +   ?

Diverse Wave ——————————————————————— Creativity
Pattern   (Rogers, 1986)
(Helicy)   (Barron, 1952, 1955)
                                 (Ference, 1986)
                                 (Cowling, 1986)
                                 (Alligood, 1986)

STUDY ELEMENTS

Hypotheses

Three hypotheses were generated:

1. Adults who are dying will experience more paranormal events than adults who are not dying.

2. Adults who are dying will manifest more creativity than adults who are not dying.

3. Adults who are dying will manifest an increase in paranormal events and creativity as the dying process proceeds.

Definitions

Rogers (1980) conceptualized the *dying process* as a developmental phase of the life process characterized by a transformation of the human-environmental field pattern of complexity and diversity.

Paranormal events were those beyond an individual's daily experience as perceived by the five senses of taste, olfaction, audition, touch, and sight (Palmer, 1979). Paranormal events examined in this study included the out-of-body and the apparitional experience.

As defined by Palmer (1979), the *out-of-body* experience involved the sensation of perceiving self in a space outside the body. The *apparitional* experience involved the sensation of seeing or hearing another being that was not due to a physical cause.

Finally, *creativity* was viewed as a multidimensional process of interaction between the person and the environment manifested as a perceptual preference for complexity (Chambers, 1969).

Related Literature

Literature relating to the dying process and paranormal events incorporates two types of dying: sudden, unexpected dying and chronic, expected dying. Within the area of sudden, unexpected dying lies a growing body of literature concerned with the near-death experience. This literature is highlighted by the early, largely anecdotal portrayal by Moody (1975, 1977), followed by the more systematic and scientific works outlined by Ring (1980) and Sabom (1982).

The near-death experience includes subjective reports of people who have come close to death and were subsequently resuscitated. During resuscitation, a pattern of experiences with remarkable similarity appears which, according to Ring (1980), is "almost as though the prospect of death serves to release a stored, common 'program' of feelings, perceptions and experiences" (p. 15). This pattern includes a feeling of peace and quiet, an out-of-body experience, entering a dark tunnel, meeting deceased beings or spirits, seeing a being of light, and experiencing a panoramic review of life. Ring interviewed 102 people who had come close to death with 48 percent of the sample recounting 104 near-death experiences. The interviews were quantified by the Weighted Core Experience Index, a systematic scoring tool, with categories developed for moderate and deep experiences. The results indicated that 26 percent of the sample recounted a deep experience while 22 percent of the sample recounted a moderate experience.

Sabom (1982) interviewed 78 persons who had come close to death with 43 percent reporting characteristics of the near-death experience. A considerable body of descriptive research continues to accumulate that validates the existence and characteristics of the near-death experience.

Greyson (1983) has grouped the characteristics of the near-death experience into four components: affective, which includes feelings of peace and joy, a sense of harmony with the universe, and feeling surrounded by light; cognitive, in which time and thoughts are accentuated, a panoramic life review is experienced along with increased understanding; paranormal, incorporating the out-of-body experience, vivid sensations, and scenes from the future; and transcendental, which includes entering an unearthly world, encountering a mystical being, seeing spirits, and encountering a border.

With a focus on chronic, expected dying, a study of experiences of people during the last hour of life was reported by Osis (1961) and Osis and Heraldsson (1977). Five thousand physicians and 5,000 nurses were surveyed about their experiences with dying patients. Only 640 questionnaires were returned, resulting in a response rate of 6.4 percent. The surveys asked the physicians and nurses to report retrospectively their experiences with dying patients. The data indicate that 4 percent of the patients experienced apparitions, 1 percent an out-of-body experience, and 1 percent an elevation in mood.

Although the previous research is certainly limited, there is some evidence of a potential relationship between dying in a chronic, expected fashion and the experience of paranormal events, and stronger support for the relationship between dying in a sudden, unexpected fashion and the experience of paranormal events. Two additional concepts in the theoretical framework include creativity and the dying process.

No formal research has been conducted to examine the relationship between creativity and the dying process. In an anecdotal manner, Kubler-Ross and Warsaw (1978) report the experiences of four terminally ill patients in the final stages of dying. During the dying process, two patients began painting, one began writing poetry, and one developed skill in building doll houses. The authors state, ". . . a new kind of existence begins for them. We have seen countless cases. These patients often become poets; they become creative beyond expectation" (p. 30). However, the relationship between dying and creativity is supported only in a limited way by previous research and remains questionable.

In summary, then, this study, in addition to accumulating support for the theory derived from the Science of Unitary Human Beings, also extends the previous work on the variables of concern. Figure 2 summarizes the previous research relating to the study variables.

Method

A comparative, longitudinal, matched pair design was used to test the hypotheses. Subjects in the dying group were 28 adults with a medical diagnosis of cancer, knowledgeable about that diagnosis, with a life expec-

Figure 2
Previous Research Relating to Study Variables

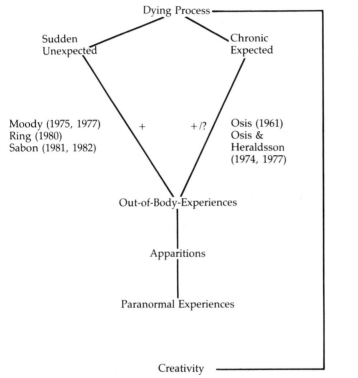

tancy of 1 month, and were able to communicate with the investigator. The non-dying group was comprised of 28 adults who were free of life-threatening disease and were able to communicate with the investigator. As age, sex, level of education, and occupation related to art, music, or acting have been reported to relate to the experience of creativity, subjects were matched on these variables. In addition, Ring (1980) found that women experienced more paranormal events as a result of illness than men, leading further support for sex as a matched variable.

Subjects in the dying group were obtained from a hospice comprised of both an inpatient and a home care unit in a large metropolitan area. All interviews were conducted in the inpatient setting. Subjects in the non-dying group were obtained from referrals from community religious and senior citizen groups in the same metropolitan area.

Subjects ranged in age from 21 years to over 80 with 39 percent between 71 and 80 years and 21 percent over 80. Thus, half the sample were over 70 years old. Sixty-four percent of the subjects were female and 36 percent were male. Sixty-four percent had a high school diploma, and only two subjects in each group indicated involvement in an occupation related to art, music, or acting. The groups were similar with respect to marital state, with the majority being either married or widowed. Seventy-nine percent of the sample was white and religious preference was almost equally divided between Catholics, Protestants, and Jews.

Instruments.   The instruments chosen reflect the operationalization of the concepts elucidated in the auxiliary theory depicted in Figure 1. Paranormal experiences were measured by the Near-Death Experience Scale developed by Greyson (1983), which uses four component subscales: cognitive component, affective component, paranormal component incorporating the out-of-body experience, and transcendental component incorporating the apparitional experience. Each component is comprised of four questions with a score range of 0 to 8. In this study, the paranormal and transcendental comprised the two components of interest. To test the hypotheses, these two component subscores were added to give a total paranormal score. Theoretical range for the total paranormal score was 0 to 16 with higher scores reflecting more paranormal experiences. Reliability was reported as .88 and .92 (Greyson, 1983). Validity was evaluated through comparison with Ring's Weighted Core Experience Index and was reported as .90 (Greyson, 1983).

Creativity was measured by the Revised Art Scale (Welsh, 1980) of the Barron-Welsh Art Scale (Barron & Welsh, 1952), which consists of 86 black-and-white forms arranged on a neutral grey background. Subjects were asked to decide for each figure whether it was liked or disliked. The theoretical score range is from 0 to 60 with lower scores indicating a perceptual preference for simplicity and higher scores indicating a preference for complexity (hence creativity). Reliability ranges from .70 (Welsh, 1980) to .96. (Barron & Welsh, 1952) were found. Validity was examined through comparing the scores obtained by artists with those obtained by non-artists. Rosen (1955) reports the scores to be statistically significantly different at the .01 level. The scale also correlates significantly with the Guilford battery of creativity tests at the .01 level of significance (Eisenman, 1969).

Data Collection

Data collection for the dying group spanned a 21-month period. During the first data collection session, written consent and background data were obtained. The Near-Death Experience Scale and the Revised Art Scale were then administered. Subjects were interviewed weekly for a minimum of 3 weeks until the time of death. In those cases in which subjects were interviewed for more than 3 weeks, only the 3 weeks prior to death were used in analysis. Seventy-eight subjects were interviewed in order to accrue the 28 needed for data analysis. The substantial subject mortality was due to the sujects becoming comatose, confused, or dying before the 3-week time period was completed.

Interviews for the non-dying group spanned 15 months. During the first session, written consent and background data were obtained. The Near-Death Experience Scale and the Revised Art Scale were then administered. During the remaining two sessions, only the Near-Death Experience Scale and the Revised Art Scale were administered. Table 2 outlines the procedure for data collection.

Results

The first hypothesis, which predicts that dying adults would experience more paranormal events than non-dying adults, was supported during the final week of life, but not during the 2 and 3 weeks preceding death. Scores on the Near-Death Experience Scale in the dying and non-dying group were compared across each of the three testing periods. Recall that the theoretical range for the total paranormal experience score was from 0 to 16, while the observed range was from 0 to 5. A score of 0 indicates that the subject did not experience a paranormal event, whereas a score greater than 0 indicates that a paranormal event was experienced.

During the first week of data collection, 3 weeks prior to death for the dying group, 26 subjects in the dying group and 27 subjects in the non-

Table 2
Procedure for Data Collection

Tool	Data Point*			
	Week 1	*Week 2*	*Week 3* . . . . . *Death*		
Consent	x			
Background data	x			
NDE scale	x	x	x x	
Revised art scale	x	x	x x	

*Data points for the Non-Dying Group comprise three consecutive weeks.

dying group had no paranormal experiences. A change in score then becomes evident during the second week of data collection, which is 2 weeks before death for the dying group, with 6 subjects in the dying group reporting a paranormal experience, while the scores for the non-dying group remain the same. During the third week of data collection, 1 week before death for the dying group, a change is again evidenced with 10 in the dying group reporting a paranormal experience and only 2 in the non-dying group reporting a paranormal experience.

Recall that the total paranormal score is comprised of the paranormal and transcendental component subscores. There was no differences between the groups in the frequencies for the paranormal component subscore, which recorded the out-of-body experience. However, the frequencies for the transcendental component subscores, which recorded the apparitional experience, were different.

During the first week of data collection, 3 weeks prior to death, two subjects in the dying group reported transcendental experiences, while no subjects in the non-dying group reported transcendental experiences. Again during the second week, the dying group begins to change with 6 subjects reporting transcendental experiences, while the non-dying group remained the same. During the week before death, the dying group further changes with 10 subjects reporting transcendental experiences, while the non-dying group stayed the same. Table 3 reports the score frequencies for the Near-Death Experience Scale.

Because the data were skewed, with the majority of subjects scoring 0, the assumption of normalcy required for parametric statistics could not be met. Hence the nonparametric Wilcoxon Rank-Sum Test was used to test the hypothesis.

Significance differences between the dying and the non-dying groups were demonstrated only during the final week of data collection for the total paranormal score ($z = 2.53$, $p < .05$). Furthermore, this significance was due to the significance obtained for the differences in the transcendental component subscale ($z = 2.80$, $p < .05$). Thus, it can be said that dying subjects had more paranormal experiences of the apparitional type than non-dying subjects during the final week of life. No significant differences were observed in the out-of-body experience. Table 4 reports the Wilcoxon Rank-Sum Test comparing the Dying and Non-Dying Groups on the Near-Death Experience Scale.

The second hypothesis predicting that dying subjects would manifest more creativity than non-dying subjects was not supported. There were no significant differences in creativity at any of the three testing periods as measured by the t-test (see Table 5).

Table 3
Frequencies of Paranormal Event Scores

Interview+	Score Frequencies			
	Dying $n = 28$		Non-Dying $n = 28$	
	0	>0	0	>0
Week 1				
Total paranormal score	26	2	27	1
Paranormal subscore	27	1	27	1
Transcendental subscore	26	2	28	0
Week 2				
Total paranormal score	22	6	27	1
Paranormal subscore	26	2	27	1
Transcendental subscore	22	6	28	0
Week 3				
Total paranormal score	18	10	26	2
Paranormal subscore	26	2	26	2
Transcendental subscore	18	10	28	0

+ Week 1 = 3 weeks before death for the Dying Group; Week 2 = 2 weeks before death; Week 3 = 1 week before death.

The third hypothesis stated that paranormal experiences and creativity would increase as the dying process proceeded. In the case of the Near-Death Experience scale scores, week to week changes were assessed by means of the Wilcoxon test (see Table 6). Indeed, significant changes were observed in the total paranormal score from week 1 to week 2, week 2 to week 3, and week 1 to week 3. Comparing the 3 weeks before death to 1 week before death, the difference was the highest at .01 level ($z = 2.67$, $p < .01$).

When the two component subscales were examined, it was clear that, as in the first hypothesis, the transcendental component was responsible for the observed differences. Significant differences in the transcendental component subscale were observed from 3 weeks before death to 2 weeks before death ($z = 2.02$, $p < .05$) and from 2 weeks before death to 1 week before death ($z = 2.20$, $p < .05$). And again, the greatest difference at the .01 level was observed when comparing 3 weeks before death to 1 week before death. Thus, it can be seen that dying subjects experienced a significant increase in the experience of paranormal events of the apparitional type as the dying process proceeded, supporting the third hypothesis. No changes were observed in creativity.

Table 4
Wilcoxon Rank-Sum Tests Comparing Dying and Non-Dying on NDE Scores
$n = 28$

Interview[+]/Scale	Pairs Where Dying Subject Has Higher Score		Pairs Where Non-Dying Subject Has Higher Score		Ties	z
	n	Mean Rank	n	Mean Rank		
Week 1						
Paranormal	1	1.00	1	2.00	26	0.45
Transcendental	2	1.50	0	0.00	26	1.34
Total	2	1.75	1	2.50	25	0.27
Week 2						
Paranormal	2	1.75	1	2.50	25	0.27
Transcendental	6	3.50	0	0.00	22	2.20
Total	6	4.08	1	3.50	21	1.77
Week 3						
Paranormal	2	2.50	2	2.50	24	0.00
Transcendental	10	5.50	0	0.00	18	2.80*
Total	10	6.15	1	4.50	17	2.53*

*$p < .05$
[+] Week 1 = 3 weeks before death for the Dying Group; Week 2 = 2 weeks before death; Week 3 = 1 week before death.

Table 5
Correlated Sample *t*-tests Comparing Dying and Non-Dying Groups on Creativity Measures
$n = 28$

Interview+	Dying Group		Non-Dying Group		t
	Mean	SD	Mean	SD	
Week 1	22.79	9.70	19.14	9.54	1.64
Week 2	23.25	9.13	19.39	9.42	1.75
Week 3	22.86	9.04	19.46	9.12	1.59

[+] Week 1 = 3 weeks before death for Dying Group; Week 2 = 2 weeks before death; Week 3 = 1 week before death.

Table 6
Wilcoxon Rank-Sum Tests for Significance of Changes in NDE Scale Scores During Dying Process
$n = 28$

Interval+	Scale	Cases Where Later Week Lower		Cases Where Later Week Higher		Ties	z
		n	Mean Rank	n	Mean Rank		
Week 1	Paranormal	0	0.00	1	1.00	27	1.00
to	Transcendental	0	0.00	5	3.00	23	2.02*
Week 2	Total paranormal	0	0.00	5	3.00	23	2.02*
Week 2	Paranormal	0	0.00	0	0.00	28	0.00
to	Transcendental	0	0.00	6	3.50	22	2.20*
Week 3	Total paranormal	0	0.00	6	3.50	22	2.20*
Week 1	Paranormal	0	0.00	1	1.00	27	1.00
to	Transcendental	0	0.00	9	5.00	19	2.67**
Week 3	Total paranormal	0	0.00	9	5.00	19	2.67**

*$p < 0.05$ **$p < 0.01$
+Week 1 = 3 weeks before death; Week 2 = 2 weeks before death; Week 3 = 1 week before death.

Table 7
Spearman Rank Correlations between NDE Scale Scores and Use of Analgesics In Morphine Equivalence
$n = 28$

NDE Scales		Measure of Analgesic Use
Interview+	Scale	Morphine Equivalence
Week 1	Paranormal	.33*
	Transcendental	.25
	Total paranormal	.26
Week 2	Paranormal	.40*
	Transcendental	.45**
	Total paranormal	.44**
Week 3	Paranormal	.40*
	Transcendental	.33*
	Total paranormal	.34*

Morphine Sulfate Equivalence (mg/week)
*$p < 0.05$
**$p < 0.01$
+Week 1 = 3 weeks before death; Week 2 = 2 weeks before death; Week 3 = 1 week before death.

Supplemental Findings

The only demographic variable that interacted with the experience of paranormal events was the use of analgesics. This may have occurred, and indeed could have been anticipated, because the two groups differed in analgesic use at the outset with all the subjects in the dying and no subjects in the non-dying group ingesting analgesics. Nevertheless, analgesic use was significantly correlated to scores on the total paranormal scale during weeks 2 and 3, on the transcendental component subscale during weeks 2 and 3, and on the paranormal component subscale during all 3 weeks (see Table 7).

CONCLUSION

The following conclusions can be drawn from this study:

1. Dying adults experienced more paranormal events of the apparitional type than non-dying adults.
2. There was no difference in creativity between dying and non-dying adults.
3. Dying adults experienced an increase in paranormal experiences of the apparitional type as the dying process proceeded.
4. Creativity did not increase as the dying process proceeded.
5. The ingestion of analgesics was the only demographic variable that correlated with the experience of paranormal events in this study.

Discussion

As this study employs the Science of Unitary Human Beings as the theoretical framework, further theoretical analysis is warranted. Figure 3 summarizes the theoretical analysis of study results.

The first hypothesis was predicted given that the Science of Unitary Human Beings describes the universe as a four-dimensional matrix of energy fields. Within four-dimensionality, modalities other than sight, taste, touch, audition, and olfaction allow for experiencing the environment. As the human field and the environmental field are engaged in simultaneous, mutual process, additional perceptual modalities may in fact be highlighted, particularly during transitional periods when the fields are expected to be most complex, as in the dying process. As those dying experienced more paranormal events than those not dying in this study, this logical formulation is supported. However, the paranormal events experienced were different.

Figure 3
Theoretical Analysis of Study Results

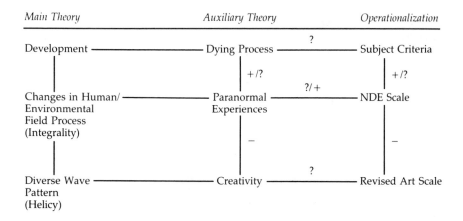

Main Theory	Auxiliary Theory	Operationalization
Development ——————— Dying Process —— ? —— Subject Criteria		
(line) +/?	?/+	+/?
Changes in Human/ —————— Paranormal ————— NDE Scale		
Environmental Experiences		
Field Process		
(Integrality) —		—
Diverse Wave ——————— Creativity —— ? —— Revised Art Scale		
Pattern		
(Helicy)		

Both paranormal events under study did not contribute in support of the hypothesis; that is, the paranormal subscale, as a measure of the out-of-body experience, did not yield significance. This subscale, however, was comprised of four questions, only one of which referred to the out-of-body experience. On close examination, it can be seen that the dying group responded "no" to the three questions that did not refer to the out-of-body experience, with three subjects in the dying group responding "yes" to only the question referring to the out-of-body experience. In contradistinction, the non-dying group responded "yes" to the three questions that did not refer to the out-of-body experience and responded "no" to the out-of-body experience question. Thus, in omitting the extraneous questions, it can be seen that three people in the dying group did indeed have out-of-body experiences while no one in the non-dying group had an out-of-body experience. Thus, the scale must be considered to contain artifact, leaving the theoretical formulation intact.

The hypothesis that the dying group would manifest more creativity than the non-dying group was not supported. This is particularly troublesome since other studies, notably Ference (1986), Cowling (1986), and Alligood (1986), have been successful in supporting creativity as an aspect of an innovative pattern profile. Additional analysis of the concept of creativity is required, both in terms of operationalization and conceptualization.

The operationalization of the concept of creativity in this study encompassed the Revised Art Scale of the Barron-Welsh Art Scale whereas previous studies used the Adjective Check List and the Simile Preference Test. The Revised Art Scale related creativity as a perceptual preference for complexity. It was reasoned that, as the human field evolves toward increased diversity and complexity, manifestations of that field would be related to those same characteristics. Hence, the tool to measure a perceptual preference for complexity was considered appropriate. However, different results may have occurred using the Adjective Check List.

In addition, consideration must be given to the theoretical underpinnings for complexity. According to Barron (1953), those pictures that are "complex, asymmetrical, and restless" in their effect yield a higher score if preferred, indicating creativity. However, the dying subjects also reported feeling calm and peaceful, which may have been in conflict with a preference for complex, restless pictures.

Further examination must also be given to the theoretical derivation and application of creativity, particularly to the meaning of an innovative field pattern that has consistently been defined in relation to creativity, as well as to a diverse wave pattern. As Ghiselin (1963) so aptly states, creativity is an elusive concept. The meaning of creativity as a characteristic, process, product or even, as Maslow (1959) terms, "self-actualizing creativeness," must be further specified in relation to an innovative field pattern.

Further theoretical analysis raises questions relating to the rate of change in the human field pattern as well as the particular constellation of correlates reflective of change. The correlates of patterning may change at different rates based on the nature of the developmental phenomenon under consideration. The pattern profile may consist of certain correlates being highlighted during particular, specific transitional periods.

In conclusion, the developmental nature of dying will be considered. Dying was conceptualized as a developmental, transitional experience. During dying, movement occurs from one aspect of development through to another, from one human field pattern through to another. However, the transition within the dying experience may take place in different ways. Three weeks were chosen as the study period to maximize the variable of paranormal events. However, this is clearly a linear time frame and heretical within the Rogerian framework. The time of dying, the transition of dying, the experience of dying, is highly variable and likely reflects the individual's ability to participate knowingly in the experience. Gathering information in a qualitative way to determine when someone is participating knowingly, and using that as the developmental criterion may indeed change the results of this study.

This study, then, has examined the experience of paranormal events and creativity in dying and non-dying individuals using the Rogerian framework of the Science of Unitary Human Beings. It was demonstrated that those dying have more apparitional experience than those not dying and that apparitional experiences increase as death approaches. Additional research, however, is clearly needed to understand the human experience of dying. In this sense, the words of Hinton (1971) still apply today:

> There are many reasons for knowing more about the state of people when they are dying. In addition to a basic preference for knowledge rather than ignorance, an increase in understanding of this particular field should lead fairly directly to further help for people whose need is often great. Experience and intuition are the frequent guides to the care of the dying, but a more exact knowledge should complement these assets, because the lessons of experience can be slanted and intuition is far from infallible. (p. 39)

Further specification of dying as a developmental phenomenon should indeed impact on the nursing care of people during their terminal life experience. Description and further research on the nature of the dying experience within the conceptual model of unitary human beings is warranted.

REFERENCES

Alligood, M. (1986). The relationships of creativity, actualization, and empathy in unitary human development. In V. Malinski (Ed.), *Explorations on Martha Rogers' science of unitary human beings* (pp. 145–154). Norwalk, CT: Appleton-Century-Crofts.

Barron, F. (1952). Personality style and perceptual choice. *Journal of Personality, 20,* 385–401.

Barron, F. (1953). Complexity-simplicity as a personality dimension. *Journal of Abnormal & Social Psychology, 48,* 163–172.

Barron, F. (1955). The disposition towards originality. *Journal of Abnormal & Social Psychology, 51,* 478–485.

Barron, F., & Welsh, G. (1952). Artistic perception as a possible factor in personality style: Its measurement by a figure preference test. *Journal of Personality, 33,* 199–203.

Cashdan, L., & Welsh, G. (1966). Personality correlates of creative potential in talented high school students. *Journal of Personality, 34,* 445–455.

Chambers, J. (1969). Beginning a multidimensional theory of creativity. *Psychological Reports, 25,* 779–799.

Cowling, N. (1986). The relationship of mystical experience, differentiation, and creativity in college students. In V. Malinski (Ed.), *Explorations on Martha*

Rogers' science of unitary human beings (pp. 131–141). Norwalk, CT: Appleton-Century-Crofts.

Crosson, C., & Robertson-Tchabo, E. (1983). Age and preference for complexity among manifestly creative women. *Human Development, 26,* 149–155.

Eisenman, R. (1969). Creativity, awareness, and liking. *Journal of Consulting and Clinical Psychology, 33,* 157–160.

Eisenman, R., & Robertson, N. (1967). Complexity-simplicity, creativity, intelligence, and other correlates. *Journal of Pyschology, 67,* 331–334.

Ference, H. (1986). The relationship of time experience, creativity traits, differentiation, and human field motion. In V. Malinski (Ed.), *Explorations on Martha Rogers' science of unitary human beings* (pp. 95–105). Norwalk, CT: Appleton-Century-Crofts.

Freedman, D., & van Nieuwenhuizen, P. (1985). The hidden dimensions of space-time. *Scientific American, 252,* 74–81.

Ghiselin, B. (1963). Ultimate criteria for two levels of creativity. In C. Taylor & F. Barron (Eds.), *Scientific creativity: Its recognition and development* (pp. 30–44). New York: John Wiley.

Golann, S. (1963). Psychological study of creativity. *Psychological Bulletin, 60,* 548–565.

Greyson, B. (1983). The near-death experience scale: Construction, reliability-validity. *Journal of Nervous & Mental Diseases, 171,* 369–375.

Grove, M., & Eisenman, R. (1970). Personality correlates of complexity-simplicity. *Perceptual & Motor Skills, 31,* 387–391.

Hinton, J. (1971). The physical and mental distress of the dying. *Quarterly Journal of Medicine, 32,* 1–21.

Kubler-Ross, E. (1969). *On death and dying.* New York: Macmillan.

Kubler-Ross, E., & Warsaw, M. (1978). *To live until we say goodbye.* Englewood Cliffs, NJ: Prentice-Hall.

Lieberman, M. (1965). Psychological correlates of impending death: Some preliminary observations. *Journal of Gerontology, 20,* 181–190.

Margenau, H. (1970). Science, creativity, and psi. In A. Angoff & B. Shapin (Eds.), *Psi factors in creativity* (pp. 78–84). New York: Parapsychology Foundation.

Maslow, A. (1959). Creativity in self-actualizing people. In H. Anderson (Ed.), *Creativity and its cultivation* (pp. 83–96). New York: Harper & Brothers.

Moody, R. (1975). *Life after life.* New York: Bantam Books.

Moody, R. (1977). *Reflections on life after life.* New York: Bantam Books.

Newman, M. (1979). *Theory development in nursing.* Philadelphia: F.A. Davis.

Osis, K. (1961). *Deathbed observation by physicians and nurses.* New York: Parapsychology Foundation.

Osis, K., & Heraldsson, E. (1977). *At the hour of death.* New York: Avon Books.

Palmer, J. (1979). A community mail survey of psychic experiences. *Journal of the American Society for Psychical Research, 73,* 221–251.

Pattison, E. (1977). The experience of dying. In E. Pattison (Ed.), *The experience of dying* (pp. 43–60). Englewood Cliffs, NJ: Prentice-Hall.

Rawnsley, M. (1986). The relationship between the perception of the speed of time and the process of dying. In V. Malinski (Ed.), *Explorations on Martha Rogers' science of unitary human beings* (pp. 77–83). Norwalk, CT: Appleton-Century-Crofts.

Ring, K. (1980). *Life at death: A scientific investigation of the near-death experience.* New York: Coward, McCann & Geoghegan.

Rogers, M. (1970). *An introduction to the theoretical basis of nursing.* Philadelphia: F.A. Davis.

Rogers, M. (1980). Nursing: A science of unitary man. In J. Riehl & C. Roy (Eds.), *Conceptual models for nursing practice* (2nd ed.) (pp. 329–338). New York: Appleton-Century-Crofts.

Rogers, M. (1986). Science of unitary human beings. In V. Malinski (Ed.), *Explorations on Martha Rogers' science of unitary human beings* (pp. 3–9). Norwalk, CT: Appleton-Century-Crofts.

Rogers, M. (1987). Rogers' science of unitary human beings. In R. Parse (Ed.), *Nursing science: Major paradigms, theories, and critiques* (pp. 139–147). Philadelphia: W.B. Saunders.

Rosen, J. (1955). The Barron-Welsh Art Scale as a predictor of originality and level of ability in artists. *Journal of Psychology, 39,* 366–367.

Sabom, M. (1982). *Recollections of death: A medical investigation.* New York: Harper & Row.

Tolstoy, L. (1960). The death of Ivan Illych. In A. Maud (Trans.), *The death of Ivan Illych and other stories.* New York: Signet Books.

Welsh, G. (1980). *Welsh figure preference test manual.* Palo Alto, CA: Consulting Psychologists Press.

Wheatley, J. (1976). The question of survival. Some logical questions. In J. Wheatley & H. Edge (Eds.), *Philosophical dimensions in parapsychology* (pp. 252–261). Chicago: Charles L. Thomas.

Reflections on Death as a Process:
A Response to a Study of the
Experience of Dying

Patricia Winstead-Fry

The impetus for these reflections was Dr. McEvoy's previous study, "The Relationships Among the Experience of Dying, the Experience of Paranormal Events, and Creativity in Adults." While Dr. McEvoy employs the standard Western scientific method to address the theory that interests her, her work makes an important contribution nonetheless and stimulated my thinking about death within Rogers' conceptual model.

These reflections can be grouped into three general areas which are addressed in subsequent paragraphs. There is no particular order to the listing and there is no necessary connection among the three areas.

PATTERN

Measurement is a hallmark and basic objective of Western empirical science. While Rogers' model deals with patterning as a process, measuring that process becomes problematic. According to Bateson and Bateson (1987), quantity does not equal pattern. In comprehending the idea of pattern vis-á-vis quantity, visualize a cup one-half full, the normal curve, and the Milky Way. Only the first pattern, the cup one-half full, is quantitative, but all three are patterns that we recognize. As a process, therefore, death probably cannot be quantified. However, such a conclusion does not lead to an impassioned plea for qualitative research. The concern is that we are asking appropriate questions. Method follows the question, not the other way around.

When dealing with death, another research problem arises as well: no one can be "objective." Death has touched or will touch each of us. As the cliche says, "One thing is for sure, none of us are going to get out of this life alive."

On the issue of appropriate questions, Wilber (1983) offers ideas that shed particular light. In writing about scientific proof, he states there are three basic "strands" for any proof to be judged acceptable. These are:

1. Instrumental injunction which refers to "If you want to know this, do this" (p. 44). For example, if you want to know the chemical composition of water, you must have certain equipment and learn to do electrolysis.

2. Intuitive apprehension refers to the cognitive grasp or experience of the data. Using the water example again, after you have performed electrolysis, you must collect the gases that are released and measure the volume of each gas.

3. Communal confirmation refers to replication. Can the community of scientists confirm or reject the findings? To continue with the water example, when other scientists do electrolysis of water, do they get two hydrogen molecules and one oxygen molecule? If the answer is yes, as it is in this case, the findings are verified. If the answer is no, then the findings are refuted.

Wilber (1983) continues to discuss three areas of study that are valued by seekers for a new paradigm with which to understand people: "sensibilia," "intelligibilia," and "transcendelia" (p. 39). Sensibilia refers to the objective world of the senses, the world where physics, chemistry, and the other empirical sciences operate successfully. For example, verification of the composition of water belongs to this realm.

When dealing with the realm of intelligibilia, we are dealing with thoughts. Verification or refutation involves the same three steps as just described. Wilber (1983) employs the translation of Egyptian hieroglyphics as an example. When the Rosetta stone was found, scientists knew that they had an opportunity to learn how to translate Egypt's ancient language and so began the process:

1. Instrumental injunction: If you want to understand a language, you look for the inner organization, or pattern, to the symbols. Usually many combinations are tried before the right one is found.

2. Intuitive apprehension occurs when the translation seems to make sense.

3. Communal confirmation requires that the translation be verified or refuted by other scholars.

Intelligibilia deals with meanings, values, and interpersonal processes. It encompasses mathematics, phenomenology, ontology, and other branches of philosophy, linguistics, and sociology. It is based upon a dialogue between the researcher and the object of study. (Empiricists don't talk with water molecules.)

Transcendelia refers to the realm of the spirit. Wilber (1983) uses Zen to illustrate the verification/refutation process within this realm, which follows:

1. Instrumental injunction: If you want to know the Buddha Nature, you must meditate and study with a certified Zen master.

2. Intuitive apprehension is the immediate perception of one's spiritual nature in a nonsensory and non-mental manner, such that the essential unity of being is experienced through contemplation.

3. Communal confirmation occurs when the community of Zen masters and meditators validate or refute the apprehension.

The empiricist who values only sense data would never allow intelligibilia or transcendelia to be considered scientific. However, to the extent that science is characterized by certain rules about proof, the argument can be made that the mental and the spiritual realms are science.

What does all of this have to do with death? Death is of concern to all three realms of human understanding. Appropriate questions can be asked in each realm. The question, "What is biological death?" gains a legitimacy in the domain of sensibilia. Within empirical-sensory science, death is the cessation of certain biophysical functions. The general acceptance of the Harvard criteria for brain death shows the success of a question asked and answered in this realm. We have quantified physiological death.

For nurses, who are charged to deal with actual and potential threats to health, a sensory understanding of death will not suffice, however. Nurses deal with the meaning of death, with death in the realm of intelligibilia. What does death mean to the person who is dying? What does it mean to the family? To the nurse? To society? These questions about meaning and interpersonal processes affect us personally and in our roles as clinician and scholar.

Rogers' (1970) concepts of energy fields and four-dimensionality fit well with the need to derive questions within the realm of intelligibilia. It should be intuitively clear that questions framed from the biomedical model, which is clearly within the realm of sensibilia, will never address the correct issues here. The concept of energy field allows us to conceptualize death as a process because fields by definition cannot end. Human beings can transform and change, but they cannot end. This is tricky, however, because so much of what we call life is really biochemical understanding of certain physiological processes or partial psychological theories that account for pathology better than they do for health. Our understanding of life as a patterned sequence of nonrepeating rhythmicities characterized by increasing diversity is just beginning. Nonetheless, the human as energy field concept is critical to understanding death. It allows us to go beyond the body (or the mind–body) and to a view of death as another developmental step characterized by increasing diversity, as are all of the other phases of life. To view death as a deviation from the principle of increasing diversity would place it outside the experience of human development.

Four-dimensionality allows us to treat time relatively. When people die, we often speak of "unfulfilled potential," "unrealized hopes," and "too little time." If time is relative, too much or too little time become fictions. The past, present, and future do not exist as discrete entities. Whether a person had enough time is not a relevant question. The question is whether the life process has been meaningful to the person.

Most nurses in their practice have met children who are about to die and who are wonderfully fulfilled. Prior to the understanding that time is relative, and, therefore, so is development, these children would have caused confusion. Yet they were able to console their parents and others and possessed a wisdom and sense of accomplishment beyond their chronological age. It is not possible, from the three-dimensional time frame, to explain these children. Obviously they had not lived long enough to express such maturity! Once it is understood that time is relative, however, the behavior of the children becomes more understandable. Development is not tied to linear time, but occurs at a pace that is "right" for the individual. These children had lived full lives because they had wisdom, compassion, and a sense of personal fulfillment. No doubt, this understanding does not erase or resolve the pain and loss consequent upon the death of such a child, but it does help when dealing with the guilt and helplessness.

Viewing death as a process and time as relative allows another question of increasing significance today: "Is there a right time to die?" Of course, people address this question in dialogue with their families and health care providers while, at the same time, courts of law are at pains to define its legality. Because some people may clearly decide that they want no extraordinary measures employed to continue physiological survival once personal meaning and interaction have ceased, the answer to this question might even prove cost effective. Allowing people to answer this question individually, rather than institutions (legal or otherwise), would certainly decrease questions about when the "plug" is to be pulled.

REINCARNATION

There is nothing so basic to Judeo-Christian culture than the idea that each of us is born with a uniquely individual soul. When the midwife slaps the newborn's bottom and the first breath is taken, we accept that an individual has arrived into this world. We then live a life that culminates in death and go on to some eternal reward; at least, that is the accepted view.

How different the view of Eastern traditions is. In these traditions, we live through a series of incarnations, as does the universe. There is hope that one will achieve enlightenment with this birth and end the cycle. However, except for rare saints, most people continue through many cycles of death and rebirth. A point of historic interest is that reincarnation was compatible with Catholic teaching until 553 A.D. when the Second Council of Constantinople repudiated it.

If one accepts reincarnation, as at least half of humankind does, then Dr. McEvoy's hypotheses make little sense. Her hypotheses were based upon the assumption that we have this one life in which to achieve whatever we are to achieve. Using Rogers' (1970) ideas that life leads to increasing diversity, McEvoy selected paranormal events and creativity as indicants of patterning and accepted Margenau's (1970) idea that the four-dimensional world is more available for some people at the time of death. Latent in the work is the idea that death is an end and that we will have more of some qualities when we reach this transitional state. But suppose death is not an end, but merely a milestone in the cycle of rebirth? Then there is no reason to think that dying persons will have more of some qualities than the non-dying. The evolution of the person occurs over millennia and changes in pattern or in quantities of characteristics may not be measurable during one lifetime.

To raise the issue of reincarnation is not an attempt to appear as a troublemaker or heretic to the scientific community. In recent years, the immigration of large numbers of oriental people to the United States makes some consideration of their beliefs and values necessary. It is also necessary to examine this concept for intellectual honesty. Death is a universal experience and there should be some universal concepts that can be derived to guide research and practice.

One of the most authoritative religious texts on reincarnation is *The Tibetan Book of the Dead*. The book offers a set of directions for the dying and for the time after death and before reincarnation (if that is to occur). For a Christian reading this book, an initial reaction could be, "This is bizarre! No one comes back from the dead, except Christ." For a Tibetan, however, everyone comes back from the dead many times. We don't remember our past deaths any more than we recall our current birth. However, our subconscious remembers everything. So it is logical that, through various meditative and yoga techniques, the subconscious can be made conscious. *The Tibetan Book of the Dead* is a synthesis and distillation of the collective experiences of generations of devout people. It may well meet Wilber's (1983) proofs for a transcendelia science.

The first part of the book deals with psychic happenings at the moment of death. Feelings of bliss and joy are described, as are the immutable light, Buddha and the shining void. One might feel as if he or she were reading Moody's *Life after Life* (1975) and question why he was not footnoted, only to be reminded that this book predates Moody by centuries. In terms of *The Tibetan Book of the Dead*, the actual process of death is most important because it is the most fortuitous time for achieving enlightenment.

The second part of the book addresses the state immediately after death. This state is dreamlike and there are predictable karmic illusions that occur. Again, the similarities to recent studies are impressive. Familiar and preferred gods may appear and there is radiant light. The third part deals with the "birth instinct," the desire to be reborn. Prenatal events are described, including guides for proper thinking such as the admonition not to be attached to worldly goods of your past life. Methods for closing the womb door on your new incarnation are offered as well.

The Tibetan Book of the Dead is fascinating from numerous perspectives. The idea that what is subconscious can be made conscious, a cornerstone of Western psychotherapy, is offered as the explanation for recalling previous lives. Descriptions are often very familiar. For example, the section in which rebirth is discussed states:

> If about to be born as a male, the feeling of itself being a male dawneth upon the Knower, and a feeling of intense hatred toward the father and of jealousy and attraction toward the mother is begotten. If about to be born as a female, the feeling of itself being a female dawneth upon the Knower, and a feeling of intense hatred toward the

mother and of intense attraction and fondness toward the father is begotton. (p. 179)

This is as clear a description of what is refered to as the Oedipal complex as can be found in an American psychology textbook.

As one reads and re-reads *The Tibetan Book of the Dead*, the profound respect for the "soul," the sensitive environment in which (ideally) one would die, and the tremendous impact and importance of the moment of death emerge clearly from the text. These concepts are compatible with Judeo-Christian beliefs and with contemporary research. As a result, these may serve as a bridge for transcultural understanding and humane care.

TRANSITION STATE

Dr. McEvoy makes an important distinction between the dying process and near-death experiences, referring to the dying process as a transitional state. In fact, when reflecting upon the research and practice in any transitional state, several similarities appear. Are they a crisis or not? Do they require medical intervention? Whether one is discussing the birth of a child or marriage, both major transitional states, the literature is replete with confusing claims about potential dangers and potential for growth. There is no doubt that a phenomenological study of transitional states that addresses both desirable states (such as marriage) and undesirable states (such as chronic illness) is needed to describe the phenomena and its characteristics. Currently, every discipline discusses these phenomena from their own purview without any real agreement about what the essential characteristics of the phenomena are.

If we could understand the basic nature of transitional states, interventions could be planned more sensitively. It is probable that education would be enhanced because each transitional state would not be treated as a totally new experience. People would be able to generalize from past experiences with other transitions to anticipate patterns. It might even be possible to decrease the fear engendered from a previous transitional experience that was negative.

In anticipation of the results of a phenomenological study, I will offer the perspective of one pattern emerging as germane to all transitional states: loss. Marriage involves loss of singleness; childbirth involves loss of some freedom; death involves loss of the ego-self. Regardless of the transition, there is some loss.

Reciprocally, whenever there is loss, there is also gain. In marriage, one gains a partner. With the birth of a child, one gains not only another family member, but a link to future generations. The gain involved with death is one that those of us in this mode of consciousness cannot experience; however, given reciprocity, the gain should be there if, that is, death itself is not an end to consciousness.

In summary, reflecting upon death raises important questions about the quality of the research questions that we ask. It challenges us to go beyond our cultural set and explore ideas such as reincarnation that will stretch our conceptualizations. I hope we can arrive at some universal concepts that will allow us to practice humanely and research wisely.

REFERENCES

Bateson, G., & Bateson, M.C. (1987). *Angels fear*. New York: Macmillan.

Evans-Wentz, W.Y. (Ed.) (1960). *The Tibetan book of the dead*. New York: Oxford University Press.

Margenau, H. (1970). Science, creativity, and psi. In A. Angoff & B. Shapin (Eds.), *Psi factors in creativity*. New York: Parapsychology Foundation.

McEvoy, M.D. (1987). *The relationships among the experience of dying, the experience of paranormal events, and creativity in adults*. Unpublished doctoral dissertation, New York University, New York.

Moody, R. (1975). *Life after life*. New York: Bantam Books.

Rogers, M. (1970). *An introduction to the theoretical basis of nursing*. Philadelphia: F.A. Davis.

Wilber, K. (1983). *Eye to eye*. New York: Anchor-Doubleday.

Response to "Reflections on Death as a Process"

Mary Dee McEvoy

Dr. Winstead-Fry's reflections, stimulated by the study "The Relationships among the Experience of Dying, the Experience of Paranormal Events, and Creativity in Adults," are thought provoking. It is interesting that she chose to concentrate on the dying experience, as opposed to creativity or paranormal experiences. The experience of dying is certainly the predominant theme of this work; its overall purpose is to describe the dying experience relative to paranormal experiences and creativity. Dr. Winstead-Fry reflects on pattern, reincarnation, and transitional states with the implication that Western science may not possess the appropriate tools to answer questions relevant to these concepts.

Certainly there can be little disagreement on this point, and her analogy of the water glass and its degree of fullness is appropriate. The fullness of dying is also of interest and may be related to transitional states. How does one know the fullness of dying? How does one know the time at which the transitional state is indeed being experienced, that is, when a dying person truly experiences dying. Few will dispute that humans respond differently to the knowledge that one is faced with a situation that will ultimately, perhaps sooner than later, bring one to experience dying. And there are multiple accounts of nurses relating that people know that death is near. Does it mean that such knowledge engages them to participate differently in the dying experience? It seems as though the concept of transitional states is intimately linked to the concept of participating knowingly. Such participation leads to the creation of an individual's transitional experience, no matter what type.

In reflecting on reincarnation, Dr. Winstead-Fry states that the hypotheses of the study imply that death is an end, at which point one will have more qualities (paranormal and creativity) than at other times. The study, however, was not to imply that death was an end, although it is true that the study was designed to determine if during dying people have different experiences of paranormal and creativity than when not in that transitional state. In fact, other researchers into the near-death experience point out that, although one can describe paranormal experiences, the meaning of them is unclear. Greyson (1983), in particular, states that near-death experiences do not reflect life after death. Paranormal researchers as well grapple with the question of proof of survival (Ducasse, 1976; Flew, 1976; Grosso, 1981). These are truly non-Rogerian concepts, however—"life after death" and "survival." The Science of Unitary Human Beings describes an energy field of wave pattern and organization. There is no survival of the energy field, one is the energy field. It is the nature of change in the field pattern that is of interest.

The concepts reflective of an experience of a field pattern of a particular type will continue to be delineated and specified by Rogerian scholars. It is my hope that dying as one example of a transitional experience will intrigue many into research, despite the difficulties. After all, a function of research is to search, and then, search again.

REFERENCES

Ducasse, C. (1976). How stands the case for the reality of survival? In J. Wheatley & H. Edge (Eds.), *Philosophical dimensions in parapsychology* (pp. 282–294). Chicago: Charles C. Thomas.

Flew, A. (1976). Is there a case for disembodied survival? In J. Wheatley & H. Edge (Eds.), *Philosophical dimensions in parapsychology* (pp. 330–347). Chicago: Charles C. Thomas.

Greyson, B. (1983). Toward a psychological explanation of near-death experiences: A response to Dr. Grosso's paper. *Anabiosis, 1,* 88–103.

Grosso, M. (1981). The cult of Dionysos and the origins of belief in life after death. *Parapsychology Review, 12,* 5–9.

17

The Relationship of Temporal Experience to Human Time

Jeanne Lynch Paletta

This study is an investigation of Rogers' (1983a, 1985) correlate of temporal patterning in unitary human beings in relation to Hugenholtz's (1959, 1972) time form, human time.

The purposes for the study were threefold:

1. To develop an instrument to measure the concept of temporal experience as a pattern representative of the developmental process of unitary human beings.

2. To test the relationship of temporal experience to human time within the framework of Rogers' (1985) *Manifestations of Field Patterning in Unitary Human Beings.*

3. To add to the base of empirically supported theory from which predictions can be made.

THEORETICAL FRAMEWORK

In Rogers' nonlinear world view, all activity is experienced as a whole in the relative present of human beings. The present is a dynamic and fluctuating experience which must be felt, sensed, and perceived as a holistic process. Rogers (1983, 1985, 1986a) proposed that the concepts of temporal experience and human time are both manifestations of the developmental process of holistic change and can be recognized by their patterns.

The construct of temporal experience was developed within the framework of human and environmental field process based upon the recognized phenomenon of subjective time awareness or time sense. This time awareness is perception of time as "passing" and evolves through a lifetime of continuous mutual processes, culminating in the individual's current pattern of time sense in relation to the environment.

Temporal development proceeds from experiencing movement in the environment in several modes: as passing slowly with time perceived as "dragging," to a more aware and complex experiencing of the change process as "time racing," to an even higher degree of complexity, where the temporal experience is perceived as "timeless" or at one with the environment rather than perceiving life events as moving past one.

As conceptualized by Hugenholtz (1959, 1972), human time is a characteristic form of interacting with the environment. It defines a time framework wherein the person is free to discover, to realize self, to broaden horizons, change, be creative, grow, expand and be flexible (Yonge, 1973, 1975). This concept presents an alternative to a clock and calendar view and allows measurement in relation to individual pattern.

Human time incorporates Rogers' postulated directions of increased diversity, creativity, innovativeness, and imagination. As a form of mutual process with the environment, it is a manifestation of the holistic developmental process. Time dragging is the least complex temporal pattern and would precede human time developmentally, whereas timelessness, which represents a more complex field pattern, is developmentally similar to human time. As time dragging and timelessness represent extreme differences in development, it was anticipated that an inverse relationship would exist in responses to these two patterns. The expected relation was postulated to range from a negative correlation of time dragging to human time, to a weak positive correlation of time racing to human time, to a strongly positive correlation of timelessness to human time.

Accordingly, this hypothesis arose: There is an increasing magnitude of relationship of temporal experience to human time from the direction of time dragging to time racing to timelessness.

Definitions

Involved in the hypothesis were these variables:

Temporal Experience. The continuous mutual process of the human field with the movement of events in the environmental field. It is measured by three independent scales which correspond to the postulated developmental direction: the Time Dragging Scale, the Time Racing Scale, and the Timelessness Scale. Collectively, the three scales are known as the Temporal Experience Scales (TES).

Time Dragging.   A human field pattern of experiencing the movement of events in the environmental field as slow, boring, tedious, leaden or dull. It is measured by the Time Dragging Scale (DRG).

Time Racing.   A human field pattern of experiencing the movement of events in the environmental field as immediate, swift, rhythmic, rapid, beating or fluctuating. It is measured by the Time Racing Scale (RAC).

Timelessness.   A human field pattern of experiencing the movement of events in the environmental field as infinite, never ending, flowing, continual or limitless. It is measured by the Timelessness Scale (TLN).

Human Time.   An experience of boundarylessness, openness, continuous change, creativity and innovation. It is measured by the Human Time Scale (HTS) of the Inventory of Temporal Experience (ITE) by Yonge (1973).

REVIEW OF THE LITERATURE

Related Literature

Review of the literature demonstrated the diversity of time, and the lack of studies with consistent results and direct relevance to this study. Temporal experience (the predictor variable) was supported conceptually.

Temporal awareness is a subjective experience with each person developing an individual rhythm. Human beings transform their experience of events into perceptions of relationships and change. In this sense, time is a construction of the human mind, relative to the process of becoming. Newman (1982) states, "as consciousness increases, an individual moves in the direction of timelessness" (p. 293).

Support for temporal experience is found in the agreement that subjective time is a unique, personal phenomenon, and not linked to objective time. The development of a subjective time sense linked to awareness is supported by Born (1965), Calder (1979), Fraisse (1963), Ornstein (1977), Piaget (1969), and Rogers (1986b). Support for the direction of temporal experience is mixed (Rawnsley, 1977; Wallach & Green, 1961), and was derived primarily from Rogers (1985).

Increasing complexity of development is associated with a changing subjective experience of time (Newman, 1982; Wallach & Green, 1961). Chronological age is not directly relevant to the subjective experience of time. The criterion is the degree of development achieved through the continuous mutual process of human and environmental fields, not age. The phenomenon of time flying by and years seeming to pass more quickly for the aged is frequently encountered in fiction and has been investigated in studies of aging and time relativity.

Problems with comparison of studies included differences in measurement techniques, the use of chronological age without measurement of developmental age, and the measurement of subjective time experiences by estimate of clock time. Conclusions of objective time supported the need to develop an instrument appropriate to subjective time and nonlinearity.

Several studies reported sex differences with females experiencing subjective time as passing more rapidly than males (t (72) $=$ 2.43, $p <$ 0.02) (Joubert, 1983). Yonge (1973) reported significantly higher scores for women on the Human Time Scale. Reports of sex differences warranted control of this variable.

The criterion variable, Human Time, emerges conceptually from the area of personality studies. In developing a link between personality and temporality, Hugenholtz (1959) formulated a theory of time to explain personal tempo as a vital factor in human existence. Four forms of time were identified as time structure differences in individuals from which personality variables and behaviors could be predicted (van Lennep, 1957): human time, animal time, vital time, and physical time.

Human time is a time of becoming. Its characteristics, as previously described, are consistent with Rogers' definition of unitary human beings (1986a).

Review of personality studies found that the majority were related to either objective time or time orientation, that is, orientation to past, present, and future—a linear framework. Support for the hypothesis was found by Barocas (1971) in a relationship of time passing slowly to high scores on the naturalistic-passive scale of the Time Metaphor Test (Knapp & Garbutt, 1958). Items from the scale were perceived as timeless by Macrae (1982). No direct relationship was found of time orientation to human time. Pedhazur (1982) states, ". . . theory is the best guide in the selection of criteria and predictors, as well as in the development of measures of such variables" (p. 137). Support for the hypothesis lies in the acceptance of the human time scale as appropriate for use in this framework by Rogers (1983b) and in the commonality of the concepts contained in the definitions of unitary human beings and of human time.

METHODOLOGY

Design

A descriptive correlational design was used in this study. Predictor variables included time dragging, time racing, and timelessness. Each of the scales contain eight metaphors rated on a five-point, equal-appearing interval scale. The criterion variable, human time, is a 34-item scale rated on a four-point, equal-appearing interval scale. Both correlational and regression techniques were used to determine the relationships among variables.

Sample

A sample of 120 volunteers who gave informed consent was used. The sample size allowed an alpha level of 0.05 and a power of 0.98, assuring the unlikelihood of either Type I or Type II errors (Cohen & Cohen, 1983).

Delimitations were based on the limited age range used in the development of both instruments, the presumption of cultural influence in temporality based on the literature, and sex, language, educational and occupational biases found during development of the temporal experience scales. Participants were limited to females, American born, ages 20–40, currently enrolled in graduate nursing courses.

Data were collected in classroom settings.

Instruments

The instruments used were the Temporal Experience Scales (TES), developed for this study, and the Human Time Scale (HTS).

Temporal Experience Scales.   Validity of the TES was established first by expert evaluation of the appropriateness of the metaphors, rating of the metaphors according to wave frequency by expert judges, classification of the items into patterns by use of the judge's mean score of the item and validation of the classification of the items included in each pattern by Dr. Rogers. The remaining items were rated by a sample of 305 male and female subjects of varied occupations. Principal factor analysis with iteration in an oblique rotation was selected to allow for the presumed conceptual correlation found in item analysis of total items. The Scree test was used to determine the strength of the factors (Thorndike, 1978, pp. 277–278). Three factors which met the criterion of an eigenvalue of 1.00 or higher after rotation were retained (Merrifield, 1983; Thorndike, 1978, p. 306). Items with maximum factor loadings above 0.30 were retained. The remaining items were reanalyzed with three factors and delta parameters of 0.00 to 0.6 calculated to compare various assumptions of factor correlation. Factor loadings, delta variations, item correlations, reliability, item-total correlations and judges' ratings were considered in selecting the final 24 items. The final factor analysis was performed using a delta parameter of 0.2 with 24 items (see Table 1).

The Time Dragging Scale (Factor 1) accounted for 50 percent of the variance. The factor eigenvalue after rotation was 4.86. Cronbach's coefficient alpha was 0.82120.

Table 1
Factor Reliability and Eigenvalues
$n = 305$

	Reliability	Eigenvalue
Factor 1	0.821	4.86
Factor 2	0.736	2.83
Factor 3	0.791	1.96

The Time Racing Scale (Factor 2) accounted for 29 percent of the variance. The eigenvalue was 2.83 and reliability was 0.73554.

The Timelessness Scale (Factor 3) accounted for 21 percent of the variance. The eigenvalue was 1.96 and reliability was 0.79108.

All scale items, in each of the scales, were significantly correlated to the total scale ($p < 0.05$ for $r = 0.15$ or higher, n of 305). Figure 1 provides a sample of the TES.

On the sample of the TES, items 1, 6, 10, and 11 represent timelessness; items 3, 4, 5 and 12 represent time racing; and items 2, 7, 8 and 9 represent time dragging. Item 2 is reverse scored as the DRG was bipolar.

Scoring is from 5 to 1 in the direction of *agree strongly* (5) to *disagree strongly* (1). Four items on the DRG are reverse scored.

The TES was tested for the influence of demographic variables (see Tables 2, 3, and 4). Language, education, and sex showed significant effects on one or more of the scales but accounted for only 2–3 percent of the variance. Professional nurses comprised 46.6 percent of the sample; sixty-three percent of the sample were female.

The most meaningful variances were found in the association of sex and occupation to all three scales. Sex shows a major effect on the DRG ($p < .001$), and accounts for 19.2 percent of the variance ($R^2 = 0.1923$). Occupation shows a stronger effect upon the TES with significant levels of $p < 0.001$ for both the DRG and TLN and $p = 0.05$ for the RAC. Occupation accounts for 30 percent of the variance ($R^2 = 0.3029$) on the DRG, 2 percent ($R^2 = 0.0217$) on the RAC, and almost 6 percent on the TLN ($R^2 = 0.0589$).

The TES showed validity within Rogers' conceptual framework and had acceptable reliability. The scales are suitable for administration to adults from 20 through 50 years with a need for control of sexual, language, educational, and occupational bias based upon the development sample. While age did not have a significant effect, data were collected for the study to validate the lack of relationship as predicted by the conceptual framework.

Figure 1
Temporal Experience Scales

Metaphors	AS	A	NO	D	DS
1. A Gull Motionless in Midair	——	——	——	——	——
2. Rolling Waves	——	——	——	——	——
3. Swinging Gate	——	——	——	——	——
4. Flame Swirling Up	——	——	——	——	——
5. Tornado	——	——	——	——	——
6. Floating Driftwood	——	——	——	——	——
7. Falling Rock	——	——	——	——	——
8. Carved in Stone	——	——	——	——	——
9. Automobile Crusher	——	——	——	——	——
10. Butterflies Hovering	——	——	——	——	——
11. Free Falling Skydivers	——	——	——	——	——
12. Space Shuttle	——	——	——	——	——

Human Time Scale. The Human Time Scale was developed by Dr. Yonge (1973) of the University of California at Davis as one of four independent scales in the Inventory of Temporal Experiences (ITE). Items were selected based upon the work of Hugenholtz (1959) at the University of Utrecht in the Netherlands, and van Lennep (1957). A sample of the items is presented in Figure 2. Content validity was established through personal consultation by Yonge with Hugenholtz (Yonge, 1984). Initially, items were written and administered to a group of 161 college students. Each item was analyzed for theoretical relevance to the scale and only items with a significant correlation to the scale were retained. The refined version was administered to 233 college students. Construct validity was established by correlation to tests measuring the concepts found in the definition of human time (Yonge, 1973). Significant ($n = 84$, $p < 0.01$) relationships

Table 2
One-way Analysis of Variance of Demographic Variables
with the Time Dragging Scale
$n = 305$

Variable	F	Significance	R^2
1. Age	0.947	0.4510	0.0015
2. Language	2.989	0.0198**	0.0307
3. Population of residence	2.316	0.0574	0.0006
4. Sex	41.813	0.0001**	0.1923
5. Education	5.683	0.0001**	0.0014
6. Occupation	11.804	0.0001**	0.3029

*$p = <.05$
**$p = <.01$

Table 3
One-way Analysis of Variance of Demographic Variables
with the Time Racing Scale
$n = 305$

Variable	F	Significance	R^2
1. Age	0.684	0.6359	0.0000
2. Language	0.729	0.5725	0.0081
3. Population of residence	0.147	0.9642	0.0009
4. Sex	4.738	0.0094**	0.0293
5. Education	1.264	0.2563	0.0001
6. Occupation	1.713	0.0283*	0.0217

*$p = <.05$
**$p = <.01$

Table 4
One-way Analysis of Variance of Demographic Variables
with the Timelessness Scale
$n = 305$

Variable	F	Significance	R^2
1. Age	0.929	0.4622	0.0046
2. Language	0.413	0.7989	0.0028
3. Population of residence	0.844	0.4983	0.0024
4. Sex	3.306	0.0380*	0.0206
5. Education	1.400	0.1875	0.0024
6. Occupation	3.189	0.0001**	0.0589

*$p = <.05$
**$p = <.01$

Figure 2
Inventory of Temporal Experiences

51. My future is what will take place "later on."

52. I have a hard time getting things done without deadlines.

53. I experience time as self-fulfillment.

54. I have an impatient craze for experiencing the ever-new.

55. My life contains a great deal of suspense.

56. I experience time as a source of freedom.

57. I experience time as everlasting growth.

58. I often find it hard to "get going" on something.

59. Very little seems stable and predictable.

60. I am often late because of trying to do too much at the last minute.

Adapted from the Inventory of Temporal Experiences (Yonge, 1973, 1975). Used with permission of the author.

---

were found of the HTS to the adjectives adaptable, imaginative, wide interests and outgoing from the Adjective Checklist (Gough & Heilbrun, 1980). The HTS showed significant correlation ($n = 62$, $p < 0.01$) to reflective thought, estheticism, and altruism on the Omnibus Personality Inventory (Heist & Yonge, 1968).

The HTS had a mean of 72.3 and a standard deviation of 15.0. Corrected split-half reliability was 0.82. Women ($n = 168$) averaged a higher score ($M_f = 74.0$, $M_m = 67.2$, $p < 0.01$)[1] than men.

The 34-item HTS is an independent scale within the Inventory of Temporal Experiences. Additional items were selected for this study from the 67 non-HTS items of the ITE scales using a random numbers table. These 26 items were randomly interspersed with the 34 HTS items resulting in a 60-question instrument. The non-HTS items were included to prevent recognition of the conceptual direction of the HTS items. As you examine these items, comparing them with the concept of human time, you can distinguish the HTS items (53–57) from the non-HTS items (51, 52, 58–60). As the scales were independent, no effect on scale reliability was anticipated.

---

[1] M_f refers to mean of female subjects; M_m refers to mean of male subjects.

The HTS provides a valid and reliable scale to measure the time structure of the individual. It is appropriate for use with young adults, male and female, of college age. It had not been used previously with older adults.

DATA ANALYSIS

Upon analyzing the data from the 120 study participants, the hypothesis received partial support. The zero order correlations (see Table 5) were in the direction and magnitude predicted: DRG to HTS, $r = -0.198$; RAC to HTS, $r = 0.141$; TLN to HTS, $r = 0.268$. Only the relationship of TLN to HTS was significant. As zero order correlations do not take intercorrelations of the variables into account, further analysis was performed.

Stepwise regression (see Table 6) was employed to test the power of the contribution of each predictor to the criterion. This method eliminates initially strong predictors that later lose their usefulness (Pedhazur, 1982; Volicer, 1984). The direction and magnitude of the relation of TLN to HTS was supported by stepwise regression analysis. TLN accounted for 7.08 percent of the variance ($n = 120$, $R = 0.266$, F (1,118) = 8.99, $p = 0.0033$). Stepwise regression neither supported nor refuted the direction and magnitude for RAC and DRG as these two variables showed a correlation of 0.448 ($p < 0.01$). DRG was inversely related to HTS as expected. DRG entered the regression equation second, rather than third, as predicted, accounting for an additional 2.74 percent of the variance ($n = 120$, $R = 0.31333$, F (2,117) = 6.36853, $p = 0.003$). RAC entered the regression equation third, or last, accounting for another 5.22 percent of the variance. In terms of the percent of variance, the magnitude and direction were: TLN, 7.08 percent; RAC, 5.22 percent; and DRG, 2.74 percent although the order of entry, or predictive strength, was TLN,

Table 5
Zero Order Correlations of Temporal Experience Scales (TES) to Human Time (HTS)
$n = 120$

TES	Correlation to HTS
Timelessness	-0.266**
Time racing	0.141
Time dragging	-0.194

**$p = <.01$

Table 6
Stepwise Multiple Regression of TLN, RAC, DRG and Age to HTS
n = 120

Variable	R	R^2	F	Significance
1. TLN	0.26608	0.07080	8.99067	.0033
2. DRG	0.31333	0.09818	6.36853	.0024
3. RAC	0.38782	0.15041	6.84526	.0003

DRG, RAC. The three predictors accounted for 15.041 percent of the variance and were significant at the 0.0003 level.

Supplementary analysis (see Table 7) indicated that age was *not* significantly correlated to either the TES or the HTS. Age did act as a moderating variable when added to the predictor variables, increasing the explained variance of the TES on the HTS by 4.01 percent to a total of 19.05 percent and increasing the significance level to 0.0001.

Reliability of the study sample was adequate for the TLN at 0.7836 and for the RAC at 0.7161. The DRG was below the acceptable level at 0.38. The reliability of the HTS was 0.88, higher than reported previously.

Cross validation of the standardized residuals indicated a significant correlation between the observed and predicted criterion scores. Shrinkage was not excessive and the distribution of the scores was close to normal, justifying the use of the regression analysis with this sample.

RESULTS

In interpreting the data analysis, the lack of a random sample precludes generalizing beyond the sample. Difficulty in interpretation of the statistical results is attributed to the strength of the negative correlation of DRG to both TLN and HTS, combined with the significant correlation of DRG

Table 7
Stepwise Multiple Regression of Age and Temporal Experience Scales (TES) on Human Time Scale (HTS)
n = 120

Variable	R	R^2	F	Significance
1. TES	0.38782	0.15041	6.84526	0.0033
2. Age	0.43650	0.19053	6.76700	0.0001

to RAC. The lack of independence of the DRG and RAC in the study sample distorted the findings. While there was unequivocal support for the relation of TLN to HTS, the predicted direction and magnitude of RAC and DRG were not confirmed. While the hypothesis was not fully supported, there is sufficient support of the relationship and of the TES to suggest that further testing is indicated.

The establishment of the DRG, RAC, and TLN supports Rogers' *Manifestations of Field Patterning in Unitary Human Beings* (1985) regarding temporal factors of time dragging, time racing, and timelessness. Factor analysis confirmed the existence of these three factors, which were further supported by the statistically significant multiple correlation of these predictors to the criterion of human time. The correlation of the TLN to the HTS provides further construct validity to both scales as it confirms the conceptual patterns developed by both Hugenholtz and Rogers.

The Time Dragging Scale is bipolar with 50 percent of its items reverse scored. Review of items indicated that the metaphors enduring, carved in stone, emptiness and rolling waves decreased reliability. The former three items may have been perceived as static by graduate nursing students familiar with the Science of Unitary Human Beings and the latter item as faster moving rather than slow.

Review of items from the Time Racing Scale indicated a decreased effectiveness of only one metaphor, a swinging gate. The image evoked may have been perceived as repetitious rather than fast moving.

Review of the items from the Timelessness Scale indicated that deletion of only one metaphor, free falling sky divers, would have raised the scale reliability from 0.79 to 0.81. Since the image of free fall seems consistent with the definition of timelessness, the experience of an external event influencing the imagery is a possible explanation. The use of metaphor in written form carries an inherent risk of change in the imagery evoked due to current events, such as the crash of the space shuttle or a recent death attributed to sky diving.

The drop in reliability of the DRG, coupled with its correlation to the RAC, demands further testing. The instrument development sample was larger and more diverse than the study sample, which may have contributed to the increased reliability with that sample. In contrast, the homogeneity of the study sample would decrease within group variance while the participants' knowledge of the Rogerian framework may have created a bias in their responses.

Analysis indicated that the outliers increased the reliability of the regression analysis. In conducting further studies, it may be advisable to consider this issue in selecting samples. In analyzing the scale statistics, it was anticipated that graduate nursing students would score higher on the Time Racing Scale, given the expected pattern of temporality for this population. Timelessness, in contrast, is the most complex form of temporality specified by Rogers, and it is probable that this pattern is less common in any population. The sample means ranged from 18.133 to 25.117 with a low mean of 18.133 for the DRG, a high mean of 25.117 for the RAC, and a mean of 19.917 for the TLN. Using Pedhazur's (1982) criterion of meaningful differences, this difference in the means of the RAC and TLN represents a meaningful difference (1.0) as does the difference between RAC and DRG (1.6). The TES does not provide a clear delineation of temporal preference, which would add further clarification to the field manifestation of temporality.

The Human Time Scale showed an upward change in reliability from 0.82 to 0.88. The mean score for the graduate nursing students was 75.2, just slightly higher than the mean score for undergraduate females in Yonge's study with a mean of 74.0 ($n = 168$). The range of age for female subjects was expanded to age 40 with effective results.

CONCLUSIONS

The conclusion drawn from this study include these elements:

1. The Temporal Experience Scales are predictive of human time ($R^2 = 0.15041$, $F (3,116) = 6.845$, $p = 0.0003$).

2. Age is not significantly related to the Human Time Scale but acts as a moderator variable. When added to the regression equation, DRG, RAC, TLN, and age account for 19.05 percent of the variance on the Human Time Scale ($R = 0.4365$, $R^2 = 0.19053$, $F (4,115) = 6.767$, $p = 0.0001$).

3. The Timelessness Scale was the most significant predictor to the Human Time Scale. TLN accounted for 47.07 percent of the explained variance using the stepwise regression model.

4. Timelessness was supported as a temporal pattern in Rogers' framework.

Recommendations

Recommendations for further study include:

1. Increase the reliability of the TES by increasing the number of items on each scale.

2. Investigate the applicability of the TES to a more diverse age range.

3. Investigate the TES for differences in males and females as reported in other studies of time experience.

4. Translate the TES to other languages to investigate possible cultural differences.

5. Investigate the relationship of the TES to constructs developed in Rogers' framework that have a logical relationship, e.g., the Human Field Motion Test (Ference, 1979). Wallis (1968), in discussing temporal experience, suggested that it may include a feeling of parallelism of internal movement with external change (pp. 18–19).

6. Construct a forced choice version of the TES to determine if there is a preferred form of temporal experience. This would provide a single score representing the dominant temporal factor.

7. As the TES is semiprojective in nature, the imagery evoked is subject to individual interpretation. A visual presentation using videotape or film would provide more consistent imagery and should add to the validity and reliability of the scales.

REFERENCES

Barocas, H.A. (1971). Temporal orientation, human response and time estimation. *Journal of Personality Assessment, 35*, 315–319.

Born, M. (1965). *Einstein's theory of relativity.* New York: Dover Publications.

Calder, N. (1979). *Einstein's universe.* New York: Viking Press.

Cohen, J., & Cohen P. (1983). *Applied multiple regression/correlation analysis for behavioral sciences.* (2nd ed.). Hillsdale, NJ: Lawrence Erlbaum Assoc.

Ference, H.M. (1979). *The relationship of time experience, creativity traits, differentiation and human field motion.* Unpublished doctoral dissertation, New York University.

Fraisse, P. (1963). *The psychology of time.* (G. Murphy, Ed.) (J. Leith, Trans.). New York: Harper and Row.

Gough, H.G., & Heilburn, A.B. (1980). *The adjective check list.* Palo Alto, CA: Consulting Psychologist's Press.

Heist, P., & Yonge, G. (1968). *Omnibus Personality Inventory Manual.* New York: The Psychological Corporation.

Hugenholtz, P.T. (1959). *Tijd en creativiteit.* Amsterdam: N.V. Noord-Hollandsche Uitgevers Maatschappij.

Hugenholtz, P.T. (1972). *Tijd en creativiteit* (Rev. ed.). Antwerpen: N.V. Noord-Hollandsche Uitgevers Maatschappij.

Joubert, C.E. (1983). Subjective acceleration of time: Death anxiety and sex differences. *Perceptual and Motor Skills, 57*, 49–50.

Knapp, R.H., & Garbutt, J.T. (1958). Time imagery and the achievement motive. *Journal of Personality, 26*, 426–434.

Macrae, J.A. (1982). *A comparison between meditating subjects and non-meditating subjects on time experience and human field motion.* Unpublished doctoral dissertation. New York University.

Merrifield, P. (1983). Personal communication.

Newman, M. (1982). Time as an index of expanding consciousness with age. *Nursing Research, 31*(5), 290–293.

Ornstein, R.E. (1977). *The psychology of consciousness* (2nd ed.). New York: Harcourt Brace Jovanovich.

Pedhazur, E. (1982). *Multiple regression in behavioral research.* New York: Holt, Reinhart and Winston.

Piaget, J. (1969). *The child's conception of time.* (A.J. Pomerans, Trans.). New York: Basic Books.

Rawnsley, M. (1977). *Relationships between the perception of the speed of time and the process of dying: An empirical investigation of the holistic theory of nursing proposed by Martha Rogers.* Unpublished doctoral dissertation, Boston University.

Rogers, M.E. (1983a). *Postulated correlates of patterning in unitary human beings.* Unpublished paper, New York University, New York.

Rogers, M.E. (1983b). Personal communication.

Rogers, M.E. (1985). *Manifestations of field patterning in unitary human beings.* Unpublished paper, New York University, New York.

Rogers, M.E. (1986a). Science of unitary human beings. In V.M. Malinski (Ed.), *Explorations on Martha Rogers' science of unitary human beings* (pp. 3–8). Norwalk, CT: Appleton-Century-Crofts.

Rogers, M.E. (1986b). Personal communication.

Thorndike, R. (1978). *Correlational procedures for research.* New York: Gardner Press, (pp. 277–278, 306).

van Lennep, D. (1957). The forgotten time of applied psychology. *Recontre, encounter, begegnung* (M. Langeveld, Ed.). Utrecht: Uitgerverij Het Spectrum, pp. 256–259.

Volicer, B. (1984). *Multivariate statistics for nursing research.* Orlando: Grune & Stratton, Inc.

Wallach, M.A., & Green, L.R. (1961). On age and the subjective speed of time. *Journal of Gerontology. 16,* 71–74.

Wallis, R. (1968). Time: Fourth dimension of the mind (B.B. Montgomery & D.B. Montgomery, Trans.). New York: Harcourt, Brace and World.

Yonge, G.D. (1973). Time experiences, self-actualizing values and creativity. *Journal of Personality Assessment. 39*(6), 601–606.

Yonge, G.D. (1975). Time experiences as measures of personality. *Measurement and Evaluation in Guidance, 5,* 475–482.

Yonge, G.D. (1984). Personal communication.

What Time Is It?
A Response to a Study of
Temporal Experience

Marilyn M. Rawnsley

This paper addresses the question of to what extent Paletta's (1988) study of temporal experience in relation to the construct of human time advances the cognitive, epistemic, and practical goals (Laudan, 1977) of the Science of Unitary Human Beings. In other words, how well does this study succeed in establishing knowledge useful in solving or identifying problems of nursing theory, research, and practice framed within the Rogerian conceptual system?

Ironically, space restrictions preclude discussion of all questions arising from my examination of this study. However, since in research, as in any open dynamic process, the impact of the whole cannot be appreciated through an analysis and summation of the parts, the holistic phenomenon of the study—the human experience of time—will constitute the focus of this response. I will also discuss the ways in which Paletta's study contributes to advancing knowledge of temporal experience relative to the constructs and principles of the Science of Unitary Human Beings with particular reference to (1) the substantive validity of the investigator's interpretations that form the theoretical basis of this study and (2) to the correspondence or "goodness of fit" between theory and method.

SUBSTANTIVE VALIDITY

Fascination with the enigma of time has been apparent since the recorded history of human thought. However, when a researcher selects to study a universal human concern like time, that researcher chooses the company not only of scientists, but also of philosophers and poets. Examining evidence gleaned through empirical objectification in the light of intuitive knowledge of philosophers and poets can be both enlightening and humbling; for to probe time's mysteries is to move in their common court. Pertinent to the study under consideration is the query of Augustine (1949) "where does time come from and by what means does it pass, and where does it go, while we are measuring it?" (pp. 276–277). This same question resonates through this investigation conducted, chronologically speaking, many centuries later.

In this study, the source of the human experience of time is said to lie in the continuous mutual process of human and environmental fields postulated by the Rogerian principle of integrality. The researcher specifies that time sense, or subjective time awareness, accounts for the perception of time passing. Such personal time sense is postulated as evolving in increasing complexity of patterning through a lifetime of continuous mutual process of human and environmental fields. This increasing complexity is said to be apparent in the subject's current pattern of time awareness which can be inferred from an individual's preference for words and phrases descriptive of the passing of time.

The researcher emphasizes that temporal experience is a function of the diversity and complexity of human field development and states that manifestations of individual development and the order of developmental change (presumably of the generic human field) can be recognized through identification of temporal patterns. These temporal patterns, taken verbatim from Rogers' correlates of unitary human fields, are stated as: time dragging, time racing, and timelessness (Paletta, 1988, pp. 4–7). Up to this point, I concur with these explanations. However, when the investigator further speculates that time dragging is developmentally precedent to human time, and that time dragging and timelessness represent a continuum of complexity in unitary human field development, we begin to part conceptual company.

It sounds strangely linear, in 1988, to propose that human time experience, conceptualized within the Rogerian framework, incorporates such a "from-to-" progression. The findings in my doctoral research (Rawnsley, 1977), in which I investigated the relationship of the speed of time in aging and dying, conceptualized within the Rogerian framework as it was written in 1970, suggested to me that perception of time passing, or temporal experience, might be a manifestation of increasing complexity of the human field. If it were such a manifestation, then it would be a rather predictable phenomenon for a given individual.

The proposition is further explicated in the following *relational statement*: If time sense is a manifestation of increasing complexity, and if the nature and direction of the development of the human field is toward increasing complexity and diversity, and if time experience is a manifestation of this maturational complexity, then, as a given human energy field matures, it will necessarily increase in complexity and diversity and time experience will proceed directionally and irreversibly from time dragging to time racing to timelessness.

That was my reasoning in 1977, and it sounds, on the surface, to be similar to the implied assumptions underlying Paletta's (1988) study. My proposition could have been tested by a longitudinal design and I considered doing so. However, Rogers (1983), true to the tenets of her theoretical system, evolved the principle of complementarity into the principle of integrality and my proposition was without meaning to the revised conceptual system.

Now, in light of the changes in the Science of Unitary Human Beings, a different proposition is warranted. Derived from the concepts and principles of the Rogerian conceptual system as explained in Paletta's (1988) study, such a proposition might read more like this *relational statement*: If persons are conceptualized as four-dimensional, unbounded, continuously patterning energy fields integral with four-dimensional, unbounded continuously patterning environmental fields, and if temporal experience is a relative phenomenon arising out of the continuous mutual process of these fields, then the reported temporal experience of a given individual is an assessment of the degree of change or intensity of patterning occurring in those integral fields at the point in space-time that the measure was taken.

To further explicate this argument, consider the insights of one of our poetic partners in time, Edna St. Vincent Millay (1941), who begins a sonnet with these words

> Time, that is pleased to lengthen out the day
> For grieving lovers parted or denied,
> And pleased to hurry the sweet hours away
> From such as lie enchanted side by side,
> Is not my kinsman; . . .
>
> (p. 101)

Now it could be argued that the poet is describing two sets of lovers; in the first set there are lovers whose individual human energy field patterning is less developmentally complex and diverse, and in the second set there are lovers whose respective human energy field patterning is developmentally more complex and diverse. With the same reasoning, it could be further argued that lovers whose fields resonate at similar frequencies are likely to fall in love. If this first set of lovers is less complex and diverse, then it can be speculated that they might have more difficulty mutually coordinating their relative space-time proximity and thus are more frequently parted and denied than their more complex and diverse counterparts who, resonating at higher frequencies, experience time as racing. This application of the Rogerian correlates of time experience not only ruins all esthetic sense of the poetry, but also strains the credibility of the conceptual system. Moreover, this explanation demonstrates the logical fallacies inherent in deducing from a false premise. It is unsettling to note that the theoretical basis of Paletta's study, with its literal interpretation of the Rogerian correlates of time experience, is consistent with this explanation.

Instead, consider St. Vincent Millay's poetry as a metaphorical illustration of integrality as previously defined in this paper. Then the time experience of these sets of lovers would be reflective of the degree of change, or intensity of patterning, in their respective human fields that occurs relative to their respective environmental fields when the patterning of the environmental field incorporates the presence or absence of the beloved. Furthermore, their reported time sense bears no connection to the complexity or diversity of their respective human fields. That is, it might be the same set of lovers being described, and relative to the environmental field conditions presented in this explanation, their temporal experience will pattern accordingly as a manifestation of the continuous mutual processing of human and environmental fields as postulated in the principle of integrality. Under the condition of blissful togetherness, the lovers perceive time as racing. In the next condition of separation, when, by conceptual definition each human field must be more complex and diverse relative to itself than in the previous condition, the same set of lovers perceive time as dragging.

It is important to note that it is not validity of the Rogerian conceptual system that is being addressed in this critique but Paletta's (1988) literal interpretation of its correlates of temporal experience. It is this literal interpretation which calls into question the substantive validity of this study. Further implications of this problem are addressed in relation to the correspondence or "goodness of fit" between the theoretical framework and the methodology.

GOODNESS OF FIT

Paletta (1988) demonstrates detailed concern for the statistical precision of her study. The data is exhaustively analyzed to substantiate the development of the instrument and to examine the findings relative to the hypothesis. The methodology is logically and comprehensively described so that an informed reader can evaluate the results and reach conclusions about the evidence for the increasing magnitude of relationship between the variables, as measured by the instruments in the sample studied.

However, the rationale presented for the selection of the sample was confusing to this respondent. Paletta (1988) states that "in Rogers' postulated patterns of development, age is not relevant to the subjective experience of time" (p. 12). If this statement is an assumption underlying the study, then why not present it as such, and dismiss it? Instead, a substantial portion of the literature review is devoted to studies in which age was a variable in time perception. Age of the present study sample was delimited to those between 20 and 40 years, and inexplicably for an irrelevant variable, its effects on human time are statistically analyzed. Also worthy of note was the lack of attention to the importance of gender and occupation apparent in the development sample of 305 subjects from whose responses the factor analysis and internal consistency of the instrument were derived. The connection among time sense, gender, and occupation were acknowledged by Paletta, yet the convenience sample of 120 in this study had a preponderance of those same demographic characteristics.

The investigator does give reasons for delimiting age to the same range used in developing the human time form and in 82 percent of the 305 subjects in the development sample who responded to the temporal movement scale. If instrument development were the sole aim of this study, then I would agree. Paletta states, however, that one study goal is to provide evidence of the validity of the Rogerian conceptual system by testing its concepts and their relationship—to which age is claimed to be irrelevant.

The dilemma here may be that the study is at cross-purposes within itself. Instrument development and verification of theoretical postulates of such an abstract conceptual system may not be feasible within a single study. Nevertheless, this study yields important considerations for future research within the Rogerian framework of nursing science.

It is clear that Paletta (1988) has provided support for concurrent validity between the instrument that she developed to assess temporal experience and the instrument measuring the construct of human time. Satisfactory reliability was demonstrated for the time racing and the timelessness scales. Paletta also claims construct validity for her tool and for the human time form. If she is restricting her definition to mean instrument construct validity, then I agree that she has done this, based on Cronbach's (1971) explanation of Nagel's views on the validity of theoretical entities as "descriptive, realist or instrumentalist" (p. 481).

In summary, the evidence for validity and reliability indicates that the temporal experience scales are measuring some variable or dimension, as is the human time form. But are they really describing Rogerian four-dimensionality? Can paper-and-pencil instruments, developed according to a method consistent with the logical positivist approach to justification of knowledge, capture the essence of such an abstract, holistic phenomenon? It seems reasonable to speculate that any paper-and-pencil measure reveals as much about Rogerian four-dimensionality as does a clock about space-time: both measures are artifacts.

This position presides here as well: The concepts and principles of the Science of Unitary Human Beings are not subject to verification by traditional methods of empirical science. This position is derived from my understanding of the processes involved in moving from an abstract conceptual system to empirical data. Briefly, the researcher working in the quantitative paradigm must develop and specifically state his or her own theoretical propositions for testing, and clearly link those propositions through explicit assumptions about reality that are logically consistent with the conceptual system. The study hypotheses are directly derived from the theoretical propositions in order to examine the degree of correspondence between the theoretical statements and the empirical data (Reynolds, 1971).

In the end, the study results can only support or fail to support the researcher's propositions about reality. Statistical significance of the findings does not in itself constitute substantive or theoretical significance. Whether or not the results of a given study have meaning for an abstract conceptual system is a function of the researcher's demonstrated skills in interpreting theoretical ambiguities of the system, in postulating relational statements that can be defended as logically consistent with its principles, and in avoiding an inherent hazard of "affirming the consequent." Managing these intellectual tasks is an impressive feat for experienced theoretical thinkers, not to mention doctoral candidates for whom a dissertation signals the commencement, rather than the conclusion, of a scholarly career.

The Rogerian Science of Unitary Human Beings, as it is currently structured, can be said to be prone to what Laudan (1977) identifies as "normative difficulties" (pp. 57–61), that is, its concepts and principles are in conflict with the methodologies of the dominant ideology of empiricism in the scientific community. Paletta's (1988) scrupulous attention to statistical procedures makes a significant contribution to clarifying cognitive and epistemic goals of the Science of Unitary Human Beings by illustrating that conflict.

What, then, is the nature of the knowledge that the Rogerian conceptual system seeks to explain? Is it really our experiences *of time* that are important to this nursing science, or is it our experiences *in time*? The answer to that question guides the choice of investigative method.

Let us look at a different domain's purpose in studying time. In his book, *A Brief History of Time,* Stephen Hawking (1988) tells us that his goal is nothing less than knowing the mind of God by breaking the code of the origins of the universe and thus of the beginnings of time. His method is the mathematics of theoretical physics, an elegant structure that does not pretend to explain the source of human wonder or the depth of human passion. So if—or when—Hawking succeeds in unraveling the mystery of how time began, the paradox of the human experience of awareness of self and mortality that emerges in, through, and perhaps beyond time, will remain unsolved.

CONCLUSION

It seems reasonable, then, to propose that unsolved problems of the mechanism *of time* properly belong in the domain of physics, while the investigations of lived experiences *in time* are appropriate for study within a human science like nursing. And while insights from one domain can be useful as analogy in another, they cannot be literally transposed, unless the foundational assumptions of the theoretical systems are the same. And if they were the same, there would be no need for separate sciences; both could be theories in the same science.

With this caution in mind, I find Hawking's (1988) proposal that spacetime may be finite yet unbounded useful, in a metaphorical sense, for suggesting questions to be explored within a Rogerian framework. For example, conceptualizing our human experience in time (i.e., our four-dimensionality) as finite but unbounded offers new ways of thinking about the construct of human memory, a patterning unique to individual fields, folding in and through itself, finite yet unbounded, contributing personal meaning to a life in time. Phenomenological and other qualitative inquiry approaches seem suited to this perspective, as do interpretative studies of classical and contemporary literature that might illuminate the four-dimensional characteristics of memory patterning that resonate across culture and generation. For researchers comfortable with quantitative analysis, a non-causal design that examines the association of memory to other nonlinear field correlates of the human experience such as creativity, compassion, diversity, or grief might generate data of heuristic value to the evolving Science of Unitary Human Beings.

Two points for further discussion are suggested here. First, insights from disciplines whose foundational assumptions about reality are different from those of the Science of Unitary Human Beings can be significant springboards for inspiration, but not suitable vehicles for determining variable definitions and hypothesis derivation within the Rogerian framework. Second, the possibilities for identifying and examining questions within the conceptual system may be finite, but they are also unbounded. Rogers' visionary thinking frees us to explore our existence without restrictions imposed by the artificial objectification of empirical methods that sacrifice individual meaning in the service of obtaining group means.

Whether a researcher chooses to pursue the study of our lived experiences in time through a qualitative or quantitative paradigm will more likely represent a field manifestation of the researcher's patterning than an index of the parameters of the Rogerian conceptual system. Regardless of choice, the concepts and principles of the Science of Unitary Human Beings are constructed to serve as guides to investigation and interpretation; they cannot be directly verified or refuted by scientific inquiry.

Bronowski's (1965) words lend fitting conclusion to this response: "Science is not a mechanism but a human progress, and not a set of findings but the search for them" (p. 63). Through this study on temporal experience and human time, Paletta (1988) has demonstrated her commitment to the human progress of nursing science. On behalf of all who are interested in advancing the cognitive, epistemic, and practical goals of the Rogerian Science of Unitary Human Beings, I applaud her achievement. Personally, I thank her for the opportunity for the intellectual challenge that has elicited this response.

REFERENCES

Bronowski, J. (1965). *Science and human values.* New York: Harper & Row.
Collected Sonnets of Edna St. Vincent Millay. (1941). New York: Harper & Row.
Cronbach, L.J. (1971). Test validation. In R.L. Thorndike (Ed.), *Educational measurement* (2nd ed.) (pp. 443–507). Washington, DC: American Council on Education.
Hawking, S. (1988). *A brief history of time.* New York: Bantam Books.

Laudan, L. (1977). *Progress and its problems*. Berkeley: University of California Press.

Paletta, J.L. (1988). *The relationship of temporal experience to human time*. Unpublished doctoral dissertation, New York University, New York.

Rawnsley, M. (1977). *The perception of the speed of time and the process of dying: An empirical investigation of the holistic theory of nursing proposed by Martha E. Rogers*. Unpublished doctoral dissertation. Boston University, Boston.

Reynolds, P.D. (1971). *A primer in theory construction*. New York: Macmillan.

Rogers, M.E. (1983). *Nursing science. A science of unitary human beings—a glossary*. Unpublished paper, New York University, New York.

The confessions of St. Augustine. (1949). (F.J. Sheed, Trans.). New York: Sheed & Ward, Book XI, chapter 21.

Response to "What Time Is It?"

Jeanne Lynch Paletta

In designing any research study, the investigator makes numerous decisions—perhaps even more so when attempting to test a postulate in the Rogerian framework. Dr. Rawnsley's critique of the study I conducted in 1988 raises questions that deserve a more extensive discussion than is possible here. However, I thank her for raising the questions on behalf of everyone who investigates phenomena within the Science of Unitary Human Beings.

This study intended to test and develop aspects of negentropic development of temporality: the postulated manifestations of time dragging, time racing, and timelessness. This required defining the concept and developing temporal experience as a construct. In so doing, the goal was to support or refute this "piece" of the framework. The decision to test temporal experience by developing and testing an instrument using psychometric theory and quantitative methodology was made with full knowledge of the difficulties in using traditional methods to investigate a complex phenomenon. Nevertheless, the use of newer and less accepted methods of investigation, which should require a more experienced researcher, were rejected in pursuit of acceptability within the values and standards of the broader scientific community. Dr. Rawnsley's (1990) suggestion that this choice is ". . . a field manifestation of the researcher's patterning . . ." raises the issue of cognitive style as a potential human field manifestation. The implication of a relationship of a logical analytic style's association with quantitative methods would be interesting to compare with whether a preference for qualitative methods is associated with a human relations, insightful, cognitive style.

The theoretical issues raised center primarily on "direction" within the Rogerian framework. Negentropy specifies a *direction* from less to more complex. This study proposes that the field manifestations *develop* in this direction. Neither the theoretical framework nor the hypothesis describe these manifestations as a continuum. While the direction of temporal development is addressed as negentropic, the complexity of the subject's patterning is placed solely within the subject's present. Time is not tested. Instead, the temporal experience of perceiving the movements of events in the environment as "time passing" is presented as a learned perception of reality as moving past one rather than the human experience of changing with environmental change. Temporal experience is described as continuously changing through the mutual process of the human and environmental energy fields. Placing temporal experience in the nonlinear present, without reference to either past or future, distinguishes this experience from a linear flow of time.

While the question of the relationship of time dragging, time racing, and timelessness to individual field pattern is of great interest, it was not possible to test this relationship within the scope of this study. Secondary analysis of the data indicates a decisive preference for any single factor does not appear. In fact, in almost all subjects in the sample data, all three factors were found. This finding is consistent with Phillips' (1988) suggestion that time dragging, time racing, and timelessness exist simultaneously. It is also consistent with the presence of multiple manifestations within the continuous patterning of the human energy field.

The possibility of a continuum of the fast to slow element was discussed in the findings (Paletta, 1988) in relation to Sanders' (1986) Time Experience Scales, which identified two factors of Fast Tempo and Slow Tempo. Additionally, the significant correlation of time dragging to time racing was discussed within a range of "possibilities" including simultaneity, scale deficiency, and failure to delineate two distinct experiences of time dragging and time racing in the study sample (in contrast to the larger and more diverse instrument development sample) (Paletta, 1988).

The instrument development sample revealed consistent differences by sex and occupation with differences due to education and language found only on the time dragging scale. The study controlled for these findings by delimiting the sample to single sex, single occupation, English-speaking, American-born, single educational level students. Age was not significantly related, as anticipated, but the age range for development for both instruments was restricted, requiring control of the sample age range.

Age was a major focus of the majority of the studies dealing with the phenomena of time passing, as was clock time. It was the mixed results, or failure, of these studies to support their hypotheses, combined with the recommendations of past studies, that led to decisions to eliminate any reference to clock time by developing a new instrument and to control statistically for the effect of age (Fraisse, 1963; Newman, 1982; Rawnsley, 1977; Wallach & Green, 1961). Age acted as a moderator variable on the effect of temporal experience on human time while chronological age was specified as "irrelevant" to Rogers' framework as a theoretical predictor. The correlation of chronological age to developmental status leads to its predictiveness, that is, age is significant not due to chronology but due to its strong association with development in the population. This indirect relationship is not predictive for an individual as the assumption of uniformity of development with age is unwarranted.

I can only conclude by thanking Dr. Rawnsley for stimulating reexamination of the conceptual relationships postulated and for creating new ideas and directions for further study.

REFERENCES

Fraisse, P. (1963). *The psychology of time*. (G. Murphy, Ed.) (J. Leith, Trans.). New York: Harper & Row.

Newman, M. (1982). Time as an index of expanding consciousness with age. *Nursing Research, 31*, 290–293.

Paletta, J. (1990). The relationship of temporal experience to human time. In E. Barrett (Ed.), *Visions of Rogers' science based nursing*. New York: National League for Nursing.

Paletta, J. (1988). The relationship of temporal experience to human time. *Dissertation Abstracts International, 49*, 05B, 1621. (University Microfilms No. 88-12-521)

Phillips, J.R. (1988, June). *Changing human potentials and future visions of nursing*. Keynote address. Presented at The Third Rogerian Conference, New York University, New York, NY.

Rawnsley, M. (1977). *Relationships between the perception of the speed of time and the process of dying: An empirical investigation of the holistic theory of nursing proposed by Martha Rogers*. Unpublished doctoral dissertation, Boston University.

Rawnsley, M. (1989). Response to "What time is it?" In E. Barrett (Ed.), *Visions of Rogers' science-based nursing*. New York: National League for Nursing.

Sanders, S.A. (1986). Development of a tool to measure subjective time experience. *Nursing Research, 35*, 178–182.

Wallach, M.A., & Green, L.R. (1961). On age and the subjective speed of time. *Journal of Gerontology, 16*, 71–74.

18

Guided Imagery within Rogers' Science of Unitary Human Beings: An Experimental Study

Howard K. Butcher
Nora I. Parker

A pretest/posttest control group design with 60 participants was used to examine the subjective feelings of timelessness, motion, boundarylessness, transcendence, and increased imagination experienced during pleasant guided imagery within Martha Rogers' Science of Unitary Human Beings. Two hypotheses were derived from Rogers' principle of resonancy, which describes "the continuous change from lower to higher wave frequency patterns in the human and environmental fields." Pleasant guided imagery was postulated to pattern the human energy field from a lower toward a higher wave frequency pattern. The hypotheses tested in this study were (a) participants experiencing an 11-minute pleasant guided imagery tape will have significantly lower time metaphor test scores than participants experiencing an 11-minute educational tape and (b) participants experiencing pleasant guided imagery will have significantly higher human field motion tool scores than participants experiencing the educational tape. Lower time metaphor test scores and higher human field motion tool scores reflect a higher wave frequency pattern of the human energy field. A significant treatment by trials interaction effect ($F = 4.358$; $df = 1/118$;

Used with permission of *Nursing Science Quarterly* Vol. 1, pp. 103–110. Copyright © 1988 Williams & Wilkins.

$p < 0.05$) provided support for the first hypothesis. The second hypothesis was not supported. On the basis of a factor analysis, the validity of the human field motion tool is questioned. The findings suggest that Rogers' principle of resonancy may provide an explanation of the subjective feelings experienced during pleasant guided imagery.

Pleasant guided imagery is one of a variety of relaxation techniques used by nurses and other health care professionals to assist patients to cope with stress, anxiety, and pain (Achterberg & Lawlis, 1982; Girdano & Everly, 1979; Guzzetta & Dossey, 1984; Korn & Johnson, 1983; Krieger, 1981; McCaffery, 1979; Sodergren, 1985). Participants experiencing pleasant guided imagery often report sensations of time standing still, or timelessness; weightlessness, or floating; motion; feelings of expansion, radiating outward or boundarylessness; and feelings of increased imagination and creativity (Dossey, 1982; Girdano & Everly, 1979; Korn & Johnson, 1983; Ludwig, 1966; Samuels & Samuels, 1975).

Although a number of studies have investigated the effect of guided imagery on anxiety (Korn & Johnson, 1983; McCaffery, 1979; Sodergren, 1985), the subjective feelings experienced during pleasant guided imagery have not been investigated. In other words, although pleasant guided imagery is used in nursing practice for the purpose of promoting relaxation, there is little understanding of the subjective feelings experienced by patients, and no theoretical interpretation is available that would guide the development of pleasant guided imagery as a nursing intervention.

The purpose of this study was to examine the experience of pleasant guided imagery within Rogers' (1970, 1980, 1986, 1987) Science of Unitary Human Beings. Specifically, this study tested two hypotheses derived from Rogers' (1987) principle of resonancy to determine the effect of pleasant guided imagery on time experience and human field motion.

PLEASANT GUIDED IMAGERY

Imagery is the basis of thought processes (Korn & Johnson, 1983). Imagery is a universal, inescapable activity integral to the life process of human beings. One can imagine daily in the form of daydreams, fantasies, and mental pictures. In the mind's eye, humans can visualize memories of past events, imagine future situations, daydream of what may be or might have been, or dream of vividly textured happenings beyond the bounds of space and time (Samuels & Samuels, 1975).

Imagery techniques in health care may be the most ancient healing techniques used by man (Samuels & Samuels, 1975). Guided imagery is defined as the purposeful or therapeutic use of mental images to achieve a specific, desired, or therapeutic goal (McCaffery, 1979). Achterberg and Lawlis (1982) define guided imagery as internal representations of events involving the senses that serve as a bridge between body and mind. All sensory modalities are involved in imagery: visual, tactile, auditory, olfactory, and kinesthetic. Scenes commonly used to promote relaxation include guiding the participant to visualize sitting on a hillside watching a sunset, lying in a field watching clouds float by, sitting on a warm beach watching the sea, sitting by a fire on a snowy evening, or floating through water or through space (Sodergren, 1985). Several pleasant images, such as a beach, mountain, or meadow scene, have been standardized by Kroger and Fezler (1976). While experiencing pleasant guided imagery, the participant is alert, concentrating intensely, and imaging all the sensory images described by the guide (McCaffery, 1979). The participant becomes totally absorbed, participating with his/her whole being, visualizing the scene as if it were real. Most often, pleasant guided imagery is designed to promote feelings of tranquility, peace, calmness, and relaxation.

THEORETICAL FRAMEWORK

Within Rogers' science, the unitary human being is viewed as a four-dimensional, negentropic, irreducible energy field engaged in a continuous, mutual process with the four-dimensional, negentropic environmental energy field. Both the human and environmental fields are identified by patterns (Rogers, 1986). New patterns emerge from the mutual process of the human and environmental fields.

The postulate of Rogers' system relating most directly to the study of the subjective feelings experienced during pleasant guided imagery is the principle that there is a "continuous change from lower to higher frequency wave patterns in human and environmental fields" (Rogers, 1987, p. 144). Rogers (1983) postulates the following seven manifestations of human field patterning, which emerge out of the human-environmental energy field mutual process:

1. Movement from lower frequency waves to higher frequency waves and then toward waves that seem continuous.
2. Movement from longer rhythms to shorter rhythms toward rhythms that seem continuous.
3. Time perceived as dragging through time perceived as racing and then toward the experience of timelessness.
4. Movement from slower through faster motion toward motion that seems continuous.
5. Sleeping through increased wakefulness toward beyond waking.

6. Movement from pragmatic through imaginative toward visionary.

7. Movement from less toward more diversity.

Given Rogers' (1987) principle of resonancy and the postulated changes in patterning that emerge from the human-environmental energy field process, the authors' hypothesized that the subjective feelings of timelessness, motion, and increased imagination experienced during pleasant guided imagery may be a manifestation of a change from a lower to a higher frequency wave pattern in the human field.

Pleasant guided imagery is a four-dimensional energy pattern, a manifestation of four-dimensional reality. Four-dimensionality is defined as a nonlinear domain without temporal or spatial attributes (Rogers, 1987). Any image is reality for the person experiencing it. According to Rogers (1970), everything is an energy field pattern. All matter is pure energy vibrating at different rates of speed and thus has different qualities, from finer to denser. Consciousness, imagery, or visualization are relatively fine forms of energy and therefore can change quickly. The evolutionary idealistic view of consciousness discussed by Sarter (1988) provides support for the Rogerian conceptualization of imagery as an energy field manifestation. The pleasant guided imagery scene that participants were guided through in this study originated in the environmental energy field. When the participant visualized the image, the visualizations occurred within the human energy field. This conceptualization views the human and environmental energy fields as being integral to one another. It is assumed that the wave frequency pattern of pleasant guided imagery, originating in the environmental energy field, resonates with the human field pattern and has a potential to participate in patterning of the human field toward a higher wave frequency pattern.

The hypothesis tested in this study was that participants who experienced pleasant guided imagery would demonstrate higher wave frequency. patterns (as measured on two instruments: the time metaphor test (TMT) and the human field motion tool (HFMT)) than the participants in a control group who experienced an educational tape on imagery. This hypothesis was reduced to two operational hypotheses as described below.

METHODOLOGY

Design

A pretest/posttest control group design was used to test the following two operational hypotheses:

1. Participants experiencing the pleasant guided imagery tape will have significantly lower posttest scores on the TMT than the participants in a control group.

2. Participants experiencing the pleasant guided imagery tape will have significantly higher posttest scores on the HFMT than participants in a control group.

Significantly lower posttest scores on the TMT and higher scores on the HFMT are assumed to reflect patterning of the human energy field toward a higher wave frequency pattern. Sixty adult subjects were randomly assigned to an experimental or control group to test the above hypotheses.

Instrumentation

Demographic Data. Each participant completed a short questionnaire identifying age, gender, and educational level.

Time Metaphor Test. Time experience in this investigation was measured by the TMT (Knapp & Garbutt, 1958), which consists of 25 metaphors. The factorial validity is evident in Knapp and Garbutt's (1958) and Wallach and Green's (1961) analyses. They report one factor described as a "swift to static" meaning of time. The factor structure remained consistent even when Wallach and Green (1961) performed a separate factor analysis on each of the four groups in their study. In assessing for the reliability of the tests, Wallach and Green (1961) obtained a Kuder-Richardson formula 20 value of 0.95. The TMT has been used in a number of studies testing hypotheses derived from the principles of Rogers' science of unitary human beings (Ference, 1979; Macrae, 1982; Rawnsley, 1986).

The loading weights reported by Wallach and Green (1961) were used for scoring the TMT in this study. Each metaphor was given a pretest rating from 25 to 1, with the weight of 25 points to the swiftest metaphor and 1 point to the most static. The method for scoring the TMT has gradually changed. Ference (1979) suggested that participants should place a check next to the five metaphors from the list that most closely reflected how time seemed to be passing at the moment. Using the weight assigned to each item by Wallach and Green (1961), each subject's total score was computed by adding up the rank number of the item. Using a similar scoring format, Ference (1979) obtained a Kuder-Richardson formula 20 value of 0.99. Macrae (1982) suggested that the simpler format allows for faster reporting so that the participant can proceed more rapidly to the HFMT, thereby minimizing the loss of valuable information as the participants return to their "normal state."

The summed scores on the TMT were considered interval data (Macrae,

1982). A high score on the TMT would indicate that time was perceived as moving quickly whereas a low score would indicate a perception of time moving slowly.

Important to note is the interpretation of low TMT scores. Within the science of unitary human beings, a low score on the TMT does not reflect time dragging but rather a sense of timelessness. The slow-rated metaphors, "a vast expanse of sky" and "a quiet motionless ocean" describe a nonlinear domain that represents the experience of timelessness and a more direct experience of a four-dimensional reality (Macrae, 1982). Thus, the lower the score on the TMT, the greater the sense of timelessness. This in turn reflects a higher wave frequency pattern of the human energy field.

Human Field Motion Tool. The HFMT developed by Ference (1979) was designed to be an indicator of the continuously moving position and flow of the human field pattern and to measure relative states of human field motion through a series of semantic differential scales judged to elicit responses ranging from lower to higher frequency. In developing the HFMT, Ference (1979) submitted 64 words that comprised 32 scales to a panel of judges who were considered to have expert knowledge of Rogers' framework. The judges were asked to determine the validity and the relative direction of the bipolar descriptors. Twenty-three of the scales were original semantic differential scales reported by Osgood and Suci (1955). Nine additional bipolar pairs that were postulated to be associated with lower and higher wave frequency patterning according to Rogers' conceptual system were added. In a pilot study, 43 subjects rated three concepts against the 32 scales. Two concepts ("my motor is running" and "my field expansion") and 13 scales were retained as a measure of human field motion. Because some scales were rated on both concepts, the total number of scales in the tool is 20. The HFMT was then submitted to 213 subjects, and the results were factor analyzed. Three factors emerged, activity, potency, and evaluation, as predicted, and each scale was loaded on at least one factor. Ference (1986) indicates that the analysis "provides factorial validity of the tool and supports the principle of resonancy" (p. 99). Barrett (1983) also factor analyzed the HFMT ($n = 266$). Initially, "my motor is running" and "my field expansion" were factor analyzed together. Five factors (eigenvalues > 1.0) were obtained. "My motor is running" loaded on factors one and three, "my field expansion" scales on factors two and four. The fifth factor had only one salient scale. Barrett (1983) states that "this provided evidence of construct validity by supporting the theoretical position that 'my field expansion' and 'my motor is running' are two different HFM [human field motion] concepts" (p. 40).

Of the instrument's 20 semantic differential scales, only 16 are actually used in the scoring. Eight scales are rated on the concept "my motor is running" and eight scales are rated on the concept "my field expansion." Three scales are incorporated as retest items and one scale is included for balance. The semantic differential scales composing the HFMT are assigned values from 1 to 7 in the direction of a shorter and higher wave frequency pattern.

The HFMT score is obtained by computing the individual's average score for the 16 semantic differential scales. A linear relationship is assumed to exist between the test score and the relative motion of the human energy field: the higher the HFMT score, the higher the wave frequency pattern of the human field.

Ference (1979) reported the test–retest reliability as 0.77 in a pilot test and 0.70 in a main study. The part-whole correlations of each scale ranged from 0.51 to 0.77. The correlation of the score of each concept to the total test score is 0.87 for both concepts of "my motor is running" and "my field expansion" (Ference, 1979). The HFMT has been used in a number of studies testing hypotheses derived from Rogers' conceptual system (Barrett, 1986; Gueldner, 1986; Ludomirski, 1984; Macrae, 1982).

Posttest Guided Imagery Questionnaire.   Participants in the experimental group completed a short questionnaire that provided verbal descriptions of their guided imagery experience.

Posttest Control Group Questionnaire.   Participants in the control group completed a short educational questionnaire consisting of five true or false questions concerning the information on the control group tape and an open-ended question asking participants to describe how they felt while listening to the tape. Participants were told that if they were in the educational group, there would be a short recall test. The test was administered as an incentive to help assure that participants experiencing the educational tape would be alert and concentrating on the information on the tape and thus limit the possibility of subjects becoming bored, falling asleep, or experiencing spontaneous daydreams.

Sample

The sample was composed of 60 volunteer adult, full-time staff members from a large community hospital; 30 were randomly assigned to each group. All participants were 18 years or older, had a minimum of a high school diploma, were able to read and speak English, were not on any mood- or consciousness-altering medications, and had no history of meditative experience. All participants were assumed to have normal hearing.

Laboratory Setting

Each participant was tested individually in a 12 × 12 × 7-foot office located in the hospital. The room was in a quiet area and had no windows or clock and few decorations. Temperature was kept constant between 72 and 74°F throughout testing of all participants. A 60-watt shaded desk lamp was kept on at all times to create a slightly darkened atmosphere. Each subject sat in a well-padded reclining chair in the upright position.

Procedure

After approval from the university ethics committee and hospital's research review committee, a notice was posted throughout the hospital briefly describing the study. Interested individuals contacted the researcher, signed the appropriate consent form, and were scheduled for testing. Participants were told that they would listen to one of two tapes. Each participant in the experimental group listened to an 11-minute tape that described a peaceful meadow and beach scene. The length of the pleasant guided imagery tapes may vary from as brief as 5 minutes to as long as 20 minutes (McCaffery, 1979). Most standardized images are 10 to 15 minutes in length. In this study, the 11-minute length was chosen because participants had not previously experienced pleasant guided imagery, and a longer tape may lessen the participants' ability to concentrate intensely on the images described on the tape. The taped image included descriptions of the pleasant smells of flowers, the gentle sounds of waves, the warmth of the sun, the coolness of water, the softness of grass, and the warmth of beach sand. The quality of the tape was judged by a qualified and highly experienced psychologist who is an expert in guided imagery techniques. The script of the tape was adapted from Turk, Meichenbaum, and Genest (1983, pp. 286–288).

Each participant in the control group listened to an 11-minute educational tape explaining the theory and practice of guided imagery. The purpose of the educational tape was to provide a controlled activity for 11 minutes and to keep the subjects from experiencing pleasant imagery. The investigator recorded both tapes; thus, each participant listened to the same voice. Participants did not know whether they were in the control or experimental group. Once in the testing room, participants were instructed to sit in the reclining chair, complete the pretest TMT and HFMT, and then listen to the tape through the headphones on the Sony Walkman. The control for the volume was constant for all participants. At the end of the tape, participants completed the post-TMT and -HFMT.

Because the TMT may be completed much more quickly than the

HFMT, Macrae (1982) had participants complete the TMT first and then the HFMT immediately after meditation in order to prevent the loss of valuable information as participants return to a more "normal" state. Since guided imagery is similar to meditation, all participants in this study completed the TMT first and the HFMT second during both pre- and post-testing. After the instructions were given, the researcher left the room and met the participant outside the room after the posttest questionnaires were completed.

FINDINGS

All 60 participants included in the study met the sample selection criteria. The participants were employed in a wide variety of hospital departments, including social work, dietary, pharmacy, housekeeping, communications, and finance, and 43 percent of the participants were employed in the nursing department. Only 4 of the 60 participants were men. The demographic data are summarized in Table 1. There were no significant differences between the two groups with respect to age, gender, or educational level. The means, standard deviations, and variance on pre- and post-TMT and -HFMT scores are summarized in Table 2. The absence of significant differences on the pretest scores gave additional assurance that random assignment had resulted in the groups' equality on the independent variables.

Both hypotheses were tested by a repeated measures analysis of variance, the most appropriate analysis for a pretest/posttest design (Gray & Rudy, 1981; Nunnally, 1975; Shelly, 1984; Volicer, 1984). In this analysis, the interaction effect examines whether there are significant differences in pretest/posttest scores between experimental and control groups (Keppel, 1982; Nunnally, 1975; Volicer, 1984; Winer, 1962).

Time Metaphor Test

The mean post-TMT score was 42.033 in the experimental group and 57.100 in the control group. The data analysis revealed (see Table 3) that the interaction effect was significant ($p < 0.05$) and thus supported the first hypothesis. Participants experiencing the pleasant guided imagery tape did have significantly lower scores on the post-TMT than those participants experiencing the educational tape. Participants in the experimental group selected more of the nonlinear, timeless metaphors and thus had significantly lower posttest scores than participants in the control group. Within the science of unitary human beings, a low score, indicating a greater sense of timelessness, reflects a higher wave frequency pattern.

Table 1
Distribution of Demographic Variables by Frequency in Total Sample and in Groups

Variable	Sample	Control	Experimental
Gender			
Male	4	3	1
Female	56	27	29
Age (years)			
18–33	21	9	12
34–49	34	16	18
50–65	5	5	0
Educational level			
High school	15	9	6
Community college	28	13	15
University	17	8	9

Human Field Motion Tool

The second hypothesis, that participants experiencing the pleasant guided imagery tape will have significantly higher post-HFMT scores than those participants experiencing the educational tape, was not supported. The mean pre-HFMT score for the experimental group was 5.244 and for

Table 2
Overall Means and Standard Deviation of Pre- and Posttest Scores on Time Metaphor and Human Field Motion by Subject Group

Group*	Mean	SD	F	p
Pretest time metaphor				
Control	68.933	24.790		
Experimental	69.133	20.656	0.001	0.9730
Posttest time metaphor				
Control	57.100	19.658		
Experimental	42.033	14.476	11.427	0.0013
Pretest human field motion				
Control	5.477	0.709		
Experimental	5.244	0.629	1.818	0.1829
Posttest human field motion				
Control	5.225	0.873		
Experimental	5.290	0.817	0.008	0.7683

*n = 30 in all groups.

Table 3
Repeated Measures Analysis of Variance on Pre- and Post-TMT Scores

Source of Variation	Sum of Squares	df	Mean Square	F	p
Total	55,242.6	239			
Between subjects	25,019.6	119			
Conditions	828.8	1	828.8	<1	NS
Error between	242,190.8	118	2,052.46		
Within subjects	30,223.0	120			
Pre-/post-TMT	5,684.3	1	5,684.3	28.34	0.001
Pre-/post-TMT × Cond.*	874.0	1	874.0	4.358	0.05
Error within	23,664.7	118	200.55		

*Conditions = guided imagery tape vs. educational tape.

the control group was 5.477. The mean post-HFMT score was 5.290 in the experimental group and 5.225 in the control group. Neither the main nor interaction effects were significant (see Table 4).

Closer analysis of the scales on the HFMT using t-tests comparing the differences between pretest and posttest scores between the experimental and control groups showed that the experimental group had significantly higher scores on only two of the scale items (dark-bright and weak-strong) under "my field expansion." In addition, although the differences were not statistically significant, this analysis also showed that the differences in scores on those scales that appeared to most closely represent Rogers' mani-

Table 4
Repeated Measures Analysis of Variance on Pre- and Post-HFMT Scores

Source of Variation	Sum of Squares	df	Mean Square	F	p
Total	5190.53	239			
Between subjects	5170.53	119			
Conditions	0.11	1	0.11	<1	NS
Error between	5170.42	118	43.817		
Within subjects	20.00	120			
Pre-/post-HFMT	0.15	1	0.15	<1	NS
Pre-/post-HFMT × Cond.*	0.36	1	0.36	2.18	NS
Error within	19.49	118	0.165		

*Conditions = guided imagery tape vs. educational tape.

festations of patterning (unimaginative-imaginative, pragmatic-visionary, limited-boundaryless, finite-transcendent) were higher in the experimental group. However, the dull-sharp, drag-propel, and passive-active scales showed lower score differences. Because of these observations, the validity of the tool seemed in question and a varimax rotated factor analysis of the pre-HFMT scores was done. In this study, factor analysis identified five factors. Ference's (1979) original factor analysis identified three factors. In addition, some of the participants expressed difficulty in understanding the terminology and directions on the HFMT. For example, participants had difficulty understanding the concepts "my motor is running" and "my field expansion." Some participants did not conceptualize "field" as a human field but rather as a "farmer's field."

On the posttest guided imagery questionnaire, subjects experiencing pleasant guided imagery reported feelings of floating, motion, timelessness, relaxation, calmness, and peacefulness. However, on the posttest control group questionnaire, participants reported feeling alert, attentive, and comfortable.

DISCUSSION

The investigators postulated that pleasant guided imagery may participate in patterning of the human energy field from a lower to a higher wave frequency pattern. The results from the study are inconclusive. Participants experiencing pleasant guided imagery scored significantly lower on the TMT than participants in the control group. The support of the first hypothesis provides empirical evidence of the anecdotal reports in the literature (Girdano & Everly, 1979; Dossey, 1982; Korn & Johnson, 1983) describing feelings of timelessness during pleasant guided imagery. The support of the first hypothesis suggests that the pleasant guided imagery tape, as an environmental wave frequency manifestation, had a significant impact in patterning the human energy field toward a higher wave frequency pattern as measured by the TMT.

On the other hand, the second hypothesis was not supported. There was no significant difference in pretest and posttest scores on the HFMT between participants experiencing the pleasant guided imagery tape and those experiencing the educational tape. Closer examination of the individual scales comparing the HFMT, as well as concerns regarding the terminology and directions expressed by subjects in the study, raised questions as to the validity of the tool. A factor analysis of the tool indicated that dimensions other than the two major concepts identified by Ference (1979) are incorporated in the tool. It is questionable whether all items on the HFMT are consistent with Rogers' Science of Unitary Human Beings. For example, the dull-sharp scale presupposes an edge or boundary. However, within the Rogerian system, pleasant guided imagery is without boundaries. Also, the active-passive and the drag-propel scales seemed confusing to participants. Relaxation suggests an active form of passivity and a stillness in motion. As Macrae (1982) pointed out, participants would tend to mark the middle of the scales to solve the paradox. Macrae (1982) used the HFMT while studying subjects who meditate and suggested that the active-passive, dull-sharp, and drag-propel scales may not be appropriate for the investigation of meditative experiences and do not seem consistent with a four-dimensional framework, an interpretation supported by this study.

Differences in the educational level of participants may have also contributed to the the lack of definitive results on the HFMT. In Ference's (1979) sample of 213 subjects, only 4 percent had no college degree. Only one participant in this study had a master's degree, whereas 60 percent of the subjects in Ference's study had either a bachelor's or master's degrees, and 24 percent had doctoral degrees. The HFMT needs to be modified for use in populations with less formal education if it is to be useful in measuring human field motion. As Clarke (1986) has pointed out, there are significant difficulties and problems of measurement when using a Rogerian framework for research. Whether human field motion is a measurable dimension and whether Ference's HFMT is a valid measure are questions raised by this study.

Perhaps the 11-minute experience of pleasant guided imagery was too short to significantly participate in a patterning of human field motion as measured by the HFMT. Also, the participants in this study were inexperienced with imagery techniques. More experienced participants are likely to have deeper and more effective experiences during pleasant guided imagery and may experience more intense feelings reflecting higher human field motion.

According to Tart (1975), one of the difficulties in studying "altered states of consciousness" is that the memory of the experience fades rapidly as participants return to the "normal" state. The possibility that participants returned to a "normal" state quickly after experiencing pleasant guided imagery may have contributed to the nonsignificant findings on the HFMT.

CONCLUSIONS AND RECOMMENDATIONS

This study demonstrates the conceptualization, operationalization, and testing of phenomena of concern to nursing within Rogers' Science of Unitary Human Beings. The study also illustrates the potential of the science of unitary human beings for providing a scientific rationale for the use of pleasant guided imagery in nursing practice. The findings suggest a new, more meaningful understanding of the therapeutic value of pleasant guided imagery as a nursing intervention. This study provides beginning evidence that the feelings of timelessness, transcendence, boundarylessness, and increased imagination experienced during pleasant guided imagery may be interpreted within Rogers' Science of Unitary Human Beings. Participants exposed to pleasant guided imagery did experience a significantly greater sense of timelessness and, although not statistically significant, did experience a greater sense of transcendence, boundarylessness, and increased imagination. Within Rogers' conceptual system, the subjective feelings reflect a patterning of the human energy field toward a higher wave frequency pattern. A higher wave frequency pattern facilitates the actualization of the human field potential and allows for transcendence beyond three-dimensional constraints such as time and space that impede motion toward harmony and well being (Rawnsley, 1985). In addition, participants reported feeling very relaxed during the experience of pleasant guided imagery. Within the science of unitary human beings, relaxation is conceptualized as expansion and increased motion in the human energy field (Scandrett, 1987). The expansion and increased field motion facilitates energy patterning, producing greater fluidity and fluctuation of the energy field, which Scandrett (1987) states may enhance patterning toward integrity of the human field and harmony with the environmental field.

To confirm the tentative findings of this investigation, further research leading to fuller understanding of the feelings of timelessness, transcendence, increased imagination, weightlessness, motion, and boundarylessness experienced during pleasant guided imagery is needed. Because a number of participants were confused by the HFMT, the tool needs to be further developed by including explanation of the meaning of "my motor is running" and "my field expansion" in the directions to the test. Scales more consistent with Rogers' four-dimensional space-time could be added to the tool. Further evaluation of the validity of the HFMT is needed. The development of additional instruments for measuring human field motion will facilitate construct validation. Future studies should consider a longer experience of pleasant guided imagery with participants who are more experienced in guided imagery techniques. Because this study raised questions regarding quantitative measurement of time experience and movement through space, perhaps these phenomena could be further explored by using qualitative research methods.

REFERENCES

Achterberg, J., & Lawlis, F. (1982). Imagery and health intervention. *Topics in Clinical Nursing, 4,* 55–60.

Barrett, E.A.M. (1983). An empirical investigation of Martha Rogers' principle of helicy: The relationship of human field motion and power. *Dissertation Abstracts International, 45,* 615A. (University Microfilms No. 8406378)

Barrett, E.A.M. (1986). Investigation of the principle of helicy: The relationship of human field motion and power. In V. Malinski (Ed.), *Explorations on Martha Rogers' science of unitary human beings* (pp. 173–188).

Clarke, P.M. (1986). Theoretical and measurement issues in the study of field phenomena. *Advances in Nursing Science, 9,* 29–39.

Dossey, L. (1982). *Space, time & medicine.* Boulder, CO: Shambhala.

Ference, H.F. (1979). The relationship of time experience, creativity traits, differentiation, and of Rogers' correlates of synergistic human development. *Dissertation Abstracts International, 40,* 5206B. (University Microfilms No. 8010281)

Ference, H.F. (1986). The relationship of time experience, creativity traits, differentiation, and human field motion. In V. Malinski (Ed.), *Explorations on Martha Rogers' science of unitary human beings* (pp. 95–106). Norwalk, CT: Appleton-Century-Crofts.

Girdano, D., & Everly, G. (1979). *Controlling stress and tension: A holistic approach.* Englewood Cliffs, NJ: Prentice-Hall.

Gray, V.R., & Rudy, E.B. (1981). Decision bases for assisting graduate nursing students in writing a thesis. *Advances in Nursing Science, 3,* 85–97.

Gueldner, S.H. (1986). The relationship between imposed motion and human field motion in elderly individuals living in nursing homes. In V. Malinski (Ed.), *Explorations on Martha Rogers' science of unitary human beings* (pp. 161–172). Norwalk, CT: Appleton-Century-Crofts.

Guzzetta, C., & Dossey, B. (1984). *Cardiovascular nursing: The body-mind tapestry.* Toronto: C.V. Mosby.

Keppel, G. (1982). *Design and analysis: A researcher's handbook.* Englewood Cliffs, NJ: Prentice-Hall.

Knapp, R.H., & Garbutt, J.T. (1958). Time, imagery, and achievement motive. *Journal of Personality, 26,* 26–434.

Korn, E.R., & Johnson, K. (1983). *Visualization: The uses of imagery in the health professions.* Homewood, IL: Dow Jones-Irwin.

Krieger, D. (1981). *Foundations for holistic health nursing practices: The renaissance nurse.* Philadelphia: Lippincott.

Kroger, W.S., & Fezler, W.D. (1976). *Hypnosis and behavior modification: Imagery conditioning.* Philadelphia: Lippincott.

Ludomirski, B.G. (1984). The relationship between the environmental energy wave frequency pattern manifest in red light and blue light and human field motion in adult individuals with sensory perception and those with total blindness. *Dissertation Abstracts International, 45,* 2094B. (University Microfilms No. 842147)

Ludwig, A.M. (1966). Altered states of consciousness. *Archives in General Psychiatry, 15,* 225–234.

Macrae, J. (1982). A comparison between meditating subjects and non-meditating subjects on time experience and human field motion. *Dissertation Abstracts International, 33,* 5362B. (University Microfilms No. 8307688)

McCaffery, M. (1979). *Nursing management of the patient with pain* (2nd ed.). Philadelphia: Lippincott.

Nunnally, J. (1975). The study of change in evaluation research: Principles concerning measurement, experimental design, and analysis. In E.L. Struening & M. Guttentag (Eds.), *Handbook of evaluation research* (Vol. 1, pp. 101–137). Beverly Hills: Sage Publications.

Osgood, C.E., & Suci, G.J. (1955). Factor analysis of meaning. *Journal of Experimental Psychology, 50,* 325–338.

Rawnsley, M. (1985). H.E.A.L.T.H.: A Rogerian perspective. *Journal of Holistic Nursing, 3,* 25–28.

Rawnsley, M. (1986). The relationship between the perception of the speed of time and the process of dying. In V. Malinski (Ed.), *Explorations on Martha Rogers' science of unitary human beings* (pp. 79–89). Norwalk, CT: Appleton-Century-Crofts.

Rogers, M. (1970). *An introduction to the theoretical basis of nursing.* Philadelphia: Davis.

Rogers, M. (1980). Nursing: A science of unitary man. In J. Riehl & C. Roy (Eds.), *Conceptual models for nursing practice.* (2nd ed.) (pp. 329–337). New York: Appleton-Century-Crofts.

Rogers, M.E. (1983). Science of unitary human beings: A paradigm for nursing. In I.W. Clements & F.B. Roberts (Eds.), *Family health: A theoretical approach to nursing care* (pp. 219–228). Toronto: Wiley.

Rogers, M.E. (1986). Science of unitary human beings. In V. Malinski (Ed.), *Explorations on Martha Rogers' science of unitary human beings* (pp. 3–8). Norwalk, CT: Appleton-Century-Crofts.

Rogers, M.E. (1987). Rogers' science of unitary human beings. In R.R. Parse (Ed.), *Nursing science: Major paradigms, theories and critiques* (pp. 139–146). Philadelphia: W.B. Saunders.

Samuels M., & Samuels, N. (1975). *Seeing with the mind's eye: The history, techniques, and use of visualization.* New York: Random House.

Sarter, B. (1988). *The stream of becoming: A study of Martha Rogers' theory.* New York: National League for Nursing.

Scandrett, S.L. (1987). Relaxation and the healing process. *Journal of Holistic Nursing, 5,* 28–31.

Shelly, S.I. (1984). *Research methods in nursing and health.* Toronto: Little, Brown.

Sodergren, K.M. (1985). Guided imagery. In M. Snyder (Ed.), *Independent nursing interventions* (pp. 103–124). Toronto: Wiley.

Tart, C.T. (1975). *Altered states of consciousness.* Garden City, NY: Doubleday.

Turk, D.C., Meichenbaum, D., & Genest, M. (1983). *Pain and behavioral medicine: A cognitive-behavioral approach.* New York: Gilford Press.

Volicer, B.J. (1984). *Multivariate statistics for nursing research.* Toronto: Grune & Stratton.

Wallach, M.A., & Green, L.R. (1961). On age and subjective speed of time. *Journal of Gerontology, 16,* 71–74.

Winer, B.J. (1962). *Statistical principles in experimental design.* New York: McGraw-Hill.

The Patterning of Time Experience and Human Field Motion during the Experience of Pleasant Guided Imagery: A Discussion

Katherine E. Rapacz

The Science of Unitary Human Beings has recognized imagery as a phenomenon of great relevance to its continuing development. Rogers (1970) first observed the importance of a person's capacity for imagery some 20 years ago. More recently, Rogers (1986), Malinski (1986a), and Cowling (1986) suggested the usefulness of imagery within this abstract system for assessing field pattern and mobilizing self-healing potentials. The need for basic research on imagery is primary to our understanding of its fullest potential in assisting individuals and in order to expand our knowledge of the nature of unitary human beings. Dr. Phillips (1988), in his concept of human field image, reminded us of the primacy of image within the Science of Unitary Human Beings.

THEORETICAL RATIONALE

The article by Butcher and Parker (1988) reprinted in this volume is based on Butcher's (1986) study (the first of its kind) to conceptualize imagery within the Science of Unitary Human Beings. Butcher's aim was to study the subjective experiences of individuals during guided imagery in order to increase understanding of the phenomenon and to provide a theoretical interpretation of these subjective experiences so as to guide the development of imagery as a nursing intervention.

Based on documented descriptions of subjective experiences during relaxation and imagery, Butcher made theoretical linkages between the experience of imagery and manifestations of higher frequency human energy field patterning. His hypotheses, based on the principle of resonancy and correlates of human field patterning, are logically sound. The principle of resonancy (Rogers, 1986) states that in human and environmental fields there is continuous change from lower to higher frequency wave patterns. Rogers' postulated correlates of patterning include the following (Malinski, 1986b):

pragmatic	imaginative	visionary
time drags	time races	timelessness
slower motion	faster motion	seems continuous

Butcher (1986) hypothesized that a higher frequency environmental field, operationalized as an 11-minute pleasant guided imagery experience, would influence patterning of the human field in a direction of higher frequency pattern manifestations as measured by the Time Metaphor Test (TMT) and the Human Field Motion Test (HFMT) (Ference, 1979).

DESIGN

The study utilized a pretest/posttest control group experimental design. Caution must be used with this approach to investigation, however, since the Science of Unitary Human Beings is a noncausal model of reality (Reeder, 1984). However, probabilistic change manifested in the human-environmental process may be captured by experimental design, particularly in a study such as Butcher's which measured manifestations of human field patterning in relation to an introduced environmental field change (Cowling, 1986). Therefore, while the design is adequate, it may be more appropriate to use a descriptive (qualitative or quantitative) design to more fully understand the phenomenon in question. This is especially desirable when new topics are investigated, as was the case with Butcher's study.

SAMPLE

Unfortunately, Butcher (1986) fails to provide a rationale for his decision to use a sample size of 30 for the experimental and control groups (n = 60). In decision making for sample size selection, a conceptual and statistical power analysis may have provided useful information in study design and sample selection. Particularly in new areas of research, all measures that can be taken to enable the researcher to capture the change process should be implemented (Volicer, 1984). The danger is in not capturing the change when it did indeed occur due to inadequate sample size or other characteristics of study participants. Availability of subjects is always a practical consideration of great importance as well. However, the decision must be balanced against the already considerable amount of time and effort invested in the research process and the impact this may have on results. In addition, a larger sample size would also have increased the probability of detecting change given that we know little about the relationship of imagery and the patterning process in the human field.

Subjects experienced in relaxation and meditation were excluded as potential study participants (Butcher, 1986). A power analysis from a conceptual perspective, however, may have suggested a different decision, that is, to recruit individuals experienced in creating vivid imagery. Participation of a group such as this would have increased the probability of capturing changes in patterning introduced through environmental change of the 11-minute guided imagery tape. While it is important to know how a group inexperienced in imagery and relaxation manifest patterning, the selection of such a group for this study did not enhance the probability of detecting changes.

Another observation related to sample size is offered here for the decision to perform a factor analysis on the Human Field Motion Test (HFMT) tool (Ference, 1979). Factor analysis procedures generally recommend that there be many more data elements (here, relating to sample size) than variables (Nunnally, 1978, p. 334). For example, it has been recommended that for every variable entered into the analysis there be 10–15 data elements (Hepworth 1988; Young, 1987). In the factor analysis of the HFMT tool there were 16 variables entered and 60 data points. Instead of a ratio of 10 or 15 to 1, in this analysis the ratio was less than 4 to 1. Thus, the results may not be statistically stable, and Butcher's criticism of the HFMT tool, based on the results of this factor analysis, cannot be considered with substantial confidence.

INTERPRETATION OF RESULTS

Results of imagery and health research to date reveals that specific content of imagery is important in relation to the nature of change that occurs (Achterberg & Lawlis, 1980, 1984; Heidt, 1978; Johnson, 1973; Norris & Porter, 1987; Simonton, Simonton, & Creighton, 1978). It is the content and suggestions inherent in the imagery sequence that provides the experience and thus influences the nature of the emerging patterning process.

The experimental condition consisted of listening to an 11-minute tape recording of a script for relaxation and pleasant guided imagery describing a beach and meadow scene. Let us examine the content of the pleasant guided imagery script in relation to the changes in the subjects' patterning manifestations of time and motion.

Consider the following passages of the script (Butcher, 1986, pp. 118–122) within the context of Human Field Motion Test (HFMT), recalling that human field motion is the "experiential, multidimensional position" of the human field (Ference, 1979, p. 4):

> . . . picture yourself *standing . . . looking* . . .
> . . . it is a perfect day and you have . . . *nothing to do, nowhere to go* . . .
> . . . you spread the blanket and *lie down* on it . . .
> . . . you *walk* into the warm water *slowly* . . .
> . . . you *slowly* walk further into the water . . . you *gently* splash . . .
> . . . you *lie down* and enjoy the sun . . .
>
> (emphasis added)

The entire last passage of the script is an image of lying languidly on the blanket in the meadow. These images would seem to promote an experiential subjective feeling that was captured on the HFMT tool by adjectives such as "drag," "sleepy," "dull," and "passive." Subjects in the experimental group in fact showed lower posttest scores on HFMT scales including these adjectives.

Returning now to the imagery content of the script, the subjects imaged themselves deeply immersed in the environment of the beach and meadow. Images included experiencing the breeze, sun, water, sand, and grass from a multisensory perspective. Expansive images included gazing at a distant sailboat, an expanse of water, a far shore, and the sky far, far above. These images seem to promote feelings of process with the environment and of a higher frequency in relation to HFMT adjectives such as "visionary," "imaginative," "boundarylessness," "transcendence," and "bright." Experimental subjects had much higher posttest scores on these HFMT scales than did control group subjects.

It appears that the script of the tape used in the experimental condition suggests images which are manifestations of mixed pattern frequencies as measured by the HFMT tool. This could promote a subjective sense of both lower *and* higher frequency patterning in relation to adjectives describing both concepts of the HFMT tool, that is, "My Motor Is Running" and "My Field Expansion." Experimental group subjects may have had subjective experiences that, when recorded on the HFMT tool, were theoretically interpreted as both lower and higher frequency.

Finally, let us consider the imagery content in relation to the Time Metaphor Test (TMT) in the following excerpts from the script:

> . . . a large lake . . .
> . . . looking out across the expanse of blue water to the far shore . . .
> . . . the sky is pale blue with clouds drifting by . . .
> . . . you look up at the sky seeing those great billowy clouds far, far above . . .
> . . . you hear the sound of a bird gently singing in a tree nearby . . .
> . . . behind you stretches a grassy meadow . . .
> . . . walking through the meadow . . .

Similarities between the wording in the imagery script and the description of metaphors on the TMT are quite striking. The most frequent posttest choices of the experimental group on the TMT included "drifting clouds," "a quiet motionless ocean," "a road leading over a hill," "a vast expanse of sky," and "a bird in flight." The changes in subjects' choices to these most frequently selected metaphors may represent subjective feelings experienced but it is more difficult to link the change in responses to a change in pattern frequency due to the confounding effect of the similarities in imagery script wording and metaphor descriptions.

This analysis leads to an alternative interpretation of the study results. Perhaps the findings reflect what the subjects actually experienced, that is, moving toward a sense of timelessness, and a mixture of lower and higher frequency manifestations of human field motion. On close examination the script contains suggestions which may have led subjects to check adjectives indicating feelings of both lower and higher frequency pattern manifestation on the HFMT tool concepts "My Motor Is Running" and "My Field Expansion." In short, the obtaining of equivocal results on HFMT was to be expected due to the combination of images presented in the script. Whereas, there was a great similarity between images of the script and metaphor choices in the TMT considered to be indicators of "timelessness" experience.

Rapacz and Cowling (1988) have recently postulated that imagery is the prototype activity involving human-environmental field patterning. It is a field phenomenon, involving more than the five physical senses, and transcends the subjective experience of person-environment boundaries usually maintained in other states of awareness. Relaxation, repetitive activities, and meditative or contemplative states which accompany imagery may change awareness and be necessary for changes in patterning during imagery, but the nature of pattern change is open and can be influenced toward either a higher or lower frequency pattern depending on the forms suggested in the specific imagery content and the level of knowing participation on the subjects' part. These notions and others related to the many as yet unknown factors of the nature of imagery undoubtedly impacted the findings of this study.

RECOMMENDATIONS

Future studies should build upon Butcher's (1986, 1988) work with special attention to imagery content, sample selection, sample size, and the inclusion of other human-environmental patterning measures, such as Barrett's (1986) power instrument. Descriptive designs and single case time series analysis (Barlow, Hayes, & Nelson, 1984) would be useful approaches in explicating the phenomenon of imagery. Greater understanding and testing of factors such as the influence of varying imagery content, the intent of both practitioner and client (subject), and the extent to which the client (subject) knowingly participates in change may be prerequisite to developing the knowledge base required to understand how this modality can be of assistance in helping individuals toward the well being they wish to achieve.

CONCLUSION

This study contributes to the body of knowledge within the Science of Unitary Human Beings through its theoretical formulations and its pioneering leap into an uncharted territory. Butcher's own patterning from pragmatic toward visionary manifested in the formulation of this study provides a good base for further investigation and may stimulate others to begin research into this most important area.

REFERENCES

Achterberg, J., & Lawlis, G.F. (1980). *Bridges of the bodymind*. Champaign, IL: Institute for Personality and Ability Testing, Inc.
Archterberg, J., & Lawlis, G.F. (1984). *Imagery and disease*. Champaign, IL: Institute for Personality and Ability Testing, Inc.
Barlow, D.H., Hayes, S.C., & Nelson, R.V. (1984). *The scientist practitioner: Re-*

search and accountability in clinical and educational settings. New York: Pergamon Press.

Barrett, E.A.M. (1986). Investigation of the principle of helicy: The relationship of human field motion and power. In V. Malinski (Ed.), *Explorations on Martha Rogers' science of unitary human beings* (pp. 173–187). Norwalk, CT: Appleton-Century-Crofts.

Butcher, H.K. (1986). *Repatterning of time experience and human field motion during the experience of pleasant guided imagery: An experimental investigation within Rogers' science of unitary human beings.* Unpublished masters' thesis, University of Toronto, Toronto.

Butcher, H.K., & Parker, N.I. (1988). Guided imagery within Rogers' science of unitary human beings: An experimental study. *Nursing Science Quarterly, 2,* 103–110.

Cowling, W.R. (1986). The science of unitary human beings: Theoretical issues, methodological challenges, and research realities. In V. Malinski (Ed.), *Exploration on Martha Rogers' science of unitary human beings* (pp. 65–77). Norwalk, CT: Appleton-Century-Crofts.

Ference, H.M. (1979). The relationship of time experience, creativity traits, differentiation, and human field motion. *Dissertation Abstracts International, 40,* 5206B. (University Microfilms No. 8010281)

Heidt, P. (1978, November). *Patients tell their stories.* Paper presented at the Second Annual Conference on Imaging and Fantasy Process. Chicago, IL.

Hepworth, J. (1988). Personal communication.

Johnson, J.E. (1973). Effects of accurate expectations about sensations on the sensory and distress components of pain. *Journal of Personality and Social Psychology, 27,* 261–275.

Malinski, V. (1986a). Nursing practice within the science of unitary human beings. In V. Malinski (Ed.), *Explorations on Martha Rogers' science of unitary human beings* (pp. 25–32). Norwalk, CT: Appleton-Century-Crofts.

Malinski, V. (1986b). Further ideas from Martha Rogers. In V. Malinski (Ed.), *Exploration on Martha Rogers' science of unitary human beings* (pp. 9–14). Norwalk, CT: Appleton-Century-Crofts.

Norris, E.A., & Porter, G. (1987). *I choose life: The dynamics of visualization and biofeedback.* Walpole, NH: Stillpoint Publishing.

Nunnally, J.C. (1978). *Psychometric theory.* New York: McGraw-Hill.

Phillips, J.R. (1988, June). *Changing human potentials and future visions of nursing.* Keynote address presented at the Third Rogerian Conference, New York University, New York, NY.

Rapacz, K.E., & Cowling, W.R. (1988, May). *Imagery and the science of unitary human beings.* Paper presented at the Annual Meeting of the Nightingale Society. Carmel, CA.

Reeder, F. (1984). Philosophical issues in the Rogerian science of unitary human beings. *Advances in Nursing Science, 6*(2), 4–23.

Rogers, M.E. (1970). *Introduction to the theoretical basis of nursing.* Philadelphia: F.A. Davis.

Rogers, M.E. (1986). Science of unitary human beings. In V. Malinski (Ed.), *Explorations on Martha Rogers' science of unitary human beings* (pp. 3–8). Norwalk, CT: Appleton-Century-Crofts.

Simonton, C., Simonton, S., & Creighton, J. (1978). *Getting well again.* Los Angeles: J.P. Tarcher, Inc.

Volicer, B. (1984). *Multivariate statistics for nursing research.* Orlando: Grune & Stratton, Inc.

Young, D. (1987). Personal communication.

Response to "Discussion of a Study of Pleasant Guided Imagery"

Howard K. Butcher
Nora I. Parker

We appreciate Katherine Rapacz's thoughtful and thorough critique of the report on our study, and we are grateful for this opportunity to respond. Since the completion of the study, there has been an accelerating and expanding awareness of the use of imagery as a patterning strategy for the promotion of well being and harmony. Recent popular books by Siegel (1986, 1989) and Borysenko (1987) illustrate this increasing awareness.

There are several points we wish to address in Rapacz's critique, however. First, Rapacz does not base her questioning of the sample size on the design of the study, but rather on the factor analysis of the Human Field Motion Tool (HFMT) (Ference, 1979). The sample size of 60 participants was actually chosen on the basis of the study's pretest/posttest, experimental and control group design. For this type of design, "preferably 20–30 participants should be selected for every subdivision of data, or each cell of the design" (Polit & Hungler, 1987, p. 220). The factor analysis was conducted only after participants reported difficulty in understanding the terminology and directions on the HFMT. We agree that the factor analysis is not statistically stable, and that a larger sample is needed for a factor analysis because of the tool's 16 scales or variables. However, the validity of the tool is not questioned by the results of the factor analysis alone. For example, some scales moved toward higher frequency, while other scales moved toward lower frequency. The concepts "My Motor is Running" and "My Field Expansion" were often not clearly understood. We would suggest repeated factor analysis of the HFMT in studies with a sample size of 160–240 or greater (meeting the 10–15:1 ratio of variables to data points suggested) to further evaluate the tool's validity.

In addition, we do suggest that a qualitative study may contribute to understanding more fully the subjective experience of guided imagery. At the time of the study's evolution, a review of the literature provided ample descriptive anecdotal reports of feelings of motion, timelessness, boundarylessness, lightness, transcendence, and increased imagination. As Rapacz noted, an experimental design was appropriate to measure a change in field patterning in relation to the experience of guided imagery. However, new research methods unique to nursing science must be designed that are in harmony with and evolve from the ontological beliefs of the Rogerian system. The development of a Rogerian research methodology would need to be consistent with the concepts of wholeness, four-dimensionality, human-environmental mutual process, and patterning. For example, Phillips (1989) suggested a new way of looking at the manifestations of patterning by collapsing them into a single column, thus connoting the multiplicity of possible potentials of the human-environmental field mutual process. In this way, pattern profiles can be researched, and specific profiles may emerge in relation to specific types of patterning strategies.

Rapacz's reinterpretation of the results based on the content of the imagery is quite interesting. It supports the principle of integrality of the human-environmental field process. The content of the tape was selected because of its relaxing content. Macrae (1982) with meditators, and Ludomirski-Kalmanson (1984) with blue light, found feelings of relaxation to be associated with higher human field motion. Thus, we hypothesized that the relaxing nature of pleasant guided imagery may also be associated with higher human field motion. It is difficult to imagine a script of pleasant guided imagery that would not include images of a calming or peaceful nature. One can conclude that the content of the image has a more significant impact on the HFMT and Time Metaphor Test (TMT), than the more generalized feelings of relaxation. Future research could explicate the patterning profiles associated with various types of imagery experiences. Images designed for energizing, empowering, calming, healing or actualizing the human field potential may each have unique patterning profiles. In addition to Barrett's (1983, 1989) Power as Knowing Participation in Change Tool, Paletta's (1988) Temporal Experience Scales provide an alternative measure of time experience developed within the Rogerian conceptual system. These tools may be used as measures of changes in human field patterning relative to guided imagery. We hope that the study along with the suggestions for future research serves as a foundation for future studies of guided imagery within the Rogerian science perspective.

REFERENCES

Barrett, E.A.M. (1983). An empirical investigation of Martha E. Rogers' principle of helicy: The relationship of human field motion and power. *Dissertation Abstracts International, 45*, 615A. (University Microfilms No. 8406278)

Barrett, E.A.M. (1989). A nursing theory of power for nursing practice: Derivation from Rogers' paradigm; In J. Riehl-Sisca (Ed.), *Conceptual models for nursing practice* (3rd ed.) (pp. 207–217). Norwalk, CT: Appleton-Lange.

Borysenko, J. (1987). *Minding the body, mending the mind.* Reading, MA: Addison Wesley.

Ference, H.M. (1979). The relationship of time experience, creativity traits, differentiation and human field motion. *Dissertation Abstracts International, 40*, 5206B. (University Microfilms No. 8010281)

Ludomirski-Kalmanson, B.G. (1984). The relationship between the environmental energy wave frequency pattern manifest in red light and blue light and human field motion in adult individuals with visual sensory perception and those with total blindness. *Dissertation Abstracts International, 45*, 2094B. (University Microfilms No. 842147)

Macrae, J. (1982). A comparison between meditating subjects and non-meditating subjects on time experience and human field motion. *Dissertation Abstracts International, 43*, 3537B. (University Microfilms No. 8307688)

Paletta, J.L. (1988). The relationship of temporal experience to human time. *Dissertation Abstracts International, 49*, 1621B. (University Microfilms No. 8812521)

Phillips, J.R. (1989). Science of unitary human beings: Changing research perspectives. *Nursing Science Quarterly, 2*, 57–60.

Polit, D.F., & Hungler, B.P. (1987). *Nursing research: Principles and methods* (3rd ed.). Philadelphia: Lippincott.

Siegel, B.S. (1986). *Love, medicine and miracles.* New York: Harper & Row.

Siegel, B.S. (1989). *Peace, love and healing: Bodymind communication and the path to self-healing: An exploration.* New York: Harper & Row.

Unit IV
Visions of Rogers' Science-Based Education

The distinguishing characteristic of professional education in nursing is the transmission of nursing's body of abstract knowledge, arrived at by scientific research and logical analysis.

Martha E. Rogers

19

The Continuing Revolution of Rogers' Science-Based Nursing Education

Elizabeth Ann Manhart Barrett

Rogers called for an educational revolution in nursing and, indeed, for the past 30 years has been an educational revolutionary. Perhaps second only to Rogers' contribution to nursing through her creation of the Science of Unitary Human Beings is her clear articulation of the tenets of professional nursing education.

> The distinguishing characteristic of professional education in nursing is the transmission of nursing's body of abstract knowledge, arrived at by scientific research and logical analysis—not a body of technical skills. This is not to deny the importance of technical skills but rather to make clear that it is nursing's organized body of theoretical knowledge that identifies nursing as a profession. It is the utilization of this knowledge in service to people that determines the nature of nursing services. It is this body of knowledge that encompasses nursing's descriptive, explanatory, and predictive principles, principles that guide its practitioners and make possible professional practice—a fulfillment of nursing's scientific humanitarianism. (Rogers, 1985a, p. 381)

As an educator, Rogers has been a living example of tenacious courage and authentic liberation. She has been a role model of participating knowingly—of changing the world by action in the world. She lit many candles to guide nursing's emergence as a discipline and a profession; she has also been known to occasionally curse the darkness. An optimist who cautions against fear mongers, she will be long remembered for what Freeman (1961) called her "uninhibited thinking" (p. v). Rogers has exemplified characteristics she deemed necessary for professionally educated nurses. Namely, in addition to being committed to people, "they must be risk takers. They must be characterized by a mutual respect for differences. They must be imaginative and creative and, above all, they need a good sense of humor" (Rogers, 1985b, p. 14).

Gioiella (1989) captured the fighting, committed spirit of Rogers when she wrote of her legacy of professionalizing nursing. "She was not alone in her vision of education for the profession but she was clearly a leader with few peers in moving her belief that nursing is a learned profession from rhetoric to fact" (p. 62). She again and again challenged, insisted, "exhorted, prodded, stimulated, and at times exasperated her colleagues and students" (p. 62).

THE REVOLUTIONARY MESSAGE

Throughout the years Rogers' thinking has evolved into more precise formulations. However, the revolutionary ideas that formed the basis for her contributions to nursing appear as themes in her earliest writings. Some cornerstones of Rogers' position on professional nursing education, as expressed in her own words, are presented here as affirmations for educators.

1. Education is for the future; yesterday's methods will not suffice for tomorrow's needs. (Rogers, 1961, p. 33)

2. Man[1] is as different from his parts as water is different from hydrogen and oxygen. (Rogers, 1964, p. 35)

3. The time is past when any one profession holds the key to man's well being. Nursing shares knowledges and skills with other professions but nursing is not dependent on any other profession for either its body of knowledge or the application of that knowledge. (Rogers, 1964, p. 39).

4. A learned profession is responsible to the society it serves. The services members provide are unique. They cannot be provided by another group. And the uniqueness of services rendered lies firmly in the body of knowledge that defines nursing's scope of service. (Rogers, 1964, p. 44)

---

[1]Note that use of the word "man" has since been changed to "human beings."

5. Nursing is a social necessity. Professionally educated nurses are indispensable to the furtherance of man's welfare. There is no room for self-doubt. The kind of morale, without which excellence in education and practice cannot exist, demands a firm belief in one's self and an equally firm belief in the vital role of nursing. (Rogers, 1964, p. 45)

6. Professional and liberal education represent an integrated whole. A collection of courses, of themselves, prepare for nothing; any more than a piece, or a pile of pieces, of a jigsaw puzzle make a picture. Only in the systematic ordering of knowledges into an intelligible whole does there emerge a professional curriculum. (Rogers, 1964, p. 51)

7. The primary purpose of professional education in nursing is to transmit a body of scientific knowledge (specifically nursing science). (Rogers, 1964, p. 59)

8. Impoverished baccalaureate degree education has too often laid a weak foundation for the education of scholars in nursing. (Rogers, 1964, p. 66)

9. The art of applying scientific knowledge with imagination and compassion is an integral aspect of professional practice. (Rogers, 1964, p. 82)

10. Nursing's contribution to the future of mankind will be no greater than the scholarly research through which the theoretical basis of nursing practice becomes explicit. (Rogers, 1964, p. 94)

11. Achievement of excellence in the art of practice is a lifetime process. (Rogers, 1964, p. 95)

12. The tools of nursing practice are specific to translating nursing knowledge into human service. (Rogers, 1985a, p. 381)

13. The baccalaureate degree is the first professional degree in nursing. (Rogers, 1985a, pp. 381–382)

14. Professional education in nursing is as concerned with maintenance and promotion of health as it is with care and rehabilitation of the sick and disabled. (Rogers, 1985a, p. 382)

15. Professionally educated nurses are independent practitioners prepared to knowledgeably provide health services to individuals, families, groups, and communities. They are accountable for their own acts and liable to the public they serve. They are peer participants in collaborative judgments made with professional personnel in other fields. (Rogers, 1964, p. 382)

16. Graduate education in nursing builds on and articulates with undergraduate education. Doctoral programs *in nursing* prepare the scholars and researchers essential to evolving and elaborating theo-

retical knowledge in nursing—knowledge that may be fed back
into the educational process and into nursing practice. (Rogers,
1985a, p. 382)

17. The term *nursing*, used to signify a learned profession, is a noun,
not a verb. By definition, then, "nursing" specifies an organized
body of abstract knowledge specific to its central purpose. (Rogers,
1985a, p. 381)

Rogers has consistently asserted that nursing is by definition a learned
profession and an academic discipline characterized by a unique and abstract body of knowledge about nursing's phenomenon of concern—people
and their world (Rogers, 1986). Her proposal in July of 1989 that there is
something to know in nursing along with her caveat that some nurses and
others still believe that there is nothing to know in nursing succinctly
summarizes her stance.

That Rogers' ideas on professional education do not sound as revolutionary today as they did is testimony to this fact: Much change has occurred in
nursing education during the more than 25 years since most of her ideas
were written. The point is the revolution has begun and continues despite
opposition; yet, it is far from over. This process is appropriately described
by Munhall's (1988) question referring to a curriculum revolution that she
believes has begun in nursing. Munhall asked, "Who is to know if the
fluttering of one's butterfly wings is not the beginning of a hurricane two
hundred years later" (p. 218). Somewhere between fluttering butterfly
wings and the hurricane, Rogers has been a consistent voice crying out
against antieducationism and dependency while crying out for nursing as a
learned profession that is unique in the phenomenon of its concern and in
its substantive theoretical knowledge base (Rogers, 1985b). She warns that
nursing does not exist for the benefit of any other profession but rather it
exists for the benefit of the society it serves through nursing services. As
a peer of other learned professions, nursing shares its knowledge and society benefits through collaboration of various health professions (Rogers,
1985a).

No discussion of Rogers' science-based education would be complete
without including her position on licensure for nursing practice. She has
continuously maintained that while there are three entry levels to practice
(vocational, technical, and professional), licensure exists for only two (practical nurse level prepared in vocational programs and registered nurse level
prepared in associate degree and hospital school technical programs).
Hence, public safety and professional credibility are jeopardized and require
the addition of a new license for the baccalaureate level of practice. This

autonomous baccalaureate prepared professional would provide direction for nurses licensed at the vocational and technical levels. Excellence and respect for differences are required for education and practice at all levels (Rogers, 1985b).

While little progress has been made toward differentiation of roles in practice or by distinct licensure of the baccalaureate graduate, Rogers has been politically active through participation in professional organizations. In fact, some may remember her primarily as a nursing politician. She was instrumental in obtaining a revision of the Nurse Practice Act in New York State in 1972 (Gioiella, 1989). This revised nurse practice act has become a national model and laid groundwork for third-party reimbursement for independent nursing services in private and employed practice of nursing as an autonomous profession.

Gioiella (1989) called Rogers a prophet and noted that "Whether she was a prophet crying in the wilderness is yet to be determined" since nursing has for the most part "ignored her message and is suffering the consequences" (p. 61). According to Gioiella, Rogers' blueprint for differentiation between vocational, technical, and professional education and practice has yet to be realized.

THE CURRICULUM REVISION IMPERATIVE

Rogers (1985b) maintains that "nursing's survival as a knowledgeable endeavor demands that the education of nurses be squarely within educational institutions" (p. 13). She proposed that valid baccalaureate nursing education requires (1) a strong liberal arts foundation, (2) additional knowledges in the humanities and sciences that facilitate understanding of humankind and environment, and (3) substantive theoretical knowledge in the science of nursing along with opportunity to demonstrate safe and effective use of this knowledge in providing nursing care to people (Rogers, 1961, 1964, 1985b).

These three areas of knowledge continue to provide the basic structure for designing curricula. What has changed, however, and requires further change is the designation of particular courses and the distribution of credits in the second area (additional knowledges) and third area (nursing science). As substantive nursing knowledge has been developed and will continue to be developed, more content and credit hours are required for nursing science. Concurrently, fewer and different courses and credits are required in the second area of additional knowledges that facilitate understanding of nursing science.

Entering the last decade of the century, most nursing educators would agree with Rogers' 1964 statement that "the instructional process must be centered on the transmission of a body of scholarly knowledge—the science of nursing" (p. 95). However, disagreement would most certainly arise concerning the knowledge that constitutes nursing science. What is the substantive body of knowledge in nursing? That is the critical question. It is exciting that the discipline has evolved to the place where we can ask this question and expect to find answers. The answers tend to reflect two different perspectives. Parse, Coyne, and Smith's (1985) differentiation of the totality and simultaneity paradigms is relevant in understanding the two perspectives of nursing science and their impact on curricular matters.

Two major ways of viewing people in their world evolved over time. Nurse theorists have "set forth systematized theoretical structures grounded in views of man and health that specify the substance of the discipline" (Parse, 1987, p. 3). These frameworks, often referred to as the conceptual models of nursing, comprise bases of nursing science knowledge and reflect two different paradigms. These competing old and new world views have respectively been named the totality paradigm and the simultaneity paradigm (Parse, 1987).

The totality paradigm views the whole person as the sum of the parts and the simultaneity paradigm views the whole person as more than and different from the sum of the parts. In the totality paradigm the person is described as a "total, summative organism whose nature is a combination of bio-psycho-social-spiritual features" (Parse, 1987, p. 4). I would also add "cultural" features. A person as a totality reacts and adapts to internal and external environmental stimuli to maintain equilibrium. "This belief," according to Parse, "is very different from the belief that man is a unitary being in continuous mutual interrelationship with the environment, and whose health is a negentropic unfolding, which is the view set forth in the simultaneity paradigm" (p. 4). The totality paradigm encompasses the conceptual models of Roy (1976), Orem (1971), King (1981), Johnson (1980), B. Neuman (1972), Leininger (1979), Peplau (1952), and others.

In 1970, Rogers "posited the first view of nursing outside the primary operating belief system" of the totality paradigm when she described the human being as "more than and different from the sum of parts, changing mutually and simultaneously with the environment" (Parse, 1987, p. 4). Parse (1981), M. Newman (1986), and J. Fitzpatrick (1983) have since proposed conceptual models, based in part on Rogers' Science of Unitary Human Beings, that fall within the simultaneity paradigm.

"The emergence of different nursing world views and congruent theories advances the . . . discipline and thus is necessary for the development of nursing science" (Parse, 1987, p. 4). Clearly, these different world views result in development and use of different knowledges and, hence, have major implications regarding the nursing science content of the curriculum as well as cognate courses that provide additional knowledges related to the nursing major. For example, if one believes that a holistic person is a combination of bio-psycho-social-cultural-spiritual features, then advanced courses in physiology, psychology, sociology, and perhaps comparative religions will be desirable. From this totality view and in-depth knowledge of components of a person arises an understanding of the whole person. However, theorists working in the simultaneity paradigm would tend to disagree here, even though they value and consider such knowledge important. From a Rogerian view knowledge of parts does not describe or lead to understanding of unitary human beings (Rogers, 1970, 1986). Rather, that understanding comes from the study of the Science of Unitary Human Beings; knowledge for this abstract system is developed through logical analysis and scientific research (Rogers, 1970, 1986). Cognate coursework would reflect areas of knowledge consistent with the unitary world view or otherwise pertinent to the conceptual model. Examples for Rogerians include astronomy, modern physics, Eastern philosophy, logic, and new world views of human development and the life process.

For both the totality and simultaneity paradigms coursework dictated by changing societal trends and health care delivery systems will be reflected in courses such as economics, ethics, critical thinking, political science, computer science, and cultural anthropology. Qualitative and quantitative modes of inquiry will also be essential.

The above discussion of suggested courses that support the nursing science major is not to be confused with introductory courses in those disciplines that provide general liberal arts and science knowledges reflective of a baccalaureate education. What then should content in this area be? Rogers (1961) suggested the following: written and spoken English, foreign language, mathematics, logic, philosophy, history, biology, microbiology, physics, chemistry, psychology, sociology, literature, music, and art. She has also proposed that baccalaureate education in nursing requires 5 years (Rogers, 1964, 1985b). Other nurse leaders in education have likewise commented on the difficulty of preparing a professionally educated nurse in 4 years (Fitzpatrick, 1985; Moccia, 1989; Watson, 1988).

For both the totality and simultaneity paradigms, an enriched baccalaureate curriculum focused on the three areas of (1) general education, (2) supportive courses that enhance the nursing major, and (3) nursing science providing a firm foundation for graduate work. Master's study will be geared toward in-depth study and use of a conceptual model to guide practice and applied research. Doctoral study will focus on theory development and basic research to develop new knowledge in the conceptual system. Electives and independent study at both the master's and doctoral levels will allow students to acquire advanced knowledges they require for enhancement of their individualized learning goals. Baccalaureate students will experience a nursing curriculum guided by one conceptual model. At the master's level students will study a broad spectrum of nursing conceptual models and will then select one to guide their specialization. At the masters and doctoral levels students may decide to change paradigms or change models within paradigms; yet they will again select one model to guide their work in theory development and research. Doctoral programs will attract students interested in particular conceptual models when their faculty have expertise in those models.

Nonetheless, the basic structure of baccalaureate education has not changed. However, since unique nursing knowledge has increased over the past 20 years, there is urgent need to spend more time studying that knowledge base and less time studying advanced knowledge from other disciplines. In addition, due to changes in society, different courses relative to nursing science are required that will reflect consistency with the totality or simultaneity world views. In some cases they will reflect particular nursing conceptual models (e.g., astronomy for Rogerians, existential philosophy for Parsians). Finally, to develop a fully educated person whose profession is nursing requires a strong and broadly based liberal arts component.

Valiga (1988) asks, "How many students may have received a degree without receiving an education?" (p. 180). This is not solely a nursing education dilemma. Bloom, in *The Closing of the American Mind* (1987), concluded that many of today's students know less and are cut off from tradition. He warns of the danger of "being closed to the emergent, the new, the manifestations of progress" (p. 29).

Currently, curriculum revision for professional education requires much discussion. We must be able to disagree without self-destructing (Fitzpatrick, 1985). These ideas for the content of curriculum revision provide a starting point for discussion. They are intended to invite dialogue not to conclude it.

PEDAGOGY FOR THE CURRICULUM IMPERATIVE

Having discussed the content of curriculum revision (what we teach), it is important to focus on pedagogy (how we teach it). What teaching–learning approaches will foster curriculum implementation in ways that allow students to evolve into graduates who are well-educated, cirtically thinking nursing professionals? How can we create learning environments that enhance power, the capacity to participate knowingly in change, in students and faculty?

Teachers are learners and learners are teachers; their shared experiences are integral to the educational process. Professional education allows us to seek our meaning, purpose, and identity as individuals, as members of a profession, and as part of a world and a universe. "To investigate the world is to study ourselves, and to investigate ourselves is to study the world" (Massanari, 1989, p. 29). This human-environment mutual process is explained by Rogers' (1986) principle of integrality.

The student-teacher interchange can promote students' liberation by avoiding prescription which transforms freedom into conformity (Freire, 1981). The student-teacher mutual process is dynamic; it is *not* "motionless, static, compartmentalized, and predictable" (p. 57). Rather, this interchange aims for dialogue. Dialogue requires an intense hope and belief in students' ability to create and transform. It requires and generates critical thinking. According to Freire, without dialogue there is neither communication nor true education.

Education is a human activity and, as such, it consists of reflection and activity; it is praxis. "And as praxis, it requires theory to illuminate it" (Freire, 1981, p. 119). Praxis is "a dance wherein ideas, concepts, theories may rise in the intellect from reading, discussions, lectures, classroom learning activities or in practice" (Bevis, 1988, p. 48). Chinn (1989) paraphrases feminist praxis:

> Nursing ideas are an integral component of nursing praxis, and are defined as an implicit set of beliefs underlying the explicit ethical/ political statements of a nursing group. Praxis and ideas are grounded in nursing theories which give philosophical explanations on frameworks for health. (p. 74)

In charting new directions for a new age in professional education, Bevis (1988) maintained that distinguishing between learning that is training and learning that is education demands abandonment of the Tyler-type model of curriculum development. The Tyler model requires "a philosophy; a conceptual framework; behaviorally defined, measurable objectives on every level (program, curriculum, course, unit or module, and learning activity); the development or selection of learning activities sorted into a program of studies; and the evaluation of learning based on the behavioral objectives" (pp. 30–31). Based in behaviorist learning theory, such a model, Bevis argues, lends itself to training and not to education. She suggests that use of the same technical training model in all types of nursing programs is a major factor in lack of differentiation between programs and graduates of vocational, technical, and professional programs. Being technically oriented toward training, such a curriculum cannot support the necessary changes required by society's changing trends and nursing as a profession and a discipline.

Bevis (1988) outlined six types of learning for "New Age" curriculum models that differentiate between training and education. Three types (item, directive, relational) comprise the focus of technical nursing programs. Three types (syntactical, contextual, inquiry) comprise the focus of baccalaureate and higher degree programs. Table 1 presents Bevis' differentiation.

As we alter the approaches to teaching nursing science content, Sykalys' and Watson's curricular recommendations that emphasize "intellectual skills such as analytic, problem-solving and critical thinking" along with "greater emphasis on essential values and attitudes" (cited in Bevis, 1988, p. 45) come to the forefront. In this regard, an American Association of Colleges of Nursing's 1986 report recommended seven values for the professional nurse: "altruism, equality, esthetic, freedom, human dignity, justice, and truth" (Bevis, 1988, p. 43).

The outstanding educator of the professional uses processes that teach students how to learn, how to think critically, how to see patterns, find meanings, and gain scholarly insights. The content may remain similar but the approach to the content is changed so that there is a "legitimization of the teaching of inquiry, reflection, criticism, independence, creativity, and caring" (Bevis, 1988, p. 50).

The curriculum imperative requires innovative teaching strategies. Laboratory and computer simulation are two major innovations used in many, if not most, programs; various other pedagogical approaches have also been developed (Fuszard, 1989).

Some pedagogical innovations and curriculum models offer options that require consideration. However, before we throw out the baby with the bath water, let us carefully consider aspects of the Tyler model that have served us well by improving the quality of nursing education.

PRACTICE SETTINGS IN NEW CURRICULA

Throughout Rogers' writings nursing practice is discussed in conjunction with the need for substantive nursing knowledge to underwrite it. Like the song, they go together and you can't have one (nursing practice) without the other (nursing knowledge). She clearly states that neither experience

Table 1
Curriculum Model: Technical and Professional Education*

Associate Degree Technical	Baccalaureate and Higher Degree Professional Education
Item Learning	Syntactical Learning
Simple relationships	Seeing wholes,
Use of equipment and tools	patterns, relationships
Lists and procedures	
Directive Learning	Contextual Learning
Rules and exceptions	Sociocultural context
Injunctions	Philosophy, values,
Do's and don'ts for tasks	ethics, esthetics
Relational Learning	Inquiry Learning
Uses theory to	Creativity
reinforce practice	Investigation
Rational for	Defining problems
interventions	and generating solutions

*Based on Bevis, 1988, pp. 39–41

nor training is a substitute for education. "Content in the nursing major is focused on transmission of an organized body of theoretical nursing knowledge. Laboratory study is an integral part of the total curriculum and must be preceded by appropriate theoretical content" (Rogers, 1961, p. 35).

The curriculum imperative also requires appropriate practice settings for optimum student learning experiences. A vital consideration in selection of practice sites is evidence that autonomous professional nursing practice exists in those settings. The influence of role models and practice activities in practice settings cannot be underestimated in terms of socialization of students as professionals and as nurses. If nursing practice is theory in action, then we must ask the hard questions of "what theories from what science" and "what actions"? The answers provide direction for designing student practice experiences.

Orlando and Dugan (1989) call for a radical independent path where nurses understand their "product and function" and, therefore, "can get on and stay on a path that permits the independent organization and delivery of service within the ever widening and competitive health services field" (p. 80). This path is prerequisite to persuading consumers and health policy makers to fully consider the necessity of nursing's professional services.

Both the need for practice settings that allow for autonomous nursing practice and the shift from hospital to home care demand that nurse educators carefully evaluate current settings where students practice. Although nursing care can and must be delivered in *all* settings where nursing services are needed, some practice environments optimize students' learning opportunities.

The issue of alternative settings for student practice is critical since the definition of nursing as an autonomous discipline demands student experiences that allow for use of the discipline's knowledge—nursing science. If we maintain that nursing's phenomenon of concern is unitary human beings, to what extent can beginning students practice nursing in settings where the primary focus is often on medical treatment of acutely diseased parts? As hospitals become intensive care facilities, practice experience in these tertiary care centers will increasingly be designed for the advanced baccalaureate student who is more firmly grounded in the science of the nursing discipline. Fewer students per faculty member will also be essential.

While the need for nursing care in hospitals is obvious, the fact of the matter is that it is becoming more and more difficult for the student to provide it. Moccia (1989) predicts an even greater complexity of needs of clients requiring acute, intensive care and proposes that it is becoming increasingly unrealistic to think that future nurses can be educated in 2- and 4-year programs. She wonders if a master's degree will be the most appropriate degree for the nursing case manager in the 1990s. Regardless, a wider variety of master's prepared specialists will be needed in many settings. Rogers, (1964, 1985b) of course, for the past 25 years has argued that the professional education of the baccalaureate graduate requires 5 years.

If we maintain that nursing's primary focus is health, then students also need opportunities to practice in settings where providers have a commitment to health promotion, illness prevention, and health maintenance during chronic disease. Health promotion programs, managed care programs, shelters for the homeless, public clinics, senior centers and clients' homes allow students to apply nursing knowledge in ways that may not be possible when clients are acutely ill. Many such student experiences in the community have been observational rather than caregiving in the recent past. However, as delivery systems shift from the critical care, high acuity hospital-based systems to home care systems, more hospital experiences will become observational. Increasingly the focus for student practice opportunities will be outside of hospitals. Simultaneously, as home care becomes more technologically complex, the need for learning sophisticated procedures in college learning laboratories and on-site faculty supervision of students providing home care also increases.

To discuss the educational experience of nursing students in the human laboratory without discussing the experiences of licensed nurses who practice in those settings is to discuss education in a vacuum. The need for nursing care in tertiary care institutions along with the increasing difficulty in providing it is somewhat paradoxical. Clients who require intensive, critical care not only are in dire need of knowledgeable nursing services, their very survival may depend on it.

The 24-hour care of the whole person through patterning the environment is a unique nursing contribution to care of clients in institutional settings. To manage such nursing care using vocational, technical, and professional nurses is indeed difficult. It is impossible without substantive nursing knowledge to guide nursing actions. Often adding to the dilemma are staffing patterns that preclude such care and management priorities that neither hold nurses accountable for autonomous nursing functions nor reward them for operationalizing nursing knowledge. Regardless of setting, to the extent that nurses are unable to provide nursing services for whatever reasons, there will be job dissatisfaction and high turnover of staff.

There is not only a shortage of *nurses*, there is a shortage of *nursing* in all types of settings although not in all settings. Could it be that this is why many consumers have difficulty understanding what nursing has to offer them beyond use of technical skills? Could it be that this is at the root of the nursing image and nursing identity dilemmas? How much longer are we going to avoid dealing with entry into practice, differentiation of nursing roles according to educational preparation, and licensure issues? Nursing cannot survive if we avoid our societal obligation to provide nursing services through knowledgeable caring.

Chinn (1989) dreams of nurses creating their own environments that comfort and heal. In this light, it may be time for nursing to create independent nursing institutions in a systematic manner so as to found a nursing care delivery system. Successful models such as Anderson's Personalized Nursing do exist (Anderson & Smereck, 1989).

The educational revolution in nursing is far from over. The crisis in nursing education today requires educators to take another look at Rogers' revolutionary message and design curriculum content revision and pedagogical approaches that reflect nursing as a learned profession and as a basic human science and art. These curriculum imperatives are essential to the education of nurses for science-based research and practice in the 21st Century.

Rogers (1985b) foretells that "the direction of change makes imperative nurses' move toward scientific identity and social responsibility. Whatever the future of nursing may be, it will be within the context of rapid change, diversity, new knowledge, and new horizons" (p. 14).

What about those butterfly wings? Are they fluttering and stirring? Perhaps if today's educators design and deliver nursing science-based education, tomorrow's nursing professionals may actualize the revolutionary message. No doubt, such a profound event will generate dramatic changes in the health and well being of people.

REFERENCES

Anderson, M., & Smereck, G. (1989). Personalized nursing LIGHT model. *Nursing Science Quarterly, 2*, 120–130.

Bevis, E.M. (1988). New directions for a new age. In *Curriculum revolution: Mandate for change* (pp. 27–52). New York: National League for Nursing.

Bloom, A. (1987). *The closing of the American mind.* New York: Simon and Schuster.

Chinn, P. (1989). Nursing's patterns of knowing and feminist thought. *Nursing & Health Care, 10*, 70–75.

Fitzpatrick, J.J. (1983). Fitzpatrick's rhythm model: Analysis for nursing science. In J.J. Fitzpatrick & A.L. Whall (Eds.), *Conceptual models of nursing* (pp. 303–326). Bowie, MD: Brady.

Fitzpatrick, M.L. (1985). Perspectives on the patterns of nursing education. In *Patterns in education: The unfolding of nursing* (pp. 3–10). New York: National League for Nursing.

Freeman, R. (1961). *Foreword.* In M.E. Rogers' *Educational revolution in nursing* (pp. v–vi). New York: Macmillan.

Freire, P. (1981). *Pedagogy of the oppressed.* (M.B. Ramos, Trans.). New York: Continuum. (Original work published in 1968.)

Fuszard, B. (Ed.). (1989). *Innovative teaching strageties in nursing.* Rockville, MD: Aspen.

Gioiella, E. (1989). Professionalizing nursing: A Rogers legacy. *Nursing Science Quarterly, 2*, 61–62.

Johnson, D.E. (1980). The behavioral system for nursing. In J.P. Riehl and C. Roy (Eds.), *Conceptual models for nursing practice* (2nd ed.) (pp. 207–216). Norwalk, CT: Appleton-Century-Crofts.

King, I.M. (1981). *A theory for nursing: Systems, concepts, process.* New York: John Wiley & Sons.

Leininger, M. (1979). *Transcultural nursing.* New York: Mason.

Massanari, R.L. (1989). Re-visioning education. *Re-Vision: The Journal of Consciousness and Change, 1*(2), 27–30.

Moccia, P. (1989). 1989: Shaping a human agenda for the nineties. *Nursing & Health Care, 10*, 15–17.

Munhall, P.L. (1988). Curriculum revolution: A social mandate for change. In *Curriculum revolution: Mandate for change* (pp. 217–230). New York: National League for Nursing.

Neuman, B. (1972). The Betty Neuman model: A total person approach to viewing patient problems. *Nursing Research, 21*, 264–269.

Newman, M.A. (1986). *Health as expanding consciousness*. St. Louis: C.V. Mosby.

Orem, D.E. (1971). *Nursing: Concepts of practice*. New York: McGraw-Hill.

Orlando, J.J., & Dugan, A.B. (1989). Independent and dependent paths: The fundamental issue for the nursing profession. *Nursing and Health Care, 10*, 76–80.

Parse, R.R. (1981). *Man-living-health: A theory of nursing*. New York: John Wiley & Sons.

Parse, R.R. (1987). *Nursing science: Major paradigms, theories, and critiques*. Philadelphia: W.B. Saunders.

Parse, R.R., Coyne, A.B., & Smith, M.J. (1985). *Nursing research: Qualitative methods*. Bowie, MD: Brady.

Peplau, H.E. (1952). *Interpersonal relations in nursing*. New York: G.P. Putnam.

Rogers, M.E. (1961). *Educational revolution in nursing*. New York: Macmillan.

Rogers, M.E. (1964). *Reveille in nursing*. Philadelphia: F.A. Davis.

Rogers, M.E. (1970). *An introduction to the theoretical basis of nursing*. Philadelphia: F.A. Davis.

Rogers, M.E. (1985a). The nature and characteristics of professional education for nursing. *Journal of Professional Nursing, 1*, 381–383.

Rogers, M.E. (1985b). Nursing education: Preparing for the future. In *Patterns in education: The unfolding of nursing* (pp. 11–14). New York: National League for Nursing.

Rogers, M.E. (1986). Science of unitary human beings. In V. Malinski (Ed.), *Explorations on Martha Rogers' science of unitary human beings* (pp. 3–8). Norwalk, CT: Appleton-Century-Crofts.

Rogers, M.E. (1989, July). *Research in the new way of thinking: The science of unitary human beings*. Paper presented at the Summer Research Conference, College of Nursing, Wayne State University, Detroit, MI.

Roy, C. (1976). *Introduction to nursing: An adaptation model*. Englewood Cliffs, NJ: Prentice-Hall.

Valiga, T.M. (1988). Curriculum outcomes and cognitive development: New perspectives for nursing education. In *Curriculum revolution: Mandate for change* (pp. 177–200). New York: National League for Nursing.

Watson, J. (1988). A case study: Curriculum in transition. In *Curriculum revolution: Mandate for change*. New York: National League for Nursing.

20

Using Rogerian Science in Undergraduate and Graduate Nursing Education

Gean M. Mathwig
Alice Adam Young
J. Mae Pepper

USING ROGERIAN NURSING SCIENCE-BASED EDUCATION AS A CONCEPTUAL FRAMEWORK: NEW YORK UNIVERSITY

When the Science of Unitary Human Beings (Rogers, 1970, 1986) serves as the conceptual framework for nursing curriculum, all relevant concepts and knowledge are analyzed within that framework. Of paramount importance here is the understanding that nursing science content is not integrated into other relevant knowledge and concepts; rather, relevant knowledge and concepts are analyzed within the context of Rogerian nursing science. In this light, we must remember that the conceptual framework provides the cognitive structure and logical basis for organizing the information and priorities in the nursing process as well.

Essentially, use of the Rogerian nursing science conceptual model accomplishes two things. First, it places the nursing process within an expanded frame of reference. Second, it makes the nursing process specific to each individual as a unitary being. When the client is viewed as an energy field, the focus is shifted to the individual-environmental field process. While the individual may have a medical diagnosis, the individual-environmental field process remains the primary focus. This idea is similar to gerontology literature that brings emphasis to the term "being old": the assessment and intervention are influenced by whether the nurse focuses on the "being" or the "old" aspect of the term.

Content to be Included

Including Rogerian nursing science content in nursing courses involves three principles: integrality, resonancy, helicy, and the building blocks (energy, fields, openness, pattern, four-dimensionality) inherent in these principles (Rogers, 1970). All of the principles involve these aspects: (1) human and environmental field process, (2) continuous change, and (3) increasing diversity of the human and environmental fields. (See Appendix A for Rogers' most recent definitions of terminology.)

The principle of helicy deals with the nature and direction of change in human and environmental fields. Human and environmental field patterns emerge out of interacting processes with field patterns that constantly gain in diversity. Thus, as individuals age they do not become simple or regress back to childhood; rather, they become more diverse and complex. For example, contemporary data indicate that there is great variation in health and functioning among the elderly of the same age groups (Andres, Bierman, & Hazzard, 1985; Calkins, 1986). Another concept inherent in the principle of helicy is that of nonrepeating rhythmicities. Much research data have been published on human and environmental rhythmic patterns. Examples of environmental rhythmic patterns include economic depression, wars, crime, and sun spots. Examples of human rhythmic patterns include sleeping and waking, flying across time zones, fluctuating work shifts, administration of medications, seasonal weather changes, changes in life process and state of well being, and peaks and troughs in the human energy field.

The principle of integrality concerns the continuous, mutual human and environmental field process. Of utmost importance is the concept that as nurses we are integral with the client's environmental energy field. At the baccalaureate level, in particular, development of the student's awareness of self as an aspect of the client's environmental energy field and the dynamic role the nurse's energy field pattern has on the client is emphasized. As energy signifies the dynamic nature of the field and as field is the unifying concept, the ramifications of integrality and inherent concepts for nursing intervention that promote client well being are of major importance. In nursing practice, such caregiver–recipient energy field processes that have been clinically demonstrated include therapeutic touch, life review, reminiscence, music therapy, therapeutic use of self, and active listening. The significant factor is that the nurse deliberately strives to pattern the environmental energy field, directing the energy flow to the client to facilitate the client's knowing participation toward well being.

Equally significant is the concept that to generate energy, one must use energy. Thus, the use of movement, exercise, or other activity programs to continuously pattern the human energy field become important. At all age groups and throughout life, attention to the human and environmental energy field process is necessary and important. An essential role of the health care provider is the identification of the human and environmental energy field process that assists clients in mobilizing their unique energy patterning to maximize well being.

The principle of resonancy deals with the continuous change of wave patterns in human and environmental fields. The pattern is perceived as a single wave and apprehended as a whole. A significant aspect is that human and environmental field characteristics are manifestations of the whole. Just as the life process derives from the functioning of the person as a whole, so does the totality of human and environmental field patterns define the characteristics of the individual and environment.

Essential to Rogerian nursing science-based education is the concept of four-dimensionality, which is defined as a nonlinear domain without spatial or temporal attributes (Rogers, 1986). Acknowledging that four-dimensionality is nonlinear, however, does not negate the relevance of subjective perceptions of traditional space-time dimensions. Personal space, territoriality, privacy, and intimacy are all inherent in the client's subjective perception. A native resident of New York City, for example, may perceive personal space and crowding in quite a different context than a native resident of rural Wyoming. The literature indicates that when individuals are deprived of their personal space or territoriality, there is an increased need to dominate (Sommer, 1969). In addition, in our Western society, the allocation of increased space indicates increased status. Thus, to deprive an individual of space is to deprive that individual of status. Considered in this same manner is the client's subjective perception of time. The relative past, present, and future are part of the client's subjective experience of time. The experience of duration, for example, when the client has pain, may involve a less diverse patterning of the human field. As a result, time may seem to drag. On the other hand, the experience of duration, when the client participates in activities that he or she enjoys, may involve a more diverse patterning of the human field. As a result, time may seem to race forward rapidly.

The Process of Implementation in the Curriculum

In the initial stages of implementing the Rogerian conceptual framework in the curriculum, it is necessary to (1) identify the concepts to be developed and incorporated and (2) to determine the organizing structure. For example, in the baccalaureate program at New York University, the faculty selected the life span, conception through the aging adult. It is also necessary to identify what other nursing knowledge and concepts need to be included and analyzed within the Rogerian conceptual framework. Because our prior program was based on a traditional medical model, the faculty from the speciality areas of community health, mental health, medical-surgical, obstetrics, and pediatric nursing identified knowledge and concepts essential to incorporate in the conceptual framework identified. They then provided an overall perspective for each nursing course in accord with the course objectives and anticipated level of student performance. At the end of each academic year, faculty further operationalized the nursing science content and evaluated the content and specific teaching–learning experiences in day-long workshops.

Of most importance to the process of implementation in nursing curriculum development, however, is the ongoing operationalization of nursing science principles and building blocks. As the Rogerian conceptual framework is an evolving body of knowledge with a limited number of publications available for reference purposes, this requires creative work on the part of the faculty. The ongoing discovery of new relationships as well as the innovative application of the conceptual framework in the theoretical and clinical experiences of the nursing curriculum remains an ongoing process. In the final analysis, it is through the application of the principles and building blocks of the conceptual framework in curriculum content, curriculum and course objectives, and the teaching–learning experiences that the conceptual framework takes on meaning and is subsequently implemented in the nursing process.

IMPLEMENTING THE ROGERIAN CONCEPTUAL FRAMEWORK IN A GENERIC AND RN UNDERGRADUATE NURSING PROGRAM: WASHBURN UNIVERSITY

Washburn University is located in the center of the United States, in the northeast section of the state of Kansas, in the capital city of Topeka. The undergraduate nursing program was founded in 1974 and developed with several features unique for its setting in "Middle America" (Young, 1987). The program was the first in the state: to (1) develop a curriculum based on a nursing conceptual model and (2) to utilize the Rogerian conceptual system, the Science of Unitary Human Beings, as the organizing framework for the curriculum. Early formulations of the framework at Washburn University were derived from the 1970 published works of Rogers and from my previous experiences as a doctoral student and faculty member in the Division of Nursing at New York University, 1968–1974. The use of Rogerian concepts in the nursing framework at Washburn has been updated over time to reflect ongoing refinements Rogers herself has made. The problem of "time lag" that occurs in curriculum implementation when using a conceptual model that is itself developing was described in an earlier publication (Young, 1985), as was the overall method of utilizing the Rogerian conceptual system in the baccalaureate nursing program at Washburn University (Young & Keil, 1981; Young, 1985).

Rogerian Concepts in Curriculum Design

Conceptual frameworks should be all-encompassing. It is the belief of the nursing faculty at Washburn University that the Rogerian framework fulfills this aspect. In our use of this framework for 15 years, we are satisfied that the major components underlying curriculum development (i.e., beliefs about human beings, health, nursing, and the educational process) are well articulated within the Rogerian framework. In the Washburn program, implementation of the Rogerian framework is comprehensively reflected in program materials, such as the statement of philosophy and program objectives, curriculum level objectives, course syllabi, course content, student learning experiences, evaluation tools, and examinations.

Various learning experiences are organized at the lower division level to introduce nursing students to the Rogerian conceptual system early in the nursing program. Through classroom lectures, use of audiovisuals, group discussions, family visits, reading assignments, reaction papers, and assessments of a family and a community, nursing students develop a beginning understanding and appreciation of the Rogerian "new world view," new terminology, and beginning applications of Rogerian concepts in nursing practice. Examples of some objectives from the syllabus of the first nursing course of the major, "Theoretical Basis of Nursing," illustrate these learnings:

> Give three varied examples from history to illustrate the dynamic relationship of human beings to the universe.

> Illustrate by examples how persons participate as unitary wholes in the continuous change process.

Identify two observed phenomena which support the concept of the human person as an energy field.

Define and use examples to describe the three homeodynamic principles.

Given specific situational examples, apply the nursing science indices in assessing the human behavior of individuals.

Utilize the nursing science indices to assess the health status of an assigned family.

Assess an assigned community for data concerning rhythms in the community.

Analyze the progress or change in pattern of an assigned community in terms of growth and compositon.

The nursing science indices of patterning, structure and function, energy distribution, rhythms, field patterns, space-time dimensions, and openness were derived from the Rogerian conceptual system by the nursing faculty as criteria for the assessment phase of the nursing process (Young, 1985). The following examples illustrate how some of the indices were applied in a community assessment assignment for a class of beginning nursing students.

Application

To achieve the community assessment objectives, the students divided into groups to examine the Topeka community from a number of perspectives using the nursing science indices. Each of the groups selected one of the indices by which to assess the city community. They gathered data from newspapers, the city Chamber of Commerce, the Kansas Historical Society, the city and state Departments of Transportation, the city Police Department, the state Department of Health and Environment, city libraries, and from interviews with community leaders and citizens. One group traced changes in Topeka's *structure and function* over time by citing increases in population; changes in growth patterns in business and industry; urban renewal projects; expansion of health care facilities and programs; the impact of political decisions of local, state, and federal governments (redistricting, urban building codes, the Brown vs. Topeka Board of Education Supreme Court decision on racial segregation); and the role of natural forces (Kansas River flood, 1951; Topeka tornado, 1966; major ice storms and fires in recent years) in defining the *patterning* of the city.

Another student group explored *field patterns* by looking at various communications networks within the city (transportation modes; television and radio stations; supermarkets; shopping malls; groupings of ethnic and historical landmark communities; distribution of apartment complexes, condominiums, high rises and private dwellings; availability of recreational facilities) and the relationship of the urban university to the community.

Students using the *energy distribution* index looked at the city's economic resources in terms of total population; numbers employed and unemployed; per capita income; health status based on numbers of persons receiving services in hospitals, clinics, nursing homes, health promotion programs and rehabilitation centers; and vital and morbidity statistics.

Space-time dimensions were explored in terms of city and state government operations. Students visited the Metropolitan Planning Commission to learn about plans for city growth over the next 10 to 20 years. They identified the population age groups within the community and the availability of housing and economic resources for the future. *Rhythms* within the community were assessed by identifying types of employment, kinds of leisure activities, and the degree of mobility within and without the city.

Students assessing the city with the *openness* index made the statement that "the boundaries of the city are very permeable" since "many people enter the city everyday from several surrounding communities and rural areas for employment, health care, and recreational activities because of its easy accessibility by car, bus, air and train." Other observations related to this index were cited in reference to geographic location, climate, terrain, educational opportunities, and housing facilities.

In sharing their assessments in class discussion, students identified that the indices are overlapping in the sense that given observations may relate to more than one of the indices. The students commented that the consistent growth and development of the city community over time was an illustration of the principle of *helicy*; they identified the principle of *resonancy* in the flux of legislative activities that occur regularly in the city of Topeka, the state capital, but which rise to intensity during the 90-day legislative session each year, taper off somewhat during the interim study periods from June to November, and reduce to a minimal frequency during the months of December and May. The students found the principle of *integrality* in the great variety of network systems operating within and without the city community, linking individuals, families, and businesses in mutual relationships.

In another lower division course of the nursing major, "Nursing Process," students were required to write nursing care plans and to perform beginning level client assessments in a hospital setting using the nursing indices. Further use of Rogerian principles and building blocks in nursing care plans and class presentations throughout the upper division courses of the major provide for both generic and registered nurse students' expanded comprehension of the Rogerian conceptual system and greater facility in applying the components in the nursing process.

A program objective to be achieved at completion of the lower division nursing courses (Level I) states that students will:

> Translate nursing process content and homeodynamic principles into nursing practice, utilizing the nursing science indices as the framework for assessing health status and meeting basic health needs of individuals and families.

Students achieve Level II program objectives (junior year) when they are able to:

> Apply the nursing process in a variety of settings by utilizing the nursing science indices for assessing and promoting the health status of individuals and families.

Level III achievement (senior level) requires students to:

> Integrate the homeodynamic principles and nursing science indices into the nursing process to facilitate health potential of individuals, families and groups in various settings and stages of the life process.

Student Testimonials

That we not only teach our students an appreciation of the Rogerian conceptual system, but also prepare nurses who can articulate and use the Science of Unitary Human Beings in their nursing care, is borne out in comments made by our students and graduates. One registered nurse student expressed this by saying, "Thank God for Martha Rogers! I am delighted to have found a conceptual framework that I feel I can not only live with and utilize effectively, but that I can evolve with." Another commented: "I find that I am very young in my understanding of this model. The concepts strike me as being incredibly abstract, and yet incredibly wonderful in their simplicity." Other comments by seniors approaching graduation were: "A major strength of the nursing program is its conceptual framework"; "The framework provides a strong foundation for nursing practice and for future educational purposes"; "It gave me a holistic look at nursing . . . I learned to assess so much more than physical, emotional, and psychological well being"; "I feel that the Rogerian conceptual framework takes into account the total human being. It gives us a strong knowledge base from which to look at the person as a whole."

Of course, beginning level students do not usually start out with such marvelous comments and insights. Many are frustrated, confused, and angry because of the "strangeness" of the framework in relation to their expectations of "what nursing would be like." We have noticed a difference between registered nurse and generic students' readiness for and appreciation of the Rogerian framework, especially at their initial exposure. Registered nurse students have commented that their background of nursing experiences have prepared them for "wanting something more," that is, a more meaningful way to organize data and view the world as an integral whole. With the generic students who do not have the same familiarity with nursing, there is a slower process of integration of the conceptual framework and appreciation of Rogerian terminology occurs more slowly, sometimes after graduation. It is encouraging to faculty, however, when seniors can say of framework implementation: "It was difficult to grasp at first, but it stays with you and enlightens your thinking—even in everyday life," or, "In the beginning it was hard to grasp, but in time it became easier to understand, and now it has become almost a habit." In contrast, a graduating registered nurse student said, "I had little difficulty with this framework because I already agreed with much of what Rogers teaches. I just called it something different." One alumna wrote in a note to the faculty recently, "I use the Rogerian framework in my clinical practice all the time." What more can we hope for?

IMPLEMENTATING THE ROGERIAN CONCEPTUAL FRAMEWORK: MERCY COLLEGE

"People (and I would like to add, *Curricula*) are conceived, born, grow, mature, and die, and life continues" (Rogers, 1970, p. 57). We can look at this statement two ways: (1) by focusing on our need to be humble, being reminded that human power is significant only in its context with the whole universe or (2) by focusing on our enormous capacities to influence and be influenced as we participate in the life process of a nursing curriculum, recognizing that the curriculum's influence continues after we no longer directly participate in it.

At Mercy College, we operate a baccalaureate program that admits registered nurses only, those who started their careers by preparation in associate degree or diploma programs. In this first professional degree program, our mission is to prepare students to feel and act like professionals in the scientific discipline of nursing. We also operate a second professional degree program, the first graduate program at Mercy College. Our graduate program has a dual purpose: (1) preparing professional nurses for advanced clinical practice as family nurse clinicians specializing with either the young expanding family, dealing with the health concerns during the child-bearing and child-rearing years, or the older contracting family, dealing with the health concerns of old age; and (2) preparing professional nurses for functional leadership roles as teachers or clinical leadership in middle management positions.

At Mercy College, we adhere rather literally to the title of "Rogerian Science-*Based* Education" rather than "Rogerian Science-*Organized* Education." That is, we do not use Rogerian concepts to organize the curriculum; rather, we use them to describe and explain our beliefs about the essential elements of all conceptual models of nursing: person (or preferably humankind), environment, health, and nursing (as a process) (Fawcett, 1984). This philosophical base then serves to direct the manner in which nursing is approached in terms of purpose, process, and strategies to achieve that purpose.

The major "organizer" used in our curriculum is the identified client system. The term "client" is used intentionally rather than "patient" to focus us as professional nurses on our primary responsibility: maximizing the health of humankind. Based on a perhaps debatable belief about learning, we organize by size and complexity of the client system, moving from an initial focus on nursing process with individuals to the process with small groups and families and finally to the process with communities. By organizing our curriculum around client systems and by planning learning experiences for those client systems of all ages, with various senses of well being and in a variety of settings, I believe that we have attended to at least two significant directives from Rogerian science. First, the purpose of nursing intervention is to participate with the person to continuously pattern the environment to achieve the maximum health potential of that person (Rogers, 1970, pp. 86, 127). This is in contrast to organizing curriculum by focusing on the types and elements of health care delivery systems that often are organized by categories of pathology or by subsystems of the biological human being. Second, health and illness are not differentiated. Very early in our curriculum development, we eliminated the notion of the health–illness continuum and began to focus on health and the perceived sense of well being, the sense of balance with the environment. (Parenthetically, I am aware that Rogers (1986) has spoken about the problems associated with even the use of the term "health," as well as "illness," since they are both value-laden.) I would like to note here that we use Rogerian science as the *base* for how we think and act in relation to nursing. We also use Peplau's (1952) ideas for guiding our communication with clients. Thus, we acknowledge two nursing models in our curricula. However, allow me to move away from the "organizers" and come back to the influence of Rogerian science on our beliefs about the essential elements of nursing.

Humans

Our curriculum is based on this primary premise: that nursing's central concern is humans in mutual process with their environment and striving for a sense of well being. Since Rogers clearly delineates humans as open systems in constant process with the environment, we have believed that it is entirely legitimate and logical to arbitrarily assign some categories to human systems and target our responsibility to three human client systems: individual human systems, family systems, and community systems. Each of those human systems engage in a mutual process with the environment, exhibit patterns of behavior, and strive for a sense of well being. And we as individual nurses, small groups of nurses, or the larger community of nurses, are integral with the total environment of the client just as clients are integral with our environment.

I realize that Rogers herself (Rogers, Meehan, & Malinski, 1988) has begun talking about the limitation of the term "interaction" and has noted that perhaps the term "mutual process" provides *greater* clarity in explaining that everything *is* integral, and keeping us out of the trap of temporality— the notion of "*if* a, *then* b." In this regard, however, I believe we have approached our "process" with clients as an interaction with a view toward our influences on clients and their influences on us being more sequentially rather than simultaneously organized. Nonetheless, we, as faculty, will need to rethink that as we continue to develop and mature our curriculum.

Whether we focus on the human system as being individual, family, or community, we use the same assumptions, clearly supported in Rogerian science (Rogers, 1970). For example:

1. The human system is an integrated organism reflecting inseparable abilities to exist as biologic, thinking, and feeling beings. This statement is just as true for family as individual. Clearly, we really cannot describe a family by describing individuals within it—it has its own unique structure, function, and pattern. Recall Rogers' early and major assumption that the whole is more than the sum of its parts. Indeed, particularly as we have focused on the family in the graduate program, we have come to understand more clearly that our efforts to maximize health in families are greatly enhanced if we focus on the family system as the client, rather than the family member as client. That is not to say that some particular

member may not be helped if we focus on individual family members, but we run the risk of playing into the development of counter-productive patterns in another member.

2. Human systems continually exchange energy with the environment resulting in ongoing patterning of both the human system and the environment as each evolves toward greater complexity and innovativeness. That view of the unlimited capacity of the human system has been particularly significant in shaping nurses' attitudes about clients. It has forced us to give up old notions of power in which the nurse is powerful and the patient is powerless, the nurse is strong and the patient is weak. We are all more simply human than otherwise (Sullivan, 1953). Whether or not we focus on the individual, family, community as client, the responsibility for both the process and the outcome of our purposeful interventions is mutually shared between the nurse and the client. Our pattern of behavior changes and our sense of well being changes simultaneously with the client's pattern changes and sense of well being.

Health

Using the notion that health represents a human ability to achieve increasing complexity and innovativeness of patterning in the forward direction of the life process (Rogers, 1970, p. 42; 1980, p. 333), our curricula have evolved a view of health as an experience of realizing potential or a condition of actualization. This, in fact, is the eudaemonistic model of health (Smith, 1981). We believe that health is primarily a measure of the human system's ability to do what one wants to do and become what one wants to become (Dubos, 1978, p. 74). Readers should note that we have included this idea promulgated by Dubos in the eudaemonistic model of health, unlike Smith, who categorizes Dubos' idea in the adaptive model of health. Well being is a subjective perception of balance, harmony, and vitality between the human system and the environment. Given this view of health, we have come to believe that nursing interventions can only be focused on restoration of a sense of well being and promotion of health, that is, promotion of optimal patterning. The old view of maintenance of health as a goal for the client seems obsolete. Using Rogerian science, maintenance seems to be a static state inconsistent with the ongoing potentiation of life and the dynamic nature of energy fields (both the human and the environment and their mutual processes). The deletion of the old goal of maintenance of health means that we always focus on promotion of health with all client systems, and, if the client system perceives and expresses an inadequate sense of well being, we focus on restoring health as well in an effort to help the client experience a perception of balance, harmony, and vitality with the environment.

Environment

From Rogers' (1970) early work, environment is essentially defined as an energy field in continuous interaction with an individual's energy field. Recently, Rogers (Rogers, Meehan, & Malinski, 1988) has more clearly described environment as the energy field that not only continuously, but *simultaneously* is in mutual process with the human energy field. That notion of continuous and simultaneous process certainly gives credence to the communication concepts so strongly emphasized in our curriculum; empathy, genuineness, and respect (Hammond, Hepworth, & Smith, 1980). The critical element of empathy is that the nurse permits him or herself to attend, experience, and respond in terms of the client's reality. The critical element of genuineness is that the nurse permits him or herself to feel and express self and does not expend or confound energy by guarding or defensive patterns. The critical element of respect is that the nurse views clients as human systems in their own right, mutually responsible for the process that occurs between them, and possessing achievements, abilities, and potential regardless of their state of health or any other human characteristics. Perhaps the most significant direction we take from Rogerian science in terms of environment is that we as nurses are integral with the client's environmental field. Thus we are given the opportunity to purposefully participate with that client system to develop patterns that maximize abilities and help clients "do what they want to do—and become what they want to become." That kind of relatedness with the client gives meaning to our existence and indeed is perhaps the strongest motivational force we have for choosing nursing as a profession.

Nursing

In our curricula, nursing is viewed as a process in which the nurse, who is integral with the client, intentionally attempts to assist the client system to maximize health, or in Rogerian terms, to achieve a greater sense of well being. The purposefulness of the nursing process is based on the knowledge we possess about human beings and their life process and the belief system that we have about health. We as professional nurses intentionally use the mutual process with the client to apply that knowledge to promote optimal well being. Thus, nursing process is viewed as including both cognitive and interpersonal elements.

It is our belief that the nursing process can be most effectively implemented to advance the client's health if the nurse actualizes three roles, all of which are operationalized from a Rogerian framework:

1. Agent of change: This role is based on the notion that effective and knowing participation in change emerges from a clear identification and utilization of the client's strengths. We try to help our students understand that we are doomed to failure if we try effect changes from focusing on deficits, disabilities or problems; rather, we assist more effective patterning (change) by focusing on the client's assets, abilities, or strengths. In addition to insisting that the outcomes of the assessment stage of the nursing process be organized by a list of client strengths rather than problems, we ask our students to consider what might be traditionally called client problems as client *concerns* and to reframe these concerns in terms of the client's motivational strengths; that is, the client's expressed desire to change. This helps the client to relinquish the need to invest energy in the problem and to be able to move on to do what he or she wants to do. This view of nursing, focusing on the strengths of the client, is not the traditional view today in our health care delivery systems that Rogers has frequently referred to as our "sick systems"—the acute-care settings particularly. However, I believe that today we do have systems that are indeed "health" systems that use the notion of building on strengths to maximize health—namely, the emergent "fitness" systems. We no longer have to "hardsell" the idea that we as human beings can knowingly participate in what happens in our lives and that health is our responsibility.

2. Advocate: The respect for clients that is so integral to Rogerian science helped us to select an advocacy role for operationalization in our curricula. The concepts essential to advocacy are mutuality, sometimes protection, and facilitation. Because mutuality is basic to the Rogerian framework, it has led us to reconsider power in the nurse–client relationship and to realize that it is equally shared. In our programs, therefore, the view is that the client is the expert on his or her situation, assets, and concerns and has full responsibility for health; the nurse has expertise on the indices and facilitators of health and has full responsibility for guiding the relationship with the client in a way that results in positive outcomes for both.

3. Contributor to the profession: We use this role in our curricula to emphasize the needed mutual process between the human professional system (nursing) and the societal environment. In this role, nurses are given the opportunity to develop their enormous potential to participate knowingly for achievement of better health for all people through public policy, decision making in health care delivery systems, and their professional advancement. One example of such a learning experience we provide is an undergraduate course, "Power Bases of Nursing," in which the nurses develop and present public testimony (to peers) on a concern related to nurs-

ing. We believe it urgent for us to prepare our graduates to be able to intentionally assist in the continuous patterning of the profession and the delivery system as well as client systems.

At Mercy College, we remain pleased with our continuing study of Rogerian science which, by its very nature, mandates a continual updating to our thinking, and our translating of that growth into philosphical directives that pattern both the content and process of our nursing curricula. Rogerian science-based education works!

REFERENCES

Andres, R., Bierman, L., & Hazzard, W.R. (Eds.) (1985). *Principles of geriatric medicine.* New York: McGraw-Hill.

Calkins, E. (1986). *The practice of geriatrics.* Philadelphia: W.B. Saunders.

Dubos, R. (1978). Health and creative adaptation. *Human Nature 1,* 74–82.

Fawcett, J.F. (1984). *Analysis and evaluation of conceptual models of nursing.* Philadelphia: F.A. Davis.

Hammond, D.C., Hepworth, D.H., & Smith, V.G. (1980). *Improving therapeutic communication.* San Francisco: Jossey-Bass.

Peplau, H. (1952). *Interpersonal relations in nursing.* New York: G.P. Putnam's.

Rogers, M.E. (1970). *An introduction to the theoretical basis of nursing.* Philadelphia: F.A. Davis.

Rogers, M.E. (1980). Nursing: A science of unitary man. In J.P. Riehl & C. Roy (Eds.), *Conceptual models for nursing practice* (2nd ed.) (pp. 329–337). New York: Appleton-Century-Crofts.

Rogers, M.E. (1986). Science of unitary human beings. In V. Malinski (Ed.), *Explorations on Martha Rogers' science of unitary human beings* (pp. 3–8). Norwalk, CT: Appleton-Century-Crofts.

Rogers, M.E., Meehan, T.C., & Malinski, V. (1988, June). *Rogerian practice perspectives: Excerpts from transcripts of dialogues among Martha E. Rogers, Therese Connell Meehan, and Violet Malinski.* (Available from *Rogerian Nursing Science News,* P.O. Box 362, Prince Street Station, New York, N.Y., 10012.)

Smith, J.A. (1981). The idea of health: A philosophical inquiry. *Advances in Nursing Science 3*(2), 43–50.

Sullivan, H.S. (1953). *The interpersonal theory of psychiatry.* New York: W.W. Norton.

Young, A.A., & Keil, C. (1981). The Washburn nursing curriculum: Interpreting Martha Rogers in the Land of Oz. *The Kansas Nurse, 56,* 7–9, 23.

Young, A.A. (1985). The Rogerian conceptual system: A framework for education and service. In R. Wood & J. Kekhabab (Eds.), *Examing the cultural implications of Martha E. Rogers' science of unitary human beings* (pp. 53–69). Lecompton, KS: Wood-Kekhabab Associates.

Young, A.A. (1987). Historical development: Washburn University school of nursing. *The Kansas Nurse, 62,* 68.

21

Concept-Integration: A Board Game as a Learning Tool

Mary Anne Hanley

A science examines relationships between concepts with a language specific to its phenomenon of concern that is used to communicate the intention and precision of the science to the members of the discipline (Rogers, 1986, 1988; Barrett, 1988). Of the many challenges facing students of Rogers' conceptual system is the ability to articulate its language of specificity. The application, use, and synthesis of the theoretical framework require an intimate understanding of the interrelationships among its concepts.

For many students, learning the language of the Science of Unitary Human Beings is similar to learning a foreign language. In fact, many sciences share this difficulty. The process can be cumbersome and dull, resulting from rote memorization, repetition, and recall activities. Nor is the reward for persistent application of these behaviors consistent. Some students gain facility with the language while others are only able to recognize terms and to recall discrete definitions without comprehending the relationships among the larger conceptual issues.

As a student of nursing science faced with the dilemma of applying and synthesizing terms central to the Rogerian framework, I developed "Concept-Integration: A Board Game" (Hanley, 1985). Believing that there was more to the "building blocks" and the principles of homeodynamics as outlined by Rogers (1970, 1983) than simply definitions, I began to explore various ways of relating the concepts to each other.

WHY A GAME?

The game, "Concept-Integration," is intended to provide students of Rogers' conceptual framework with a means of gaining practice and experience in the purposeful verbalizations of the terms and concepts that underlie the Rogerian nursing science paradigm. Especially attractive was the possibility of playing the game in or out of the formal classroom setting, which would enhance student-centered learning (Knowles, 1984).

From a Rogerian perspective, learning is a continuous mutual process involving student and teacher, where the teacher, being integral with the student's environment, facilitates the deliberative patterning of the student's cognitive skills in a dynamic and innovative way. Learning may also be perceived as a manifestation of the change occurring through the relationship between student and teacher (Knowles, 1984).

The concept of play represents a natural medium for learning. Games, according to Orlick (1982), "involve people in the process of acting . . . feeling, and experiencing" (p. 3). Cooperative games serve to promote environments where people play with rather than against one another, where the challenge of the game is paramount, and the structure of the game contributes to enjoying the experience. In playing "Concept-Integration," as with other cooperative games, the players find that cooperation is essential to achieve the objective: articulation of the relationships among Rogerian concepts. This game also provides an additional modality that encourages the student to express his or her fullest potential by promoting an integration of new concepts with personal life experience.

While learning manifests through increasing knowledge and diversity of thought, the process as experienced by a student and guided by objectives determined by educators (de Tornay & Thompson, 1982; Knowles, 1984; Reilly, 1980) may be outlined as follows, where the student is able to:

1. Recognize symbols or terms.
2. Recall definitions of terms.
3. Express concepts related to specific definitions.
4. Relate concepts to own experience.
5. Verbalize or write understanding of concepts.
6. Relate one concept to another.
7. Integrate concepts in order to enlarge on the scope of the original terms or concepts.
8. Synthesize relationships among concepts in order to create theories or hypotheses.

I devised a game to assist the student in moving deliberately through the first seven aspects of learning as outlined above. The eighth phase is frequently expressed as an intuitive recognition of insight or an extension of knowledge already assimilated. By providing the student with particular learning opportunities, the game promotes the assimilation of new knowledge or verification of previously learned skills (de Tornay & Thompson, 1982; Gagne, 1965). The student's expertise, however, emerges within the continuous mutual process between student and environment. In this way the game and its processes may be viewed as a learning laboratory (Jaques, 1984).

The incorporation of play during early stages of learning contributes to the ease with which the student integrates information. In early phases of learning most educators use highly structured methods, for example, the lecture and discussion format supported by readings. They then have the student write about what he or she has learned. The words, phrases, and conceptual relationships that roll so easily off the teacher's tongue seem clumsy on the lips of the student, however. Practiced vocalization of terms and phrases can be related to the physical skills practiced in a teaching laboratory (Infante, 1985) and can assist in developing a sense of competence and accomplishment with the material being studied. Feedback from players serves to provide evaluation regarding the mastery of material (de Tornay & Thompson, 1982).

STRUCTURE AND PROCESS OF PLAY

"Concept-Integration" may be played by one or more persons, individually and as teams. The game consists of a playing field or board, concept symbols, and concept statements. Guided by a basic set of rules, students are encouraged to expand their thinking, make logical connections, and express their perceptions of terms and concepts in the most imaginative way possible. Furthermore, the experience of play has demonstrated that the process of socialization and collaboration that occurs among the players stimulates understanding (de Tornay & Thompson, 1982) and a desire to explore the framework more thoroughly.

The playing field (Hanley, 1987) shown in Figure 1 is conceptualized as a space matrix which serves as the unifying theme for the elaboration of the relationships between the individual concepts and the larger scope of the Rogerian nursing science framework. Contextually open, the matrix allows for motion and change as experienced by the players, continuously reflecting the potentialities of patterning implied by the paradigm (Rogers,

Figure 1
The Playing Board

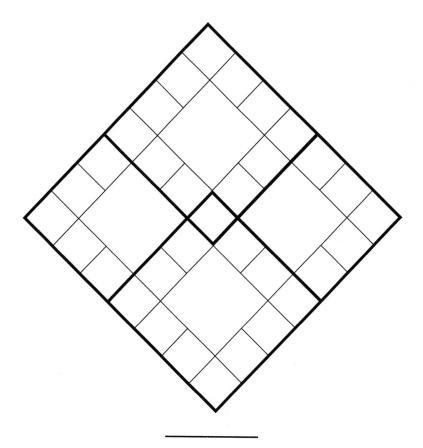

1986). Concept symbols, as seen in Figure 2, are glyphs used to signify the abstract meaning or image of the concepts (Hanley, 1987).

Concept statements derived from the building blocks, principles of homeodynamics, and other underlying concepts as discussed by Rogers (1970, 1983, 1986, 1988) act as the impetus for encouraging the student(s) to examine and expand upon previously understood relationships. Several examples include:

1. A fundamental unit of unitary human beings and the environment.
2. Energy fields are infinite and continuously open.

Figure 2
Examples of Concept Symbol Glyphs

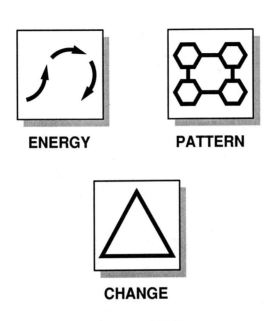

ENERGY   PATTERN

CHANGE

3. A characteristic of the human energy field that is always changing and emerges as increasingly diverse.
4. The continuous mutual process of human and environmental fields.

Employing the intentional use of chance, players select glyphs from a container not knowing what glyph they will select. With each turn, they select a statement that was previously turned face down on the playing surface. The use of chance provides the players with the opportunity to address concepts that they might not otherwise use. The decision as to where to place the glyphs on the playing board constitutes problem-solving behavior. Discussion of choices and perceptions of relationships among the concepts permits students to explore the framework in a safe and open environment.

PLAYING THE GAME

Players make statements regarding their understanding of the concept statements as represented by the glyphs and their rationale for placing any

Figure 3
Glyph Placement by the First Player

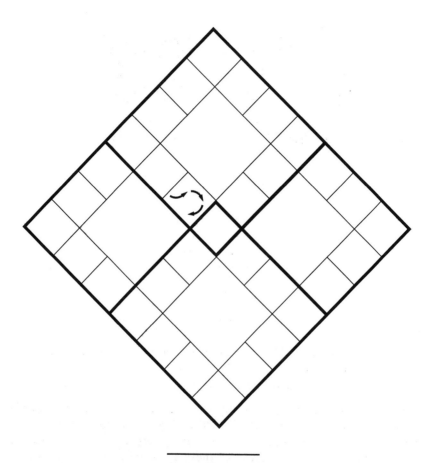

one glyph on a particular space on the game board in order to complete a turn. Other players comment in response, stating their own understanding of the glyphs, concept statements, and board placement.

The examples below represent players' perceptions about concepts and the relationships among the concepts under study. It is important to remember that students are encouraged to explore unfamiliar terrain and to become comfortable with vocalizing the language, its terms, phrases, definitions, and concepts; to integrate these within their current knowledge base; and to begin to explore the depths of the Rogerian conceptual system.

Figure 4
Glyph Placement by the Second Player

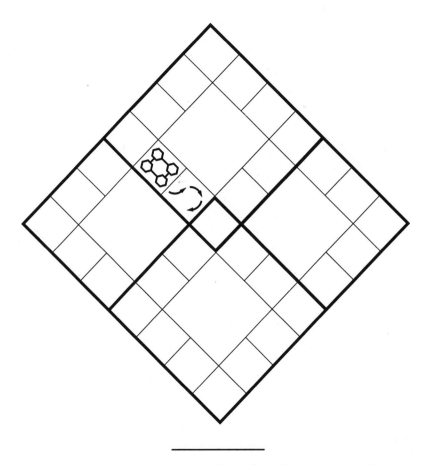

Therefore, the responses herein may be awkward or wordy to the experienced reader.

A Sample Play

Player 1, using the statement, "A fundamental unit of unitary human beings and the environment," places the glyph for energy in the space adjacent to the center space of the playing field's left upper axis (see Figure 3), stating, "Energy field is the fundamental unit of unitary human beings. By placing it next to the center I'm indicating that energy has an essential

Figure 5
Glyph Placement by the Third Player

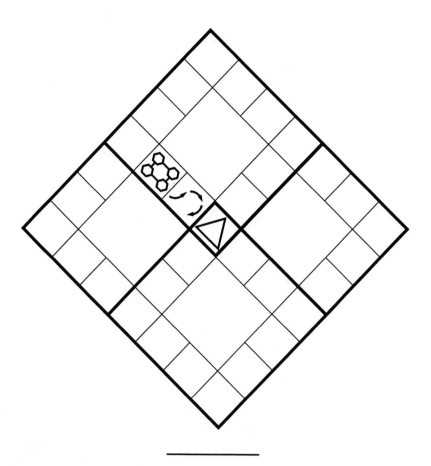

relationship with all other concepts but is not necessarily the central concept."

Player 2, referring to the statement, "A characteristic of the human energy field is always changing, and emerges as increasingly diverse," places the glyph for pattern next to the symbol for energy (see Figure 4) stating, "Pattern characterizes the human energy field. Since energy fields are open and continuously changing, patterns that emerge are understood to be innovative and increasingly diverse."

Player 3, selecting the statement, "The continuous mutual process of human and environmental fields," places the glyph for change on the playing board in the center space (see Figure 5), stating, "The relationship between energy field patterns and change are manifested in the continuous mutual process between the human and environmental fields. The process of change facilitates the rhythmic and predictable nature of our universe and is central to human field and environmental field patterning."

These examples demonstrate the direction in which play proceeds from less to more diverse responses. Suppose that you are the final player of this game. How would you discuss the overall configuration of the symbols as laid out by your colleagues in Figure 5? Do you see a pattern emerging? Can you imagine the dialogue that would take place between yourself and the other players as you each found ways to express your differing perceptions of the evolutionary pattern on the playing field's matrix? How could you utilize this pattern of play to discuss a patient care situation?

The use of "Concept-Integration" in an educational setting increases the student's learning opportunities. As a tool, the game expands the resources available to students and teachers, creating a more diverse and innovative environment in which learning might manifest. As play, the game contributes to the student's sense of enjoyment in acquiring basic and advanced understanding of the complex language of the Science of Unitary Human Beings. Participation in this medium of cooperative, student-centered learning generates a sense of collaboration among players. The creativity, enjoyment, and community engendered by this particular approach to learning can only enhance the future articulation of Rogers' paradigm of nursing science within the nursing profession.

REFERENCES

Barrett, E. (1988). Using Rogers' science of unitary human beings in nursing practice. *Nursing Science Quarterly, 1,* 50–51.

de Tornay, R., & Thompson, M. (1982). *Strategies for teaching nursing* (2nd ed.). New York: John Wiley & Sons.

Gagne, R. (1965). *The conditions of learning.* New York: Holt, Reinhart & Winston.

Hanley, M.A. (1985). *Headwerks: A game of concept-integration.* Unpublished manuscript.

Hanley, M.A. (1987). *Concept-Integration: A board game* (Patent pending No. 049,589). Washington, DC: U.S. Patent Office.

Infante, M.S. (1985). *The clinical laboratory in nursing education* (2nd ed.). New York: John Wiley & Sons.

Jaques, D. (1984). *Learning in groups.* London: Croom-Helm.

Knowles, M. (1984). *The adult learner: A neglected species* (3rd ed.). Houston: Gulf Publishing.

Orlick, T. (1982). *The second cooperative sports and games book*. New York: Pantheon Books.

Reilly, D. (1980). *Behavioral objectives: Evaluation in nursing* (2nd ed.). New York: Appleton-Century-Crofts.

Rogers, M. (1970). *An introduction to the theoretical basis of nursing*. Philadelphia: F.A. Davis.

Rogers, M. (1983). *Postulated correlates of patterning in unitary human beings*. Unpublished manuscript, New York University, New York.

Rogers, M. (1986). Science of unitary human beings. In V.M. Malinski (Ed.), *Explorations on Martha Rogers' science of unitary human beings* (pp. 3–8). Norwalk, CT: Appleton-Century-Crofts.

Rogers, M. (1988). Nursing science and art: A prospective. *Nursing Science Quarterly, 1,* 99–102.

22

Issues in Dissertation Proposal Development

Ardis R. Swanson

There are numerous points in question and matters of dispute in dissertation proposal development, irrespective of whether or not the doctoral candidate chooses to prepare a research proposal consistent with Rogers' conceptual system. In this paper, therefore, I will enumerate several issues generic to doctoral education across all programs, discuss each issue in general terms, and present points of view within Rogerian perspectives.

Among the issues of significance in doctoral education are the following: (1) What is the purpose of the dissertation for the doctoral degree, and how does its purpose articulate with the specific degree that the doctoral program offers (i.e., PhD, EdD, or DNS?). (2) If the dissertation proposal is a research proposal to extend the knowledge base for nursing, what qualifies as "knowledge"? (3) Does the dissertation require theory testing, or is the generation of theory of equal acceptability? (4) Should the dissertation product be obviously useful to nursing practice, or do studies that focus on human beings, without clear foresight of how the knowledge will be applicable to nursing, equally qualify for a dissertation? (5) Can the process of the dissertation be expected to produce substantive knowledge, or is the process basically a learning experience preparatory for postdoctoral research?

THE PURPOSE OF THE DISSERTATION

The dissertation is so universal a doctoral degree requirement that a sense of *why* it is a requirement can easily fade or be lost from awareness. What it *is* reveals *why* it is. The dissertation is an original and creative work that requires of the candidate an independence and scholarship beyond that required for prior degrees. The dissertation provides evidence to the degree-granting institution that the candidate has met the objectives of the program and has earned the highest degree the institution has to offer in academic achievement.

The central objective of the doctoral program in nursing at New York University is to prepare its candidates in research, theory development, and leadership. The dissertation that completes the requirements for the PhD degree in nursing provides the candidate a means of demonstrating acquired ability to systematically work through a problem or question relevant to nursing, from the clear conception of the question or problem to the ultimate conclusions, demonstrating an understanding of the philosophical assumptions on which the study was based, and the ability to apply an appropriate research method to the problem, such that confidence can be placed in the conclusions.

These statements relative to purpose of the dissertation declare a standard for doctoral education. They may reflect the position of various doctoral programs. It is, in fact, the standard aspired to by the doctoral program in nursing at New York University where the opportunity to develop research within the Rogerian framework is available.

However, how strongly should an academic unit in which the Rogerian conceptual framework is its major conceptual basis encourage or require that dissertations be developed within that framework? One position reminds us that the major commitment of such a program should be the development of dissertations derived from the proclaimed conceptual framework. Other positions allow more latitude. No one, to this author's knowledge, believes that the Rogerian conceptual framework can be "required." The spirit of inquiry and the principle of fostering students' intellectual capacities and pursuits renders a requirement of holding a particular world view unacceptable. It can also be argued that closing out other models would be incongruent with the Rogerian position of openness. As a result, dissertations have been and are being completed in the nursing program at New York University with a variety of conceptual frameworks. The program does, however, do much to provide opportunities for the student to be knowledgeable regarding the Rogerian system, especially its underlying assumptions or world view: It provides exemplars of studies based on the system and assigns exercises in deriving theorems from the system. These opportunities, currently extant in the research and theory development program in nursing science, may be provided in other programs as well. In fact, an increasing number of research studies are being conducted within the Rogerian system in such other programs. The position at New York University is that theory can be developed in several ways. These are outlined following the next section on knowledge and ways of knowing.

KNOWLEDGE AND WAYS OF KNOWING

Research builds a body of knowledge. But what qualifies as knowledge? Knowledge is generally considered to be more than information. Yet information may become knowledge if it is organized in some fashion. Theory, of course, is comprised of concepts that are "organized" to show relationships among concepts. At that point, theory becomes knowledge.

More than ever before, current nursing literature is addressing the epistemological questions of what knowledge is and how knowledge comes about (Carper, 1978; Chinn & Jacobs, 1987; Meleis, 1985; Sarter, 1988). Nursing research texts now regularly outline various sources of knowledge, including personal knowledge and intuition. Most outlines also acknowledge the range of possible methods by which nursing scholars build the knowledge base, including methods that discover or generate theory and methods that construct and test theory systematically. The qualitative methodologies of discovery also emphasize the necessity for systematic rigor.

It must be remembered that systematic rigor in qualitative methodologies has assisted these studies to gain respect from a wider scientific community, including previous strongholds of "quantitative" methodology.

A dissertation developed within a Rogerian framework certainly requires a systematic and rigorous approach. While all researchers acknowledge the value of intuition, it can be said that a Rogerian perspective has high regard for thought processes that put things together in new ways. The Rogerian conceptual system is itself a creative synthesis. Theories that develop within the system require concept identification and analysis consistent with the system's world view. Relationships among these concepts may be hypothesized. By this process concepts and theories are not borrowed from other fields, but rather are "derived" from within the system. While some fields of inquiry acknowledge only data that is identifiable through the five senses, a Rogerian perspective expects that information is transmitted by routes additional to the five senses. While some researchers require that data be validated by other than the subjects, a Rogerian perspective accepts as evidence that which a subject reports thinking or feeling.

Since the Rogerian system is highly abstract, research within it is an exceptional challenge. For research to be credible today, it must be comprehensibly translated from conception to empirical evidence (or in the case of qualitative studies, a comprehensible translation from raw data to abstractions). The presentation must also be logical and adhere to the other rules of the method chosen to answer the question. Faculty members on the dissertation committee guide the student, but the final approval of the dissertation stands on the candidate's ability to meet the above criteria.

THEORY BUILDING, THEORY TESTING, AND THEORY GENERATION

At New York University the doctoral sequence of courses presents the position that nursing theory can be developed in one of three ways:

1. By derivation from a conceptual framework. In this approach the framework is identified, the assumptions specified, and the concepts selected that are consistent with the system. Within the Rogerian system the interest is always unitary human beings in the context of environment; however, the choice is broad within that context. The interest might be something high on the level of abstraction, such as integrality or helicy, or something less abstract, providing the assumptions of the system are honored. The higher the level, the greater the problems of measurement, there being few instruments yet appropriate to the Rogerian system. In two recent examples of successful work, Barrett (1983) and McEvoy (1987) developed their dissertations within a Rogerian perspective derived from the principle of helicy.

2. By developing a substantive theory. This is done by identifying concepts of interest on which considerable literature exists, extracting the linkages that have been claimed, assessing the strength of the evidence on linkages, and logically proposing linkages for testing. It is important to ascertain whether instruments exist for measuring the concepts and, if so, whether they are compatible with the researcher's conceptual framework and conception of the phenomenon of interest. This way of developing theory is entirely acceptable for studies in the doctoral program, and may or may not be within a Rogerian framework.

3. By utilizing an inductive approach for the generation of theory. This is viewed as an appropriate method when very little is known about a subject or when tests of linkages have been inconclusive. The product of this approach is a theory or model, or an interpretation which is an extraction of meaning from the data obtained in naturalistic settings.

The first of the three ways described above is consistent with a Rogerian perspective. For a nursing study to be consistent with a Rogerian perspective within the second way requires that concept/constructs from the literature be thoughtfully critiqued for their assumptions and definitions. Modification may be required, or new instruments devised, to be consistent with the conceptual basis of the nursing study.

Studies by inductive methods are viewed by some as atheoretical at the outset, in the sense that the phenomenon of interest is approached without preconceptions about the phenomenon of interest. However, a study from a naturalistic point of view does not preclude a theoretical frame of reference. The emptiness desired is of *bias*, not an emptiness of objective and rational *thought*. (There are several methods available to reduce bias.) For example, data gathered by qualitative methods are subjected to systematic methods of processing. A theory may be generated which has yet to be tested. Much of the quality rests on the interpretation of the data. A researcher who is knowledgeable in the Rogerian system could finally interpret data from the frame of reference of the Rogerian system.

What makes an approach congruent with a Rogerian point of view is whether the assumptions of the Rogerian world view are evident either in the research design or in the interpretation of the inductively produced data. It is a difficult task to design a dissertation congruent with a Rogerian world view, however. Considering the limitations of current methodologies, complete consistency is not even possible yet.

Although inductive studies have become increasingly visible in nursing literature, it is too early to tell the relative significance of their contribution to nursing knowledge compared to knowledge via other approaches. The compatibility of the second and third way with a Rogerian perspective has been debated and in some details remains problematic. One point of congruence is conspicuous: in naturalistic studies the focus is on a *phenomenon in context*; in Rogerian studies the focus is on *unitary human beings in environment*.

The case study has been the method in several dissertations completed at New York University—several more are in process. By virtue of having spelled out Rogerian assumptions, and having focused on persons in the context of their environment, or having interpreted data with the assistance of the Rogerian system, some can be termed Rogerian. An important assumption underlying qualitative methods is that a phenomenon can only be understood in its context. This assumption is congruent with the Rogerian principle of integrality. Oliver (1987), for example, approached her study with a Rogerian perspective, and she did not compromise the rigor of case methodology.

The traditional "scientific method" proposes relationships among concepts/constructs and tests for the existence and strength of the relationships. Qualitative approaches, on the other hand, have as their objective the discovery or generation of theory. There are doctoral programs in nursing in the United States that have reputations of particular strength in one or another of these approaches (e.g., Teachers College, Columbia University, in historical research; University of Colorado in qualitative approaches—ethnographic and phenomenological, etc.).

The doctoral program at New York University has been nationally recognized for its strength in theory development. The majority of its dissertations have tested theory by adhering to "the scientific method." The program has capitalized on the strength of its sibling departments. Recall the reputations of Drs. Kerlinger and Pedazur, for example. Yet, from a Rogerian perspective, it is a troublesome fact that the studies have only focused on a selection of few variables, whereas the Rogerian paradigm conceives of human beings as irreducible wholes. Students, for the most part, realize this tension between wholeness and focus. Despite the assumption of wholeness, a single study requires focus. In an effort to comprehend the complexity of any human phenomenon the students construct a picture display of all the variables that are possibly linked to the one of central interest. If a qualitative study is appropriate to the question, the display model can serve to identify preconceptions (for bracketing); if a quantitative study is chosen, the researcher attempts to "hold constant" as many of the variables as possible while focusing on the few. In addition, the present age of computer capabilities and availabilities has made the inclusion of a multitude of variables possible, so that the whole of the situation is more nearly approximated.

APPLICABILITY OF DISSERTATION OUTCOMES TO NURSING PRACTICE

There is great need in society for improved nursing practice and considerable focus in nursing literature on the application of research findings to practice. While no one would challenge the desirability of applying substantiated theory to practice, there is good reason to express concern about the pressures to apply research prior to adequate replication of each original study. Because doctoral students are sensitive to social need, it follows that they tend to wish for a research question that will have an immediate practical applicability. Some students follow a question that makes a real contribution to solving a current problem, but if all studies were of this nature it would be short-sighted for the profession. From a Rogerian perspective, much is yet to be learned about human beings and their patterning in the context of environment. Wearing Rogerian "glasses" (i.e., wearing the assumptions) one sees human beings in a less time-bound sense. Groundwork has only begun in building a knowledge base for further investigation and application to nursing practice. Therefore, it is unwise to give greater emphasis to research that tackles immediate practice problems than to research that can give long-term meaning for society.

THE DISSERTATION'S VALUE: CONTENT VS. PROCESS

The profession is still so young, so new in the development of its own body of knowledge, that it is understandable that so much attention is placed on the findings of dissertations. But the dissertation is only a researcher's first effort. The idea of entire careers focused on conducting nursing research is new to the profession. The major nursing journals still contain a high percentage of reports based on dissertations. It can be expected that such journals will also contain more reports of postdoctoral studies. Perhaps then the dissertation can be viewed more as a valuable stepping stone to career-long research attitudes and achievements. No doubt, doctoral students knowledgeable in the Rogerian conceptual framework have their place in the direction of research and its products, perhaps increasingly in the years to come.

REFERENCES

Barrett, E.A.M. (1983). An empirical investigation of Martha E. Rogers' principle of helicy: The relationship of human field motion and power. *Dissertation Abstracts International, 45*, 615A. (University Microfilms No. 8406278)

Carper, B.A. (1978). Fundamental patterns of knowing in nursing. *Advances in Nursing Science, 1*(1), 13–23.

Chinn, P.G., & Jacobs, M.K. (1987). *Theory and nursing: A systematic approach* (2nd ed.). St. Louis: C.V. Mosby.

McEvoy, M.D. (1987). The relationship among the experience of dying, the experience of paranormal events, and creativity in adults. *Dissertation Abstracts International, 48*, 2264B. (University Microfilms No. 8720130)

Meleis, A.I. (1985). *Theoretical nursing: Development and progress.* Philadelphia: Lippincott.

Oliver, N.R. (1987). Processing unacceptable behaviors of co-workers: A naturalistic study of nurses at work. *Dissertation Abstracts International, 49*, 75B. (University Microfilms No. 8803598)

Sarter, B. (Ed.). (1988). *Paths to knowledge: Innovative research methods for nursing.* New York: National League for Nursing.

Unit V

Visions of the Future

Whatever the future of nursing may be, it will be within the context of rapid change, diversity, new knowledge, and new horizons.

Martha E. Rogers

23

Visions of Rogerian Science in the Future of Humankind

Elizabeth Ann Manhart Barrett

The 21st Century will arrive with a plethora of manifestations of change. Rapid acceleration will be evident in every aspect of life. Diversification and synthesis will grow as new world views multiply to encompass the extraterrestrial. Nursing's abstract system signifies a new reality as nurses participate in the process of change to benefit people. The future demands flexibility, imagination, and a sense of humor.

Martha E. Rogers, 1988

The Science of Unitary Human Beings is for the future and is about change (Rogers, 1970, 1986, 1988, 1989). While Rogerian science has been useful in understanding the Space Age to date, it promises to be even more useful in anticipating a future where nursing can make a contribution to the well being of people in this newly explored world of space. Nursing provides health services that will continue to involve patterning the environment to promote comfort, health, well being, and healing. However, the discipline needs a global perspective in order to design nursing therapeutics at the planetary level.

The author acknowledges Violet M. Malinski for her thoughtful critique of an earlier draft of this manuscript.

EARTH AND SPACE AS ENERGY FIELDS

Rogers' concept of energy fields provides a new world view to describe humankind in mutual process with space. She proposed that there are two energy fields: the human and the environmental (Rogers, 1970). Both fields are irreducible, four-dimensional wholes identified by pattern. In this system *all* that is *not* a particular human field is that field's unique environmental field. "Each environmental field is specific to its given human field" (Rogers, 1986, p. 5). The human field can be conceptualized as a person, a family, any group of people; all else is environment. "The human and environmental fields are infinite and integral with one another" (Rogers, 1986, p. 5). Therefore, humankind is integral with Earth, with space, with the universe.

Rogers' science postulates that change is accelerating. In 1903 the Wright brothers were the first to fly a plane. In 1927 Lindbergh flew across the Atlantic. In 1957 the Space Age began with the satellite Sputnik orbiting the Earth. In 1969 humans first walked on the moon. Considering that it took the entirety of history for humans to leave the earth and enter the sky in 1903 and only 66 more years to enter space and walk on the moon, there is evidence to support Rogers' theory of accelerating change. In the past 20 years, 200 people from 20 countries have seen Earth from space (Kelley, 1988). The Apollo missions from 1969 to 1972 may be "remembered as the 20th century's legacy to future generations who may expand out into the solar system" (Wilford, 1989, p. 7). The Soviet space program has also had a wide range of projects and they have set records with cosmonauts who have been in space for nearly a year (*Red Star*, 1988). Both astronauts and cosmonauts talk of falling in love with the Earth and describe awesome, visionary experiences of wonder and joy (Kelley, 1988).

HUMAN HISTORY IN TRANSITION

In a universe believed to be approximately 12 billion years old, our world and solar system is believed to be approximately 4.5 billion years old—the same age as some of the rocks found on the moon (Coates, 1975; Hart, Haupt, & Hollister, 1989). Considering the appearance of the human species in this time span, Stephen Jay Gould provides a particularly clear view of evolution:

> The human species has inhabited this planet for only 250,000 years or so—roughly .0015 percent of the history of life, the last inch of the cosmic mile. Human evolution is not random. . . . The pathways that

have led to our evolution are quirky, improbable, unrepeatable and utterly unpredictable. . . . We cannot read the meaning of life passively in the facts of nature. We must construct the answers ourselves—from our own wisdom and ethical sense ("Meaning of Life," 1988, p. 84).

One wonders if there are other places (or spaces) where life exists. If so, how many? The universe is vast. Nobel laureate Wald (1989) reminds us that our galaxy, the Milky Way, contains about 100 billion stars and yet is only a tiny spot in the universe. If 1 percent of the stars of the Milky Way have a planet that could support life, there could be a billion such places in our home galaxy. With a billion such galaxies in the already observed universe, there could be "a billion billion—10^{18}—places" that could support life (p. 11). Wald believes that life arises when given enough time wherever conditions that make life possible exist. One wonders, is humankind the only kind?

Although certainly not a random sample, 35 leading scientists were asked whether life exists in space. Twenty-six said they believed it does exist in some form in our galaxy. Astrophysicist Drake claimed that "by 2089 we will have succeeded in learning about other civilizations" ("Is Anyone Out There," 1989, p. 50). Others say that while it is very likely that life exists, it is not likely that intelligent life like humans exist.

Whether or not there are other forms of intelligent life in our galaxy, one must consider the changes in humankind that will accompany space travel. Rogers (1988) foretells of transition from humankind to spacekind. No one really knows in any great detail what will happen in the future—it is unpredictable (Rogers, 1989).

FUTURE EVOLUTIONARY EMERGENTS

It is planned that by 1998 people will work and live on the National Aeronautics and Space Administration's (NASA) permanent space station Freedom (New Frontiers, 1988). A permanent moon base that could be operational by 2005 would allow testing of space habitats, construction approaches, and ways to mine lunar ore for fuel and building materials. Attempts would be made to extract breathing gas from moon rocks that are about 41 percent oxygen (Broad, 1989).

Astronaut Michael Collins considers colonization of Mars as a long-term goal. He sees the moon as a "stepping stone to more interesting places like Mars and perhaps Titan, one of Saturn's moons" (cited in Wilford, 1989, p. 7). Most experts predict human travel to Mars in the early decades of the next century.

Space colonies are proposed as "artificial worlds moving in orbit between the moon and Earth. These artificial worlds won't be a round ball with people living on the outside of them, like Earth" (McGowen, 1987, p. 59). Most scientists propose that they would be in the shape of a "huge ring, about a mile wide, with six spokes leading to a hub in the center, like a wheel . . . Some 10,000 people could live in such a wheel in space" (p. 59).

Science fiction is fast becoming science fact. Weather and communications satellites have been operating in space for a decade. Proposals for construction projects, power plants, mining of ore, research projects, business opportunities in transportation, materials processing, and remote sensing are being discussed by major corporations and governments. Robots will play an important role in space exploration and space industry. Make no mistake about it, commercial payloads will be big business in the 21st century (*New Frontiers*, 1988).

To date more than 30,000 applications of space technology transferred to commercial or private use have been reported by NASA. Many pertain to health care. Some NASA spin-offs "allow the deaf to see sounds and the blind to feel images" (Maurer, 1989, p. 58). The eyeglasses for the deaf translate sounds into images by a microcomputer. Other research led to voice-operated wheelchairs and wheelchairs so light they can be lifted with one hand. Laser technology and fiber optics seek noninvasive treatments to replace various surgical procedures.

Knowledge of such activities is essential for nursing's future. Rogers (1988) maintains that "the study of nursing is the study of human and environmental fields" (p. 100), and that nursing is integral with the rapidly changing world. Rogers is currently developing her thinking on space in relation to the Science of Unitary Human Beings. The University of Alabama at Huntsville, College of Nursing, publishes the *Space Nursing Newsletter* and will present the second "Nursing in Space Conference" in 1990. There is potential for nursing knowledge to contribute to understanding unitary humans in the space environment.

As explained by the principle of integrality, space exploration provides evidence that humans change as the environment changes. Perhaps Rogers' postulated manifestations of field patterning (Madrid & Winstead-Fry, 1986) suggest precursors of transformation of humankind to spacekind. These postulated manifestations raise provocative questions concerning the cosmic leap of humans from Earth to space. Will the highly innovative environment of space reveal humans with field rhythms so rapid as to seem continuous? Will transition toward spacekind be characterized by greater diversity and higher frequency wave patterning than humankind? Will transition be a four-dimensional reality without spatial or temporal attributes where experience is timeless? Will highly imaginative, beyond waking, visionary experiences be the norm rather than the exception?

HEALTH IN SPACE

Nursing's purpose is to promote the health and well being of people wherever they exist. Now is the time for nursing to begin raising meaningful questions framed in a new world view that will seek to understand unitary humans in new environments. How will they eat, sleep, recreate, procreate, exercise, rest, and carry out activities of daily living?

What will nursing as a discipline contribute to the scientific understanding of human betterment in the Space Age? How will nursing knowledge be used to promote the health and well being of those in space? Will nurse scientists travel to space to conduct research on human field pattern manifestations in environments such as space stations and the moon? Will nurse scientists study the meaning of various lived experiences that will occur in space, for example, giving birth in space, the childhood of those born in space who have never been to Earth, the multigenerational families with Earth-born and space-born members? What nursing knowledge and nursing services will be required by a multiplanetary species? What will be the relationship of lifestyle and health in space? What can we discover in space that will promote health and well being on Earth? When space travelers return to Earth, what nursing services will they require?

While resistance to change is as old as human life itself, if we in nursing are awake to what is happening around us, we can begin seeking answers in nursing to such questions as those posed above. "The life of the future lies in space, and that life may be so different from what we have now that we can scarcely imagine it" (McGowen, 1987, p. 59). A pioneering spirit and cosmic leap thinking set the stage for the days ahead. The future is now as well as tomorrow and nurse scholars and leaders can knowingly participate in its creation. This is professional power.

REFERENCES

Broad, W.J. (July 17, 1989). New phase on the moon: U.S. weighs a return. *The New York Times*, pp. 1, 12.

Coates, John B.S. (1975). *The last quarter of the century*. Adyar, India: Theosophical Publishing House.

Hart, L., Haupt, D., & Hollister, A. (1989, July). Moonrocks. *Life*, pp. 58–59, 62–63, 66–67.

Kelley, K.W. (Ed.). (1988). *The home planet*. Reading, MA: Addison-Wesley.

Maurer, A. (1989, January). They came from outer space. *Modern Maturity*, 57–61.

Madrid, M., & Winstead-Fry (1986). Rogers' conceptual model. In P. Winstead-Fry (Ed.), *Case studies in nursing theory* (pp. 73–102). New York: National League for Nursing.

McGowen, T. (1987). *Album of spaceflight*. New York: Checkerboard Press.

Rogers, M.E. (1970). *An introduction to the theoretical basis of nursing*. Philadelphia: F.A. Davis.

Rogers, M.E. (1986). Science of unitary human beings. In V. Malinski (Ed.), *Explorations on Martha Rogers' science of unitary human beings* (pp. 3–8). Norwalk, CT: Appleton-Century-Crofts.

Rogers, M.E. (1988). Nursing science and art: A prospective. *Nursing Science Quarterly*, *1*, 99–102.

Rogers, M.E. (1989, July). *Research in the new way of thinking: The science of unitary human beings*. Paper presented at the Summer Research Conference, College of Nursing, Wayne State University, Detroit, MI.

Staff. (1989, July). Is anyone out there? In *Life Magazine*, pp. 48–57.

Staff. (1988, December). The meaning of life. In *Life Magazine*, pp. 82–84, 86, 89–90, 93.

Staff. (September 26, 1988). The new frontiers. *U.S. News & World Report*, pp. 48–60.

Staff. (May 16, 1988). Red star rising. *U.S. News & World Report*, pp. 46–54.

Wald, G. (1989, Spring). The cosmology of life and mind. *Noetic Sciences Review*, 10–15.

Wilford, J.N. (July 16, 1989). 20 years after the moon landing, a sense of mission is gone. *The New York Times*, Section 4, pp. 1, 7.

24

The Rogerian Science of
Unitary Human Beings as a Knowledge
Base for Nursing in Space

Violet M. Malinski

Rogers' (1970, 1986, 1987) Science of Unitary Human Beings offers a new world view, a way of perceiving and experiencing humans and their world that is radically different from much of contemporary nursing. This science enables nurses to derive theories about the continuous, creative process of change and to develop human field modalities for participation in this change process. It is a progressive view, in the sense of moving and evolving, and one that encompasses outer space as environmental field.

THE SCIENCE OF UNITARY HUMAN BEINGS

Rogers defines nursing as a basic science having a philosophy of wholeness. Nursing focuses on people and their world with the aim of assisting people to achieve their own potentials, to help them participate knowingly in the process of change. The Science of Unitary Human Beings offers a view of people and their world as an integral whole evolving or changing together via a continuous, mutual process. Humans are in mutual process with the total patterning of the environment. Rogers (1986) uses the term "field" to convey "a means of perceiving people and their respective environments as irreducible wholes" (p. 4). Within the continuous, mutual process of human and environmental fields, the person participates in the nature of change.

The person-environmental field process is characterized by energy patterning of low or high frequency. Rogers (1986) defines pattern "as the distinguishing characteristic of an energy field perceived as a single wave" (p. 5). The nature of the patterning is continuously changing and always creative. Health or well being, patterning which is optimal for the person, would be one manifestation of the field process. The principles of homeodynamics (Rogers, 1986) postulate the nature of the human-environmental field process. According to the principle of resonancy, human and environmental field patterning changes continuously, flowing in higher frequencies. The principle of helicy identifies the innovative and probabilistic (noncausal) increasing diversity of this field patterning. Integrality specifies the continuous mutual process of human and environmental fields; person and environment are unitary (whole) rather than separate entities.

Manifestations of field patterning emerge from this continuous mutual process (see Table 1). For example, Rogers has identified motion, time, and sleep as examples of such manifestations. They are postulated to flow as slower motion, faster motion, seems continuous; time experienced as slower, as faster, as timelessness; and as longer sleeping, longer waking, beyond waking.

Three theories focusing on the continuous, creative change process have been derived from the Science of Unitary Human Beings. Rogers (1987) identified two: accelerating change and the emergence of paranormal phenomena. Barrett (1984, 1986) derived a theory of power as knowing participation in change.

According to the theory of accelerating change, change is continuous, innovative, probabilistic, and characterized by higher frequency field patterning. This theory suggests, for example, that hyperactive children manifest accelerated field patterning rather than symptoms necessitating medical intervention (Malinski, 1986), and that the process of aging is rich in potentials for freedom, learning, and creative participation rather than decay and decline. It suggests that what we call "norms" are only averages; also, norms imply stasis rather than change.

The theory of the emergence of paranormal phenomena suggests that experiences labeled "paranormal," such as precognition, clairvoyance, or healing at a distance, may indicate higher frequency field patterning. A basic concept in the Science of Unitary Human Beings is four-dimensionality, defined as "a nonlinear domain without spatial or temporal attributes" (Rogers, 1986, p. 5). As it is without time and space constraints, four-dimensionality suggests nonordinary experiencing.

Table 1
Manifestations of Field Patterning in Unitary Human Beings.

The nature of unitary field patterning is probabilistic and creative. Change is relative and increasingly diverse. Some manifestations of relative diversity of field patterning are:

lesser diversity		greater diversity
longer rhythms	shorter	seems continuous
slower motion	faster	seems continuous
time experienced		
as slower	as faster	timelessness
pragmatic	imaginative	visionary
longer sleeping	longer waking	beyond waking

Madrid & Winstead-Fry, 1986, p. 79; reprinted with permission © National League for Nursing.

Unitary human beings, integral with the environment, can participate knowingly in change, actualizing some potentials rather than others (Rogers, 1970, 1986, 1987). Barrett (1984, 1986) identified this natural potential as power, defining power "as the capacity to participate knowingly in the nature of change characterizing the continuous patterning of human and environmental fields" (1986, p. 174). Manifestations of power include awareness, choices, freedom to act intentionally, and involvement in creating changes. Unitary humans *participate* in the patterning process; they do not adapt to or alter the environment. Knowing participation means that individuals can "share in the creation of their human and environmental reality" (1983, p. 119). This concept of sharing suggests that "reality" is dynamic and continuously changing rather than static, that it is a participatory experience rather than an objective one.

The ideas discussed above as illustrative of Rogers' world view can be contrasted with what she identified as older views (see Table 2).

NURSING IN SPACE

Older World Views Represented in the Space Literature

A review of the literature indicates the predominance of the older world view described in Table 2. For example, a major theme is adaptation. In the dichotomous view of person and environment, space is perceived as a hostile environment to be adapted to simulate earth. This older world view is reflected in the following themes.

1. Conceptual engineering studies indicate that space settlements can be designed to incorporate earth-like characteristics of sunshine, gravity, the

Table 2
Some Differences between Older and Newer Views of Persons and Their World*

Older Views	Newer Views
cell theory	field theory
entropic universe	negentropic universe
people: three-dimensional	people: four-dimensional
people: homeostatic	people: homeodynamic
person/environment: dichotomous	person/environment: integral
causation: single and multiple	mutual process
adaptation	mutual process
closed systems: feedback	open system: innovation
dynamic equilibrium	innovative growing diversity
waking: people's basic state	waking: an evolutionary emergent
spacialization of time	dynamization of space
present: point in linear time	present: four-dimensional
being	becoming

*Revised from Rogers' 6/83 version.
Madrid & Winsted-Fry, 1986, p. 77; reprinted with permission © National League for Nursing.

day/night cycle, and areas for flowers, trees, and grass (National Commission on Space, 1986).

2. A remote health care delivery system for outer space must be developed. Consideration should be given to implementing a system similar to the terrestrial medical care system. This includes concerns such as ways to perform surgery and dynamics of drug actions in microgravity conditions (National Commission on Space, 1986).

3. Hall (1985) identified the following technical concerns as problems awaiting solutions:

> Personal hygiene. Astronauts need to be able to bathe their entire bodies every 3 days, supplemented with multiple daily hand and face washes. Showers seem preferable to sponge baths, as the Skylab crew reported feeling more invigorated after the former.
>
> Disposal of waste water and body wastes.
>
> Lighting. Astronauts need appropriate lighting for performing work tasks as well as for maintaining activities of daily living, including sleep and recreation.
>
> Health maintenance. Although astronauts understand the importance of exercise in preventing muscle atrophy and bone decalcification, following through can be difficult unless the psychological aspects of exercising and timing are considered. The Skylab crew suggested placing ergometers in front of the window to provide a view, preventing

monotony. Hall (1985) suggested the development of bicycle ergometers with monitors tunable to feature films or videos of bicycle paths on earth.

Food and water. Food plays a role in psychological well being. The major challenge is to delay the point at which foods become monotonous.

Housekeeping tasks as they affect human productivity (e.g., trash management and cleaning).

4. From one third (Oberg, 1984) to one half (Seddon, 1988) of all space travelers experience space sickness, called Space Adaptation Syndrome, for the first few days. This is similar to motion sickness and includes nausea following movement of the head. Because there is no satisfactory etiological explanation for why this happens to some people, there is no known cure or method of prevention; however, the syndrome fades away after a few days (Oberg, 1984). Members of the Skylab crew found that deliberately experiencing the movements associated with the symptoms helped to eradicate them faster than taking medications (Whitby, 1986).

5. Long-term adaptation to space poses threats to health upon return to earth (e.g., bone decay, heart muscle atrophy) (Oberg, 1984; Whitby, 1986).

6. Isolation and confinement results in problems of boredom, irritability, depression, anxiety, fatigue, hostility, and social withdrawal. As these are general symptoms of stress, McNeal and Bluth (1981) recommended teaching astronauts stress reduction techniques like progressive relaxation.

7. "Astronauts and cosmonauts have frequently spoken rapturously of the beauty of space, but have never said they experienced an altered state of consciousness or anything like pilot breakoff" (Oberg & Oberg, 1986, p. 251).

Newer World Views Represented in the Space Literature

Rather than a problem-oriented perspective, discussions of space reflecting a newer world view focus on diversity and creative potentials for change. This world view is often reflected in comments from astronauts themselves. For example, Skylab astronauts reported heightened visual acuity and individual differences in perceptual abilities, each one finding different features of earth and detecting subtle ranges of colors and textures (Oberg & Oberg, 1986; White, 1987).

Charles Berry, former Director of Life Sciences at NASA and personal physician to the astronauts, is quoted in Bluth (1979) as commenting that all the astronauts were changed in some way by their experiences in space. Contrary to Oberg and Oberg's (1986) observation regarding altered levels of consciousness, Bluth found evidence of what he described as "deep intuition in an altered state of consciousness" (p. 531) in many astronauts' accounts of their experiences. Edgar Mitchell phrased it this way:

> Something happened to me during the flight, that I would say it was a peak experience, if you will. I flipped out, or whatever, and the next two years I spent in resettling my entire thought process, because as a result of that experience virtually all of the philosophies, ideas, scientific truth, and so forth, that were dear to me and were part of my scientific paradigm got tossed right up into the air. . . . (cited in Bluth, 1979, p. 525)

Out of this experience, Mitchell was moved to found the Institute of Noetic Sciences for the explorations of human potentials. In 1985, supported by the institute, space explorers from 13 countries including the USSR, formed the Association of Space Explorers to explore the "sometimes transformative experiences of flying in space and experiencing the home planet as a whole" (Schweickart, 1985–1986, p. 17).

Rusty Schweickart (cited in Bluth, 1979) observed that, because it was not space flight per se but the ability to open oneself to new experiences, similar changes could occur on earth for those who opened themselves to perception of new meanings (e.g., a trip to the Grand Canyon). Charles A. Lindbergh (1974), reflecting on his 1927 nonstop flight over the Atlantic in the Spirit of St. Louis, commented, "my awareness seemed to be above my body to expand on stellar scales. There were moments when I seemed so disconnected from the world, my plane, my mind and heartbeat that they were completely unessential to my new existence" (p. xi). He followed with:

> Is it remotely possible that we are approaching a stage in evolution when we can discover how to separate ourselves entirely from earthly life, to abandon our physical frameworks in order to extend both inwardly and outwardly through limitless dimensions of awareness? In future universal explorations, may we have no need for vehicles or matter? (pp. xii–xiii)

Lindbergh also experienced profound change upon his return. Gradually he moved into studies of mystical and supersensory phenomena and ecological concerns. In 1972 Lindbergh wrote,

> . . . I think the great adventures of the future lie—in voyages incon-
> ceivable by our 20th century rationality—beyond the solar system,
> through distant galaxies, possibly through peripheries untouched by
> time and space. . . . I believe early entrance to this era can be attained
> by the application of our scientific knowledge not to life's mechanical
> vehicles but to . . . the infinite and infinitely evolving qualities that
> have resulted in the awareness, shape and character of man [sic]. (p.
> 310)

According to White (1987), the core experience of space flight involves changed perceptions of space and time, silence, and weightlessness. Rather than regarding these as problems, they can be seen as creative potentials. For example, according to John Glenn, weightlessness is pleasant: "You feel completely free" (cited in White, 1987, p. 23). Upon returning home and experiencing the weight of gravity again, Skylab 3 scientist Don Lind said, "I'm going to feel crippled the rest of my life" (cited in Oberg & Oberg, 1986, p. 14). Soviet cosmonaut Gherman Titov described weight-lessness: "It is marvelous; the body astoundingly light and buoyant" (cited in Strughold & Hale, 1975, p. 537).

Robinson and White (1986) highlight the uniqueness of space migration and space societies, suggesting that there may be changes in behaviors, perception, and consciousness that we cannot anticipate or imagine for the emerging "spacekind." Thus, spacekind and humankind may one day be taxonomically different from each other, with spacekind the evolutionary emergent. Robinson and White call for the openness to explore new global paradigms and the recognition that diversity is prerequisite to "healthy transformative survival" (p. 103). White (1987) also views space explo-ration as a mutual transformation involving humans and space, not as a process of shaping space to mimic earth's characteristics. Change is a partic-ipatory process.

The Science of Unitary Human Beings as the Framework for Nursing in Space

Discussion of older and newer views does not imply "right and wrong." It does, however, guide the identification of appropriate phenomena within a particular framework. Space medicine focuses on the body and adaptation to space. Space nursing within the Science of Unitary Human Beings has a different perspective, focusing on creative change potentials and know-ing participation in the nature of that change. Theories derived from this science focus on participation in creating the future, not predicting or con-trolling the future. They offer new vistas of transformative evolution for humankind and guide nurses in providing knowledgeable service along the trajectory of human exploration in outer space.

The theories of accelerating change, the emergence of paranormal phenomena, and power as knowing participation in change flow from the principles of homeodynamics. The principle of integrality specifies the unitary (whole) nature of this process. The principle of resonancy describes the human-environmental field patterning as changing continuously, flowing in higher frequencies. The principle of helicy identifies the innovative and probabilistic increasing diversity of this field patterning. The focus is the field, not the physical body, the mind, or the interaction of the two.

The body is only one manifestation of human-environmental field patterning. The field is the reality. For example, patterning is not adaptation to the presence of disease or an altered environment. Dying is moving beyond the range of visible wavelengths; the patterning continues. In the words of the Sufi mystical poet, Jalal ad-Din Rumi (1207–1273),

> The body came out of us,
> Not we from it.
> The body is a beehive
> And we are its bees.
> And cell by cell we made the body.

The manifestation of field called "body" for spacekind may bear little resemblance to what humankind has known. As we venture into space, human-environmental field patterning fluctuates with changing environmental patterns. We can expect different manifestations of "body" as we evolve into the environment of space.

Also to be expected is increasing diversity of field patterning (see Table 1). Experiences such as those reported by Mitchell, Schweickart, and other astronauts who found themselves changed upon their return to earth can be understood in this light. Field patterning is creative and increasingly diverse, flowing in higher frequencies. To return to "business as usual" once back on earth would not be possible or desirable within this framework.

Unitary field modalities, such as therapeutic touch, meditation, and imagery, provide examples of knowing participation that focus on innovative potentials of accelerating change and emergence of paranormal phenomena. For example, all three involve centering, traditionally described as a process of focusing oneself, experiencing the emptiness that contains all things (Naranjo, 1971). Although such descriptions suggest a drawing in, experiences of centering actually reflect expansion, a transcendence of so-called "boundaries" of time and space. In the Science of Unitary Human Beings this suggests a higher frequency phenomenon. According to manifestations of patterning, examples of higher frequency patterning include time experienced as timelessness and imaginative or visionary experiences. The three unitary field modalities of therapeutic touch, meditation, and imagery embody this mode of experiencing.

Meditation can be seen as a higher frequency field process, four-dimensional experiencing where time and space do not exist. The meditator experiences timelessness and interconnectedness, a world without boundaries (Govinda, 1976; Macrae, 1982). Imagery also is four-dimensional experiencing of the field. What is imaged is perceived as "real" (Epstein, 1986). Imagery is a form of knowing participation in the change process. According to Epstein, "the image is the appearance in a human being of his or her movement toward wholeness" (p. 29). Therapeutic touch (Krieger, 1979) involves both meditation and imagery; it has been called a healing meditation (Peper & Ancoli, 1979; Borelli, 1981; Macrae, 1988). Therapeutic touch involves experiencing wholeness and unity (Macrae, 1988).

Meditation and imagery, once taught to space travelers and their significant others on earth, could change the nature of participation in perceptions of confinement, isolation, and loneliness. The physical boundaries of the space capsule and distance separating people are one manifestation of reality which could be transcended via these field modalities. Participants in mutual meditations could experience unity rather than separation, as boundaries of time and space do not exist in four-dimensional experiencing. The space traveler could transcend the physical boundaries of the space capsule; people apparently separated by space could experience field integrality.

For example, Lindbergh's (1974) speculation, noted earlier, that humans may discover how to extend awareness both inwardly and outwardly without constraints of the physical body and environment captures the possibility of this simultaneity of experiencing where inner space is outer space, and outer space is inner space. There is no here, no there. "The further out we look, the further in we see" (White, 1987, p. 67). There is no inner, no outer, only integrality.

Imagery, meditation, and therapeutic touch have potentials for health and healing as nondrug and noninvasive field modalities. Therapeutic touch, for example, is a mutual process involving nurse and client in the nature of the human-environmental field patterning, where the change is patterning "most commensurate with well being" (Rogers, 1988, p. 4). This well being could encompass strengthening the immune system of the space traveler, perhaps even stabilizing calcium levels for the space traveler who plans a return to earth. Therapeutic touch also facilitates relaxation and is a calming, integrating process (Krieger, 1979; Macrae, 1988). Space travelers who have learned and practice it may not be subject to the irritability, boredom, depression, hostility, and anxiety identified earlier as problems of confinement.

Other field modalities to incorporate in knowing participation in the nature of change include the wave phenomena of light, color, and music. Like therapeutic touch, meditation, and imagery, the three flow with each other. Color is a manifestation of light wavelength. It is possible to elicit both chords and color spectra from atoms, to hear the "music in light" (Wilczek & Devine, 1988, p. 14). They can be varied in the environment of the space capsule or space station to facilitate the experiences of well being, healing, relaxation, and meditation.

CONCLUSION

Space exploration has contributed to the development of a new mythology for humankind, what Campbell (1985) described as "the myth of this unified earth as of one harmonious being" (p. 17). For Campbell, too, outer space is inner space. Reflecting on Armstrong's walk on the moon, he said, ". . . our knowledge is the earth's knowledge. And the earth, as we now know, is a production of space" (p. 28). Thus, our knowledge is the knowledge of space.

This cosmic perspective is the experience of integrality. We move from seeing ourselves as citizens of one country, to citizens of the planet, to citizens of one small sector of the universe, to citizens of the universe.

For the space travelers who plan to make their home in space, the theories of accelerating evolution and the emergence of the paranormal open the door of transformation. The possibilities are endless as humans open themselves to participation in a continuous, mutual human-environmental field process characterized by patterning of greater diversity, timelessness, and visionary experiences.

REFERENCES

Barrett, E.A.M. (1984). An empirical investigation of Martha E. Rogers' principle of helicy: The relationship of human field motion and power. *Dissertation Abstracts International, 45*, 615A. (University Microfilms No. 8406278)

Barrett, E.A.M. (1986). Investigation of the principle of helicy: The relationship of human field motion and power. In V. Malinski (Ed.), *Explorations on Martha Rogers' science of unitary human beings* (pp. 173–188). Norwalk, CT: Appleton-Century-Crofts.

Bluth, B.J. (1979). Consciousness alteration in space. In J. Grey & C. Krop (Eds.), *Space manufacturing 3: Proceedings of the fourth Princeton/AAIA conference on space manufacturing facilities, May 14–17, 1979* (pp. 525–532). New York: American Institute of Aeronautics and Astronautics.

Borelli, M.D. (1981). Meditation and therapeutic touch. In M.D. Borelli & P. Heidt (Eds.), *Therapeutic touch* (pp. 40–46). New York: Springer.

Campbell, J. (1985). *The inner reaches of outer space: Metaphor as myth and as religion.* New York: Alfred van der Marck Editions.

Epstein, G. (1986). The image in medicine: Notes of a clinician. *Advances, Journal of the Institute for the Advancement of Health, 3*(1), 22–31.

Govinda, L.A. (1976). *Creative meditation and multidimensional consciousness.* Wheaton, IL: The Theosophical Publishing House.

Hall, S.B. (Ed.). (1985). *The human role in space: Technology, economics, and optimization.* Park Ridge, NJ: Noyes Publications.

Krieger, D. (1979). *The therapeutic touch: How to use your hands to help or to heal.* Englewood Cliffs, NJ: Prentice-Hall.

Lindbergh, C. (1972). Man's potential. In C. Muses & A.M. Young (Eds.), *Consciousness and reality: The human pivot point* (pp. 305–312). New York: Avon Books.

Lindbergh, C. (1974). Foreword. In M. Collins, *Carrying the fire: An astronaut's journeys* (pp. ix–xiii). New York: Farrar, Straus, & Giroux.

McNeal, S.R., & Bluth, B.J. (1981). Influential factors of negative effects in the isolated and confining environment. In J. Grey & L.A. Hamdan (Eds.), *Space manufacturing 4: Proceedings of the fifth Princeton/AAIA conference on space manufacturing facilities, May 18–21, 1981* (pp. 435–442). New York: American Institute of Aeronautics and Astronautics.

Macrae, J. (1982). *A comparison between meditating subjects and non-meditating subjects on time experience and human field motion.* Doctoral dissertation, New York University.

Macrae, J. (1988). *Therapeutic touch: A practical guide.* New York: Alfred A. Knopf.

Madrid, M., & Winstead-Fry, P. (1986). Rogers' conceptual model. In P. Winstead-Fry (Ed.), *Case studies in nursing theory* (pp. 73–102). New York: National League for Nursing.

Malinski, V.M. (1986). The relationship between hyperactivity in children and perception of short wavelength light. In V.M. Malinksi (Ed.), *Explorations on Martha Rogers' science of unitary human beings* (pp. 107–116). Norwalk, CT: Appleton-Century-Crofts.

Naranjo, C. (1971). Meditation: Its spirit and techniques. In C. Naranjo & R. Ornstein, *On the psychology of meditation* (pp. 3–132). New York: The Viking Press.

National Commission on Space. (1986). Pioneering the space frontier: The report of the national commission on space (1986). New York: Bantam.

Oberg, J.E. (1984). *The new race for space.* Harrisburg, PA: Stackpole Books.

Oberg, J.E., & Oberg, A.R. (1986). *Pioneering space: Living on the next frontier.* New York: McGraw-Hill.

Peper, E., & Ancoli, S. (1979). Appendix II: The two endpoints of an EEG continuum of meditation—alpha/theta and fast beta. In D. Krieger, *The therapeutic touch: How to use your hands to help or to heal* (pp. 153–164). Englewood Cliffs, NJ: Prentice-Hall.

Robinson, G.S., & White, H.M. Jr. (1986). *Envoys of mankind: A declaration of first principles for the governance of space societies.* Washington, DC: Smithsonian Institution Press.

Rogers, M.E. (1970). *An introduction to the theoretical basis of nursing.* Philadelphia: F.A. Davis.

Rogers, M.E. (1986). Science of unitary human beings. In V. Malinksi (Ed.), *Explorations on Martha Rogers' science of unitary human beings* (pp. 3–8). Norwalk, CT: Appleton-Century-Crofts.

Rogers, M.E. (1987). Rogers' science of unitary human beings. In R.R. Parse (Ed.), *Nursing science: Major paradigms, theories, and critiques* (pp. 139–146). Philadelphia: W.B. Saunders.

Rogers, M.E. (1988, June). Rogerian practice perspectives: Excerpts from transcripts of dialogues among Martha E. Rogers, Thérèse Connell Meehan, and Violet Malinski, January, February, and March, 1988. *Rogerian Nursing Science News, Newsletter of the Society of Rogerian Scholars*, pp. 4–5, 8. (Available from the Society of Rogerian Scholars, P.O. Box 362, Prince Street Station, New York, NY 10012.)

Schweickart, R.L. (Winter 1985–1986). Cosmonauts, astronauts found global organization. *Institute of Noetic Sciences Newsletter*, pp. 1, 17–20. (Available from The Institute of Noetic Sciences, 475 Gate Five Road, Suite 300, Sausalito, CA 94965.)

Seddon, M.R. (1988, April). *Keynote address.* Paper presented at the First National Conference on Nursing in Space, Huntsville, AL.

Strughold, H., & Hale, H.B. (1975). Biological and physiological rhythms. In M. Calvin & O.G. Gazenko (Eds.), *Foundations of space biology and medicine, joint USA/USSR publication, Vol. II, Book II, NASA special publication #374* (pp. 535–548). Washington, DC: U.S. Government Printing Office.

Whitby, M. (1986). *Tomorrow's world: Space technology.* London: BBC Books.

White, F. (1987). *The overview effect: Space exploration and human evolution.* Boston: Houghton Mifflin.

Wilczek, F., & Devine, B. (1988). *Longing for the harmonies: Themes and variations from modern physics.* New York: W.W. Norton.

25

A Conversation with Martha Rogers on Nursing in Space

Martha E. Rogers
Maureen B. Doyle
Angela Racolin
Patricia C. Walsh

Dr. Martha E. Rogers conversed with doctoral students on June 27, 1989 at New York University to explore her ideas on nursing in space, as well as her projections for the art and science of nursing within a new world view of transcendent unity and continuously escalating evolutionary change, and for the next evolutionary phase of human diversity—Homo spatialis. The authors are grateful for this opportunity and for Dr. Rogers' willingness to let us explore with her.

TRANSCENDENT UNITY

Martha Rogers: The main thing I want to get across is that we are talking about nursing in a whole new world of transcendent unity. We are not talking about planet bound anything, but rather, nursing in a universe where space encompasses the planet Earth. The spinoff in space is going to spell nursing on planet Earth as well as in space.

Maureen Doyle: You have said very clearly that we are integral with space. We cannot impose our view of Earth onto space. Rather, Earth is integral with the larger view.

Martha Rogers: We are changing our vision. It won't be one of causality. (You know me and causality.) One will not affect the other. Rather, we will be integral with this enlarged universe.

Angela Racolin: Could you elaborate more on the idea of transcendent unity?

Martha Rogers: It's a nice phrase. Actually, I think what this is getting at is perhaps how people's advent into space will happen. It's really a transition from humankind to spacekind and it's really about how a space-directed people change, how the world changes, and how our view of the world changes. Because it does. Actually this is not different from the Science of Unitary Human Beings. It gives it more generality, and it extends it further.

When we talk about environment, man is not the only species on this planet. In fact, we are talking about an enlarged transcendent universe in which planet Earth is integral with outer space. After being space dwellers for a couple of generations, and generations are generally considered to be 25 years, one may propose that in approximately 50 years Homo spatialis may transcend Homo sapiens. There will evolve a new kind of species. What will this mean? I don't know.

Angela Racolin: In your presentation at the Third Rogerian Conference, you made a statement that today's realities would transcend traditional averages. When talking about space and space environment, you talked about the realities transcending traditional averages. I wonder—is that talking about similarities.

Martha Rogers: Oh yes. You are really asking, "What will tomorrow's norms be like?"

Angela Racolin: Yes. What will the norms and realities be like, what would you envision? Will there be any?

Martha Rogers: You see, we are moving into living in space and we will have Homo spatialis. How necessary is it to try to transfer Earth's atmosphere to outer space? How soon will people need support systems in reverse to visit planet Earth? Just as we have to have support systems in reverse if people play around under the ocean, there are people who will have to have support systems for living in space. However, the norms will be in the enlarged universe, not planetary. It's going to be entirely different. Today the astronauts are the precursors of Homo spatialis.

Angela Racolin: When you say the norms will be the norms of the enlarged universe, would that be synonymous with saying they would be universal or interplanetary?

EVOLUTIONARY CHANGE

Martha Rogers: No, actually what I'm talking about is norms for continuously escalating evolutionary change and innovative, growing diversity. The speed of change has not only accelerated, it has gone up exponentially. There is a lot of evidence, of course, that the more change, the faster it speeds up itself; it's quite normal. It is a fantastic time to be alive because we are on the edge of a new world, just as when life moved out of the waters onto dry land. We are at a major change. Perhaps it happened before, I don't know. The point is that right now I have no doubt that out in the cosmos there is something. I don't know what to call it, call it intelligent life, it is not like us.

Things we frequently hear about are proposed to be abnormal or pathological; for example, when they talk about the astronauts and the loss of calcium. Well, why is that considered bad? Maybe it is normal in space. If it is normal and healthy, maybe if you're out there you don't need all that calcium. I consider physical bodies to be manifestations of field. This is a whole different way of looking. But if you take just our ability to see, we see within a very narrow range of the spectrum. Who's to say that there are not all sorts of intelligent fields out there outside our visible light spectrum. Just because our eyes don't see something doesn't mean it's not there.

Change just is. For example, back in the 1950s Lee DeForest, the father of modern electronics, just 12 years before the Apollo landed on the moon, asserted that this could never possibly happen. Now that's also particularly interesting because early on when he first got into electronics, he was the one who proposed a cable across the ocean. He was sued and brought to court for lying to the public, for saying that such a thing could be done. Well, fortunately the courts said it was fine. Now here is a man who dared himself and then could not face up to a thing like man on the moon. So don't think for a minute that the status quo is going to continue or that this isn't going to happen. It's already happening.

Now we are talking about a whole new breed. When I talk about Homo spatialis I'm serious and so are others. Robinson and White, the authors of *Envoys of Mankind,* use the term frequently. I think it's a marvelous term. I didn't know what to call it, now I know.

Patricia Walsh: How would you define Homo spatialis?

Martha Rogers: It's the great big question in the sky. It's the next evolutionary phase of human diversity.

Maureen Doyle: Do you think Homo spatialis will require food as we normally eat currently?

Martha Rogers: I don't know, and to me, it really doesn't matter. The point is, what is food? You see, it's not input/output, but rather we're talking about the integralness of fields and how it might be manifest in some small way. Who's to know.

Maureen Doyle: We were wondering what they might sell in a galactic grocery store.

Martha Rogers: Right off they will sell potatoes and whatever. Maybe they won't need food, maybe they'll get food from the environment somehow.

Patricia Walsh: How do you see our expansion into space taking place?

Martha Rogers: The first space islands are being built and they will be inhabited by the year 2000. It is projected that they will only hold about 20 people. But the day will come very quickly that things will change. When emigration to space begins, the demand here and on the moon and on wherever is going to happen very fast. There are thousands of people longing to get up there already.

Initially, in a space island, the designs are such that they set up motions that will involve gravitational ties similar to those on Earth; however, they are set up in such a way that the heavier gravitational ties will be toward the center. As you move out, there will be less and less gravitational pull in the island. Now this can be great if you are talking about people with cardiac conditions, or emphysema, or the like because they will not have to battle against gravity. Now take the average person who is an astronaut on a space island and spends his life on the outer edges. Pretty soon he may be in trouble if he moves to the middle of the island. And let's say he takes his wife and children, and they begin to have children. These children won't know what it's like to weigh a ton. You see, all our patterns about what things weigh, a ton of lead or a ton of feathers, all depends on how you're looking at it. So it means the whole set of categories that we've grown up with are going to be gone. Think of the excitement!

ROLE OF NURSE IN SPACE AND THE BODY OF NURSING KNOWLEDGE

Patricia Walsh: What do you think the role or function of the nurse will be on a space island?

Martha Rogers: I think the real purpose will be to promote human/space-kind well being, whatever that may be. Well being is a value, it is not an absolute. I think ways in which this will be done will be noninvasive in general, but I think it will involve modalities of which we have not yet even dreamed.

If one looks at allopathic medicine as we know it right now, it's going down the drain and going very rapidly, the reason being it is based on old world views. It is a historical absolute that somehow got the money and the prestige. There are many other medical areas equally important with allopathic medicine; for example, there are homeopathic, oriental medicine, American Indian medicine, as well as herbalism. Various modalities other than medicine are under way—such as, noninvasive modalities, holistic trends, unconditional love, etc. These are being tried in many ways, and we're finding that they have potential in relation to health and well being. We don't know what will be involved in spacekind health promotion or what these new modalities will be. They are unpredictable.

Patricia Walsh: Would nurse astronauts be actual mission specialists or would they be Earth support systems?

Martha Rogers: I think that they will not be astronauts or mission specialists at all, unless nurses decide that there is a body of scientific knowledge specific to nursing. The Science of Unitary Human Beings is the only proposal that has been made of that sort. Now people who are mission scientists have been very blunt about this issue when asked directly. If a nurse writes them to say she is interested, she will be informed that they are looking for scientists and they do not perceive nurses as scientists. I think they see a nurse as someone who can monitor machines, that all nurses do is a technical, quasitechnical job and they have plenty of those sorts of people. They ask for engineers for their pilots, and there is no end to the support personnel for their pilot/engineers. These are people who essentially have graduate degrees. The pilots mostly have degrees in engineering, and the scientists particularly in mathematics, physiology, philosophy, and aeronautics. They have a broad-based vision. To be included in this, nurses have to be committed to having a body of knowledge specific to nursing that they will be willing to transmit and for which they will be responsible.

Maureen Doyle: If science is open ended and constantly changing, how do you think our experience in space will influence the body of knowledge in nursing?

Martha Rogers: I don't think it will influence it at all. I think the Science of Unitary Human Beings provides the overall world view for an enlarged transcendent universe. Science tries to understand and describe reality.

Angela Racolin: We talk about a body of knowledge that is a science and which by definition is an organized abstract system. Something that I'm picking up on makes me question whether or not there is a contradiction in the whole idea of saying that we can have a science and a body of knowledge, which translates into the idea of research and theories, which ideally predict. But you are saying there is no predictability. So how does any of this fit?

Martha Rogers: When you say that, you see science is changing. But this is not going to throw out the physical world and biological world and all of that, just because things are unpredictable. There is no causality either, but there are relationships. Yes, I think a lot of these things are going to go, but I don't think it is important to be concerned with struggling with it. A science is identified by the phenomena of its concern. No other science has been concerned with people as irreducible energy fields. The Science of Unitary Human Beings is a new way of looking at people. Now this view of humans is neither more, nor less, nor bigger, nor greater, nor anything. It is a different phenomenon.

What is true about science is that it is an organized abstract system from which to derive theories. Now when nurses derive theories from sociology, those are not nursing theories, they are sociological theories. And a nurse might do excellent research in sociology, but it doesn't make it nursing just because a nurse does it, any more than if a physicist derived a theory from sociology, it would not be a physical theory; it would be sociological. Now here we have nursing as a basic science dealing with a phenomenon that is clearly unique to nursing; it is an organized system from which to derive multiple theories. A science generates many theories. There is no such thing as *the* theory of nursing anymore than there is *the* theory of biology. For example, we have gotten caught up in this, and we have a lot of unlearning to do, since we confused research in other fields and thought if a nurse did it that made it nursing. When we begin to look at nursing with this enlarged rapidly changing world view, the foundations and the principles of the Science of Unitary Human Beings are even more useful than before—they fit.

But science is never finished. It is always open ended. Physics, which is so long established, can be offered as an example. It is undergoing stresses that as severe as science has ever experienced. Probability replaced absolutism and now there is unpredictability. A whole world of cards is falling apart. But we have lived through absolutism, we have survived probability, and even Einstein didn't accept probability for a long time. He said, "I don't think God plays dice with the universe." And then there was quantum theory. Now we find that probability is no longer in. In addition, it is now known that black holes don't just swallow everything. It seems that they also spit things back. And the idea of worm holes is fascinating; there are now some scientists who have come up with the recognition that there are ways that can be developed, practical ways of shooting through the universe instead of having to go around the long way. In other words, you may go off to another galaxy in almost no time flat. All we are dealing with here is time within our capacity to perceive it, and Homo spatialis will not be caught in that kind of thing. It's all relative. All around us we are seeing manifestations of change; they are part of the evolutionary process.

COMPLEXIFYING WHOLENESS

Patricia Walsh: You have spoken of complexification. Could you explain what you are referring to?

Martha Rogers: You know, I think back to the 1940s when Wendell Wilkie was running for president. One day he gave a talk about "one world." I think he was referring to peace, but then I don't know. The point is people got excited, nobody wanted one world. And yet look at the changes from clans and tribes, to cities and states, to nations and now to one world—it's going to happen. And with this there is growing simplicity in the complexification.

Patricia Walsh: I presume nursing has to follow along with this to keep up with it.

Martha Rogers: We don't follow along. We are integral with it. It's a matter of "Do we want to be around or not and, if so, how?" I think if we are going to claim that nurses have something important to contribute to people, then we are going to have to deal with complexification. Now sometimes I think that we are ahead of the game. And the more I get into it, the more I know we are. And certainly we are by no means the only ones who are trying to look at this sort of thing. There are David Bohm, Renee Weber, Rupert Sheldrake, and Fritz Capra among many others. In other words, we're moving to different concepts but with the same basic philosophical approach.

Maureen Doyle: When you talk about complexifying wholeness via a new world view, which evolves out of nonequilibrium, is that like saying that order emerges out of chaos?

Martha Rogers: No, I don't think so. I think we get caught up in what we mean by chaos. Now I think in one sense, yes; for example, the whole idea of unpredictability really emerged out of some of the work that was going on in mathematics in the new field called "chaos." We grew up in absolutism, and that's part of the trouble now. People haven't even moved to a probabilistic universe. The thing is no matter what one may believe, the status quo is gone, it won't stay. Whatever one believes, now in terms of evolution and change, there is no going back. You know we've had pulsating universes and all different things. Of course, the "big bang" is the "in" thing now and has been for a while. I think that too will pass, when it's going to pass I don't know. At this point I'm willing to let anybody have it who wants it.

I do not think that whether or not the universe began as a "big bang" or some other way is going to make any difference in terms of how we try to explain the way things are. And it's going to change very rapidly. By the time we have large numbers of people emigrating into space and evolving into Homo spatialis, we are going to find many things we could never even have imagined.

I think what is important is to keep an open mind and to be able to come to grips with how things seem to be moving now. This is where the Science of Unitary Human Beings has much to recommend it, since the principles of homeodynamics apply to the new world as well as today's world. I agree that helicy needs a little bit of rewording, it's somewhat verbose, but I'm working on that. The principles represent a complete departure from old world views, but are consistent with the universe as we begin to know it now. The Science of Unitary Human Beings postulates unpredictability; it does allow for all these other things.

NOSOPHOBIA: IMPLICATIONS FOR NURSING EDUCATION

Maureen Doyle: You use the word "nosophobia." Do you think that perhaps we are going to take some of our problems into outer space?

Martha Rogers: You see, the thing about nosophobia, the morbid dread of disease, is that it is generated by greed. MDs and hospitals and multiple health professionals plus drug houses and the like are generating most of it and we are helping. The news media is very active in this also. For example, with AIDS everyone got excited. Of course, it's a horrible thing, but so was cholera. AIDS has not begun to be as massive as cholera was. Cholera decimated three quarters of the European population in the 13th century. There is also very good evidence that part of this is directly traceable to the destruction of the immune system through the use of antibiotics and immunizations.

Maureen Doyle: What would you recommend that nurse educators do to prepare nurses for nursing in space? Would this be an integral part of a nursing curriculum, or would you see it as a specialization?

Martha Rogers: I think that if you are talking about right this minute, then we need doctorally prepared nurses who are qualified in nursing as a science. There may well be nurses with doctorates in other fields who are interested in space. Now many of those are not scientists in the sense of a mission specialist. I would also note that within one generation or less, the parameters of physiology, psychology, sociology, physics, etc. will not be appropriate or acceptable for determining human health and well being, or describing humans. They are simply not going to work. There is going to be a rapid change that we are going to see. It's going to happen. I don't think it is negative; I think it is exciting. The person who is flexible and who goes with the flow will have an advantage. There are people in other fields, and some in medicine, who are interested in this sort of thing. There is a growing move toward synthesis, toward unity, and toward transcendence. I suggest you read Robinson and White's *Envoys of Mankind*. It's quite a readable book.

Maureen Doyle: I came across a statement in *Omni* by a woman who is a NASA research physician who claimed that they are developing criteria to measure an astronaut's sensitivity to self and others. Among other things, they feel this is important so that people will be able to function in tight quarters, for long periods of time, performing routine demanding tasks. Is it possible that studies being done by nursing doctoral students would be relevant to NASA and nursing in space?

Martha Rogers: If these studies are derived from the Science of Unitary Human Beings, then there would be some justification. There is no question NASA has already indicated that they need more studies about people and their relationships.

I would caution any researcher to be careful, that when you begin to split humans into pieces you are not studying people. There is all sorts of evidence that these things don't work, even when superficially they look like they are working. Many tests have been tried to predict who is going to be successful in space. They even get into something as pragmatic as motion sickness, which has no physiological parameters. No matter what has been tried, it cannot be predicted. Also, when someone goes up and has motion sickness, you can't predict if they will or will not have it again.

The Science of Unitary Human Beings is a new world view that more and more is being recognized. It does have a frame of reference that no other discipline has, and that also has a potential of encompassing space. It's not a question for space, but it is a question for human life. The whole idea of where we are within the overall picture has had to be changed, and I think the same thing is happening now.

Patricia Walsh: What then would you recommend that we could do to start to participate in creating the future?

Martha Rogers: The first thing I would like to do is to commit ourselves to a world view that is consistent with the most up-to-date knowledge available. We have to commit ourselves to nursing as a science, a peer of other sciences. We are in desperate need of basic research, and we also need applied research. If we really teach nursing as a science to undergraduate students, students themselves would use it that way. Now there is a great deal of interest in using this science in employment. We have done a lot of talking about theory-based practice. What people don't realize is that it's nursing science-based practice. This is where our focus has to be.

Patricia Walsh: Do you feel this commitment to nursing as a science and working within this framework will ensure having nursing as a major health presence in space?

Martha Rogers: Well, certainly everybody needs a broad general education, including astronomy. The science of nursing should be taught to encompass the whole, starting at the undergraduate level. Now if you are talking about the immediate, I am hoping that the United States Air Force will invite me to go to NASA and do concentrated workshops with doctorally prepared nurses to begin to see what we can do about building a scientific base. They might not buy it, I don't know, but I'm available. The point is that we will not go into space unless we do something like that. And there is no other field equipped to provide the broad base of health promotion than yourselves from the Science of Unitary Human Beings. We are going to have to devise and define new modalities, because the business of the old procedure book just will not work.

Maureen Doyle: Do you think having a baby in outer space would be feasible?

Martha Rogers: Nobody really knows what it would be like. Now there is research going on, but it is limited to the primary mission objective. Research in the life sciences has not been the primary mission of any space program so far. The NASA technical memorandum #58280 is a compilation of the Detailed Supplemental Objectives conducted by the space shuttle from 1981 through 1986. They can do no research in space of this sort on the life sciences or any thing else, except as it is consistent with the primary mission objective.

Patricia Walsh: How do you feel people knowledgeable in the Science of Unitary Human Beings, specifically nurses, can add to this?

Martha Rogers: I think it is essential that people who are involved in space travel, space immigration, and serving as mission specialists are people who are concerned with irreducible human beings. This is going to happen, whether it is nurses or somebody else. Right now we are ahead of the game and we have a responsibility to do something about it and to participate and share with others. One of the things the whole astronaut effort is strongly about is team work, in which there is mutual respect for differences. There is no one who runs the show. These teams are literally sharing, nobody thinks they have all the answers, or that they are going to tell everybody else what to do. They all have wide experience and vision and, of course, they are all committed.

We need more risk takers in nursing. If the doctoral student is going to go up into space, she or he needs to be thoroughly knowledgeable and articulate in nursing as a science. The student needs to know the cosmos, to be widely read, to have a pilot's license, and to dream big. In research we are still trying to use deductive and inductive thinking without recognizing that the pressures and trends of holistic thinking demand new ways of thinking. The chances to be creative are unlimited, you can shoot the works.

THE IMPOSSIBILITY OF "GOING HOME AGAIN"

Maureen Doyle: I've heard you speak about when astronauts reenter Earth's atmosphere that they are never the same. It's like you can't really go home again because you have been so changed.

Martha Rogers: It is quite true, you know we never go back. You can't walk in the same river twice. I think what we are dealing with here is something where what happens is very dramatic. I may fly to another city and I will never be the same again no matter what, but it does not have the same impact as going into space would have. It's funny, there are people that think that if you go up in your own capsule, and take your own atmosphere with you, that it should not make any difference. But we know that's not true. Everybody who has gone up has had all sorts of experiences. They are never the same. Some of them had startling experiences, certainly beyond normal.

Maureen Doyle: What I seem to hear from you is not only that you can't walk in the same river twice, or that you can't go home again, but why would you want to?

Martha Rogers: I wouldn't, but look at all the people who are trying so desperately to maintain the status quo. While some of it may be tied to greed, overriding that is a fear of change. It isn't just space. The whole idea of one world is very threatening to people. Look back on the interrelationships of tribes to cities to states. There are all sorts of things making it clear that we live in one world. The European economic community is already around and growing, a United States of Europe has been talked about for years, and there are reports that within 3 years a partial United States of Europe is expected to exist. If you look at how things are shaping up in different continents and different countries, it is clear that it is all moving toward this growing complexification. It looks like the wall in Germany might fall and the one in China is already cracked in a lot of places. Now if we have some of these strange little green men coming around here, it might unite people faster than you might think.

We have all these sorts of things going on that represent the continuous moving mass of interrelationships. I think it was Marilyn Ferguson who spoke of synthesis in pattern-seeing being essential for the 21st century. The whole concept of complexifying wholeness is where we are.

Patricia Walsh: I have a question specifically for you. How did you evolve from the slinky to space?

Martha Rogers: You see the slinky was just an aide to thinking. It was one way of dealing with ideas. The slinky signified open-endedness and nonrepeating rhythmicities. But the slinky had no meaning, except as a way to stimulate ideas. Once you get stimulated, then you no longer need the slinky, you just keep on thinking and keep on going. It is extremely exciting!

REFERENCES

Bohm, D. (1980). *Wholeness and the implicate order.* Boston: Routledge & Kegan Paul.

Boslough, J. (1985). *Stephen Hawking's universe.* New York: William Morrow.

Capra, F. (1975). *The tao of physics.* New York: Bantam Books.

Capra, F. (1982). *The turning point.* New York: Bantam Books

Capra, F. (1989). *Uncommon wisdom.* New York: Bantam Books.

DeForest, L. (1950). *Father of radio: The autobiography of Lee DeForest.* Chicago: Wilcox & Follett.

Ferguson, M. (1980). *The aquarian conspiracy.* Los Angeles: J.P. Tarcher.

Hawking, S. (1988). *A brief history of time.* New York: Bantam Books.

National Aeronautics and Space Administration. (1987, March). *Results of the life sciences detailed supplemental objectives conducted by the space shuttle: 1981–1986.* Technical memorandum (No. 58280). Houston, TX: Lyndon B. Johnson Space Center.

Oberg, A.R. (1989, April). N.A.S.A.'s next generation. *Omni,* pp. 28, 80.

Robinson, G., & White, H. (1986). *Envoys of mankind.* Washington, DC: Smithsonian Institute Press.

Rogers, M. (1988, June). *Health in space.* Paper presented at the Third Rogerian Conference, New York City.

Sheldrake, R. (1988). *The presence of the past.* New York: Times Books.

Weber, R. (1986). *Dialogues with scientists and sages: The search for unity in science and mysticism.* London: Routledge, Chapman, & Hall.

Appendix A: Glossary
Nursing Science: A Science of Unitary Human Beings

Martha E. Rogers

GLOSSARY

Learned Profession: A science and an art.

Science: An organized body of abstract knowledge arrived at by scientific research and logical analysis.

Art: The imaginative and creative use of knowledge.

Negentropy: Increasing heterogeneity, differentiation, diversity, and complexity of pattern.

Energy Field: The fundamental unit of the living and the non-living. Field is a unifying concept. Energy signifies the dynamic nature of the field. A field is in continuous motion and is infinite.

Pattern: The distinguishing characteristic of an energy field perceived as a single wave.

Multidimensional:[1] A nonlinear domain without spatial or temporal attributes.

---

[1]Formerly titled Four-dimensionality.

Conceptual System: An abstraction. A representation of the universe or some portion thereof.

Unitary Human Being (Human field): An irreducible, indivisible, multidimensional energy field identified by pattern and manifesting characteristics that are specific to the whole and which cannot be predicted from knowledge of the parts.

Environment (Environmental field): An irreducible, four-dimensional energy field identified by pattern and integral with the human field.

Principles of Homeodynamics

Principle of Resonancy: Continuous change from lower to higher frequency wave patterns in human and environmental fields.

Principle of Helicy: Continuous innovative, unpredictable, increasing diversity of human and environmental field patterns.

Principle of Integrality:[2] Continuous mutual human field and environmental field process.

---

[2]Formerly titled Principle of Complementarity. Updated September, 1989.

Appendix B: Reading List

Aggleton, P., & Chalmers, H. (1984). Rogers' unitary field model. *Nursing Times, 80*(50), 35–39

Allanach, E.J. (1988). Perceiving supportive behaviors and nursing occupational stress: An evolution of consciousness. *Advances in Nursing Science, 10*(2), 73–82.

Allen, V.L. (1988). *The relationship among time experience, human field motion, and clairvoyance: An investigation in the Rogerian conceptual system.* Unpublished doctoral dissertation, New York University, New York. (University Microfilms No. 891062)

Alligood, M.R. (1989). Applying Rogers' model to nursing administration: Emphasis on environment, health. In B. Henry, M. DiVencenti, C. Arndt, & A. Marriner (Eds.), *Dimensions of nursing administration. Theory, research, education, and practice* (pp. 105–111). Boston: Blackwell Scientific Publications.

Barrett, E.A.M. (1984). An empirical investigation of Martha E. Rogers' principle of helicy: The relationship of human field motion and power. *Dissertation Abstracts International, 45,* 615A. (University Microfilms No. 8406278)

Barrett, E.A.M. (1986). Investigation of the principle of helicy: The relationship of human field motion and power. In V.M. Malinski (Ed.), *Explorations on Martha Rogers' science of unitary human beings* (pp. 173–188). Norwalk, CT: Appleton-Century-Crofts.

Barrett, E.A.M. (1988). Using Rogers' science of unitary human beings in nursing practice. *Nursing Science Quarterly, 1,* 50–51.

Barrett, E.A.M. (1989). A nursing theory of power for nursing practice. Derivation from Rogers' paradigm. In J. Riehl-Sisca, *Conceptual models for nursing practice,* 3rd ed. (pp. 207–217). Norwalk, CT: Appleton and Lange.

Boyd, C. (1985). Toward an understanding of mother-daughter identification using concept analysis. *Advances in Nursing Science, 7*(3), 78–86.

Bradley, D.B. (1987). Energy fields: Implications for nurses. *Journal of Holistic Nursing, 5*(1), 32–35.

Butcher, H.K., & Parker, N.I. (1988). Guided imagery within Rogers' science of unitary human beings: An experimental study. *Nursing Science Quarterly, 1,* 103–110.

Compton, M.A. (1989). A Rogerian view of drug abuse: Implications for nursing. *Nursing Science Quarterly, 2,* 98–105.

Conner, G.K. (1986). The manifestations of human field motion, creativity, and time experience patterns of female and male parents. *Dissertation Abstracts International, 47,* 1926B. (University Microfilms No. 8616985)

Cowling, W.R., III. (1984). The relationship of mystical experience, differentiation, and creativity in college students: An empirical investigation of the principle of helicy in Rogers' science of unitary man. *Dissertation Abstracts International, 45,* 458A. (University Microfilms No. 8406283)

Cowling, W.R., III. (1986). The relationship of mystical experience, differentiation, and creativity in college students. In V.M. Malinski (Ed.), *Explorations on Martha Rogers' science of unitary human beings* (pp. 131–141). Norwalk, CT: Appleton-Century-Crofts.

Cowling, W.R., III. (1986). The science of unitary human beings: Theoretical issues, methodological challenges, and research realities. In V.M. Malinski (Ed.), *Explorations on Martha Rogers' science of unitary human beings* (pp. 65–77). Norwalk, CT: Appleton-Century-Crofts.

Crawford, G. (1985). A theoretical model of support network conflict experienced by new mothers. *Nursing Research, 34,* 100–102.

Daffron, J.M. (1989). Patterns of human field motion and human health. *Dissertation Abstracts International, 49,* 4229B. (University Microfilms No. 8827484)

Dzurec, L.C. (1986). The nature of power experienced by individuals manifesting patterning labelled schizophrenic: An investigation of the principle of helicy. *Dissertation Abstracts International, 47,* 4467B. (University Microfilms No. 8701004)

Fawcett, J. (1975). The family as a living open system: An emerging conceptual framework for nursing. *International Nursing Review, 22,* 113–116.

Fawcett, J. (in press). Spouses' experiences during pregnancy and the postpartum: A program of research and theory development. *Applied Nursing Research.*

Ference, H.M. (1979). The relationship of time experience, creativity traits, differentiation, and human field motion. *Dissertation Abstracts International, 40,* 5206B. (University Microfilms No. 8010281)

Ference, H.M. (1986). The relationship of time experience, creativity traits, differentiation, and human field motion. In V.M. Malinski (Ed.), *Explorations on Martha Rogers' science of unitary human beings* (pp. 95–105). Norwalk, CT: Appleton-Century-Crofts.

Ference, H.M. (1986). Foundations of a nursing science and its evolution: A perspective. In V.M. Malinski (Ed.), *Explorations on Martha Rogers' science of unitary human beings* (pp. 35–44). Norwalk, CT: Appleton-Century-Crofts.

Ference, H.M. (1989). Comforting the dying: Nursing practice according to the Rogerian model. In J. Riehl-Sisca (Ed.), *Conceptual models of nursing practice* (3rd ed.) (pp. 197–205). Norwalk, CT: Appleton and Lange.

Fitzpatrick, J.J. (1988). Theory based on Rogers' conceptual model. *Journal of Gerontological Nursing, 14*(9), 14–19.

Floyd, J.A. (1983). Research using Rogers' conceptual system: Development of a testable theorem. *Advances in Nursing Science, 5*(2), 37–48.

Gaydow, L.S., & Farnham, R. (1988). Human-animal relationships within the context of Rogers' principle of integrality. *Advances in Nursing Science, 10*(4), 72–80.

Gueldner, S.H. (1983). A study of the relationship between imposed motion and human field motion in elderly individuals living in nursing homes. *Dissertation Abstracts International, 44,* 1411B. (University Microfilms No. 8320597)

Gueldner, S.H. (1986). The relationship between imposed motion and human field motion in elderly individuals living in nursing homes. In V.M. Malinski (Ed.), *Explorations on Martha Rogers' science of unitary human beings* (pp. 161–171). Norwalk, CT: Appleton-Century-Crofts.

Gueldner, S.H. (1989). Applying Rogers' model to nursing administration: Emphasis on client and nursing. In B. Henry, M. DiVencenti, C. Arndt, & A. Marriner (Eds.), *Dimensions of nursing administration. Theory, research, education, and practice* (pp. 113–119). Boston: Blackwell Scientific Publications.

Guthrie, B.J. (1987). The relationship of tolerance of ambiguity and preference for processing information in the mixed mode to differentiation in female college students: An empirical investigation of the homeodynamic principle of helicy. *Dissertation Abstracts International, 49*, 74B. (University Microfilms No. 8803587)

Hanchett, E.S. (1979). *Community health assessment: A conceptual tool kit.* New York: John Wiley & Sons.

Hanchett, E.S. (1988). *Nursing frameworks and community as client. Bridging the gap.* Norwalk, CT: Appleton and Lange.

Hektor, L.M. (1989). Martha E. Rogers: A life history. *Nursing Science Quarterly, 2*, 63–73.

Johnston, R.L. (1981). Temporality as a measure of unidirectionality with the Rogerian conceptual framework of nursing science. *Dissertation Abstracts International, 41*, 3740B. (University Microfilms No. 8107215)

Johnston, R.L. (1986). Approaching family intervention through Rogers' conceptual model. In A.L. Whall (Ed.), *Family therapy theory for nursing. Four approaches* (pp. 11–32). Norwalk, CT: Appleton-Century-Crofts.

Katch, M.P. (1983). A negentropic view of the aged. *Journal of Gerontological Nursing, 9*, 656–660.

Laffrey, S.C. (1985). Health behavior choice as related to self-actualization and health conception. *Western Journal of Nursing Research, 7*, 279–295.

Ludomirski-Kalmanson, B. (1984). The relationship between the environmental energy wave frequency pattern manifest in red light and blue light and human field motion in adult individuals with visual sensory perception and those with total blindness. *Dissertation Abstracts International, 45*, 2094B. (University Microfilms No. 8421457)

McDonald, S.F. (1981). A study of the relationship between visible lightwaves and the experience of pain. *Dissertation Abstracts International, 42*, 569B. (University Microfilms No. 8117084)

McDonald, S.F. (1986). The relationship between visible lightwaves and the experience of pain. In V.M. Malinski (Ed.), *Explorations on Martha Rogers' science of unitary human beings* (pp. 119–127). Norwalk, CT: Appleton-Century-Crofts.

McEvoy, M.D. (1988). The relationships among the experience of dying, the experience of paranormal events and creativity in adults. *Dissertation Abstracts International, 48*, 2264B. (University Microfilms No. 8720130)

Macrae, J.A. (1982). A comparison between meditating subjects and non-meditating subjects on time experience and human field motion. *Dissertation Abstracts International, 43*, 3537B. (University Microfilms No. 8307688)

Madrid, M., & Winstead-Fry, P. (1986). Rogers' conceptual model. In P. Winstead-Fry (Ed.), *Case studies in nursing theory* (pp. 73–102). New York: National League for Nursing.

Malinski, V. (1981). The relationship between hyperactivity in children and perception of short wavelength light: An investigation into the conceptual system proposed by Martha E. Rogers. *Dissertation Abstracts International, 41*, 4459B. (University Microfilms No. 8110669)

Malinski, V. (1985). Martha E. Rogers' science of unitary human beings: Implications for cross-cultural nursing. In R. Wood & J. Kekhababh (Eds.), *Examining the cultural implications of Martha E. Rogers' science of unitary human beings* (pp. 25–42). Lecompton, KS: Wood-Kekhababh Associates.

Malinski, V.M. (1986). The relationship between hyperactivity in children and perception of short wavelength light. In V.M. Malinski (Ed.), *Explorations on Martha Rogers' science of unitary human beings* (pp. 107–117). Norwalk, CT: Appleton-Century-Crofts.

Malinski, V.M. (1986). Further ideas from Martha Rogers. In V.M. Malinski (Ed.), *Explorations on Martha Rogers' science of unitary human beings* (pp. 9–14). Norwalk, CT: Appleton-Century-Crofts.

Malinski, V.M. (1986). Contemporary science and nursing: Parallels with Rogers. In V.M. Malinski (Ed.), *Explorations on Martha Rogers' science of unitary human beings* (pp. 15–24). Norwalk, CT: Appleton-Century-Crofts.

Malinski, V.M. (1986). Nursing practice within the science of unitary human beings. In V.M. Malinski (Ed.), *Explorations on Martha Rogers' science of unitary human beings*. Norwalk, CT: Appleton-Century-Crofts.

Malinski, V.M. (in press). The meaning of a progressive world view in nursing: Rogers' science of unitary human beings. In N.L. Chaska (Ed.), *The nursing profession: Turning points*. St. Louis: C.V. Mosby.

Miller, F.A. (1984). The relationship of sleep, wakefulness and beyond waking experience: A descriptive study of Martha Rogers' concept of sleep-wake rhythms. *Dissertation Abstracts International, 46*, 116B. (University Microfilms No. 8505438)

Moccia, P. (1980). A study of the theory-practice dialectic: Towards a critique of the science of man. *Dissertation Abstracts International, 41,* 2560B. (University Microfilms No. 8101984)

Oliver, N.R. (1988). Processing unacceptable behaviors of coworkers: A naturalistic study of nurses at work. *Dissertation Abstracts International, 49,* 75B. (University Microfilms No. 8803598)

Paletta, J.L. (1988). The relationship of temporal experience to human time. *Dissertation Abstracts International, 49,* 1621B. (University Microfilms No. 8812521)

Phillips, J.R. (1989). Science of unitary human beings: Changing research perspectives. *Nursing Science Quarterly, 2,* 57–60.

Quinn, J.F. (1984). Therapeutic touch as energy exchange: Testing the theory. *Advances in Nursing Science, 6*(2), 42–49.

Quinn, J.F. (1989). Therapeutic touch as energy exchange: Replication and extension. *Nursing Science Quarterly, 2,* 79–87.

Raile, M.M. (1982). The relationship of creativity, actualization, and empathy in unitary human development: A descriptive study of Rogers' principle of helicy. *Dissertation Abstracts International, 44,* 449B. (University Microfilms No. 8313874)

Rawnsley, M. (1977). Relationships between the perception of the speed of time and the process of dying: An empirical investigation of the holistic theory of nursing proposed by Martha Rogers. *Dissertation Abstracts International, 38,* 1652B. (University Microfilms No. 77-21,692)

Rawnsley, M. (1985). H-E-A-L-T-H: A Rogerian perspective. *Journal of Holistic Nursing, 3*(1), 26.

Rawnsley, M. (1986). The relationship between the perception of the speed of time and the process of dying. In V.M. Malinski (Ed.), *Explorations on Martha Rogers' science of unitary human beings* (pp. 79–89). Norwalk, CT: Appleton-Century-Crofts.

Reed, P.G. (1986). The developmental conceptual framework: Nursing reformulations and applications for family therapy. In A.L. Whall (Ed.), *Family therapy theory for nursing. Four approaches* (pp. 69–91). Norwalk, CT: Appleton-Century-Crofts.

Reed, P.G. (1987). Spirituality and well being in terminally ill hospitalized adults. *Research in Nursing and Health, 10,* 335–344.

Reed, P.G. (1989). Mental health of older adults. *Western Journal of Nursing Research, 11,* 143–163.

Reeder, F. (1984). Philosophical issues in the Rogerian science of unitary human beings. *Advances in Nursing Science, 6*(2), 14–23.

Reeder, F. (1985). Nursing research, holism, and philosophies of science: Points of congruence between Edmund Husserl and Martha E. Rogers. *Dissertation Abstracts International, 45*, 2498B. (University Microfilms No. 8421466)

Reeder, F. (1986). Basic theoretical research in the conceptual system of unitary human beings. In V.M. Malinski (Ed.), *Explorations on Martha Rogers' science of unitary human beings* (pp. 45–64). Norwalk, CT: Appleton-Century-Crofts.

Rogers, M.E. (1961). *Educational revolution in nursing.* New York: Macmillan.

Rogers, M.E. (1963). Building a strong educational foundation. *American Journal of Nursing, 63*(6), 94–95.

Rogers, M.E. (1963). Some comments on the theoretical basis of nursing practice. *Nursing Science, 1*(1), 11–13, 60–61.

Rogers, M.E. (1964). *Reveille in nursing.* Philadelphia: F.A. Davis.

Rogers, M.E. (1970). *An introduction to the theoretical basis of nursing.* Philadelphia: F.A. Davis.

Rogers, M.E. (1980). Nursing: A science of unitary man. In J.P. Riehl & C. Roy (Eds.), *Conceptual models for nursing practice* (2nd ed.) (pp. 329–337). New York: Appleton-Century-Crofts.

Rogers, M.E. (1981). Science of unitary man: A paradigm for nursing. In G.E. Laskar (Ed.), *Applied systems and cybernetics, Vol. IV.* New York: Pergamon.

Rogers, M.E. (1982). Beyond the horizon. In N.L. Chaska (Ed.), *The nursing profession: A time to speak* (pp. 795–801). New York: McGraw-Hill.

Rogers, M.E. (1983). Science of unitary human beings: A paradigm for nursing. In I.W. Clements & F.B. Roberts (Eds.), *Family health: A theoretical approach to nursing care* (pp. 219–227). New York: John Wiley & Sons.

Rogers, M.E. (1983). The family coping with a surgical crisis: Analysis and application of Rogers' theory to nursing care. (Rogers' Response). In I.W. Clements & F.B. Roberts (Eds.), *Family health: A theoretical approach to nursing care* (pp. 390–391). New York: John Wiley & Sons.

Rogers, M.E. (1985). A paradigm for nursing. In R. Wood & J. Kekhababh (Eds.), *Examining the cultural implications of Martha E. Rogers' science of unitary human beings* (pp. 13–23). Lecompton, KS: Wood-Kekhababh Associates.

Rogers, M.E. (1985). The nature and characteristics of professional education for nursing. *Journal of Professional Nursing, 1,* 381–383.

Rogers, M.E. (1985). Nursing education: Preparation for the future. In *Patterns in education: The unfolding of nursing* (pp. 11–14). New York: National League for Nursing.

Rogers, M.E. (1986). Science of unitary human beings. In V.M. Malinski (Ed.), *Explorations on Martha Rogers' science of unitary human beings* (pp. 3–8). Norwalk, CT: Appleton-Century-Crofts.

Rogers, M.E. (1987). Nursing research in the future. In J. Roode (Ed.), *Changing patterns in nursing education* (pp. 121–123). New York: National League for Nursing.

Rogers, M.E. (1987). Rogers' science of unitary human beings. In R.R. Parse (Ed.), *Nursing science: Major paradigms, theories, and critiques* (pp. 139–146). Philadelphia: W.B. Saunders.

Rogers, M.E. (1988). Nursing science and art: A prospective. *Nursing Science Quarterly, 1,* 99–102.

Sanchez, R.O. (1987). The relationship of empathy, diversity, and telepathy in mother-daughter dyads. *Dissertation Abstracts International, 47,* 3297B. (University Microfilms No. 8625654)

Sarter, B.J. (1985). The stream of becoming: A metaphysical analysis of Rogers' model of unitary man. *Dissertation Abstracts International, 45,* 2106B. (University Microfilms No. 8421469)

Sarter, B. (1987). Evolutionary idealism: A philosophical foundation for holistic nursing theory. *Advances in Nursing Science, 9*(2), 1–9.

Sarter, B. (1988). *The stream of becoming: A study of Martha Rogers' theory.* New York: National League for Nursing.

Sarter, B. (1989). Some critical philosophical issues in the science of unitary human beings. *Nursing Science Quarterly, 2,* 74–78.

Schodt, C.M. (1988). *Patterns of parent-fetus attachment and the couvade syndrome: An application of human-environment integrality as postulated in the science of unitary human beings.* Unpublished doctoral dissertation, New York University, New York.

Schodt, C.M. (1989). Parental-fetal attachment and couvade: A study of patterns of human-environment integrality. *Nursing Science Quarterly, 2,* 88–97.

Schorr, J.A. (1983). Manifestations of consciousness and the developmental phenomenon of death. *Advances in Nursing Science,* 6(1), 26–35.

Smith, M.C. (1987). An investigation of effects of different sound frequencies on vividness and creativity of imagery. *Dissertation Abstracts International,* 47, 3708B. (University Microfilms No. 8625655)

Smith, M.C. (1988). Testing propositions derived from Rogers' conceptual system. *Nursing Science Quarterly, 1,* 60–67.

Smith, M.J. (1986). Human-environment process: A test of Rogers' principle of integrality. *Advances in Nursing Science,* 9(1), 21–28.

Smith, M.J. (1989). Four-dimensionality: Where to go with it. *Nursing Science Quarterly, 2,* 56.

Trangenstein, P.A. (1989). Relationships of power and job diversity to job satisfaction and job involvement: An empirical investigation of Rogers' principle of integrality. *Dissertation Abstracts International, 49,* 3110B. (University Microfilms No. 8625655)

Uys, L.R. (1987). Foundational studies in nursing. *Journal of Advanced Nursing, 12,* 275–280.

Whelton, B.J. (1979). An operationalization of Martha Rogers' theory throughout the nursing process. *International Journal of Nursing Studies, 16,* 7–20.

Wright, S.M. (1989). Development and construct validity of the energy field assessment form. *Dissertation Abstracts International, 49,* 3113B. (University Microfilms No. 8821431)

Young, A.A. (1985). The Rogerian conceptual system: A framework for nursing education and service. In R. Wood & J. Kekhababh (Eds.), *Examining the cultural implications of Martha E. Rogers' science of unitary human beings* (pp. 53–69). Lecompton, KS: Wood-Kekhababh Associates.

This list is based in large part on the citations compiled by Jacqueline Fawcett for her 1989 book, *Analysis and evaluation of conceptual models of nursing* (2nd ed.), published by F.A. Davis, and on an addendum provided by Dr. Fawcett dated 6/12/89; used with permission.

An excellent source of information related to the Science of Unitary Human Beings and containing material written by Dr. Rogers is *Rogerian Nursing Science News, Newsletter of the Society of Rogerian Scholars* (P.O. Box 362, Prince Street Station, New York, NY 10012).

EPILOGUE

Knowingly and, at times, unknowingly participating in this labor of love energized us, and a bittersweet joy marks the completion of our efforts. In publishing our book with the National League for Nursing, we pause in gratitude and acknowledge that something special has transpired.

We affectionately called ourselves "The Book Club." Our monthly meetings engendered a spirit of optimism and purpose. A web of late night phone calls and endless mailings connected us between meetings. We united to sustain our deceptively simple belief inspired by Martha E. Rogers that nursing is not only a science, but a unique science. This book is our way of acting on that belief.

The process of developing this book also provided a backdrop for the fears, hopes, growth, and change in our private lives. During its 18-month life span, "The Book Club" rekindled attempts at doctoral work and hopes for future studies; sustained commitments to Rogerian-based research, practice, and education; witnessed the joy of a pregnancy and birth, and the sorrow of painful illness and family distress; shared the excitement of a new home, and the uncertainty of a new job; and consolidated our identities as part of the growing current of hope for nursing and the health of humanity.

During the early phase of this challenge as well as in the sinking moments of despair that we would ever receive the promised manuscripts on time or juggle our own schedules to fulfill our obligations, it was helpful to recall the notion that stars are still present during the daylight hours of work even though they are not visible to us. Martha E. Rogers' star guided us throughout this adventure. Mere thanks pale against such a debt, but we do thank her for sharing so abundantly with us her light and vision.

We thank our NLN editors, Allan Graubard and Janice Weisner, for their encouragement and support with our work. And finally, we thank our families for putting up with our sporadic absences while obsessed with the book, and love, despite it all.

Elizabeth Ann Manhart Barrett, PhD, RN
and the *Editorial Review Panel*

Permission Credits

Excerpts from bibliography in *Analysis and Evaluation of Conceptual Models of Nursing,* by J. Fawcett, copyright © 1989 by F.A. Davis Co., reprinted with permission of the publisher.

Excerpt from Sonnet XXXII of "Fatal Interview," by Edna St. Vincent Millay, in *Collected Sonnets,* revised and expanded edition, Harper & Row, 1988. Copyright © 1931, 1958 by Edna St. Vincent Millay and Norma Millay Ellis, reprinted with permission.

Excerpt from "Nursing Story," by M.E. Rogers, in *Education Violet,* June 1966, copyright © 1966, New York University, reprinted with permission of the publisher.

Excerpts from pages 35, 36, 39, 44, 45, 51–53, 55, 59, 66, 68, 82, 88, 89, 94, and 95 of *Reveille in Nursing,* by M.E. Rogers, copyright © by F.A. Davis Co., reprinted with permission of the publisher.